ALLE · ZEIT · WACH · 1842

E. Alt · S. S. Barold · K. Stangl (Eds.)

Rate Adaptive Cardiac Pacing

With 160 Figures and 30 Tables

Springer-Verlag
Berlin Heidelberg New York London Paris Tokyo
Hong Kong Barcelona Budapest

Prof. Dr. med. Eckhard Alt
I. Medizinische Klinik, Klinikum rechts der Isar
Technische Universität München
Ismaningerstr. 22
8000 München 80

Prof. Dr. med. S. Serge Barold
Genesee Hospital, University of Rochester
School of Medicine and Dentistry
224 Alexander Street
Rochester, New York 14607, USA

P.D. Dr. med. Karl Stangl
Bereich Medizin (Charité)
Humboldt-Universität Berlin
Schumannstr. 20
1040 Berlin

ISBN-13:978-3-642-76651-0 e-ISBN-13:978-3-642-76649-7
DOI: 10.1007/978-3-642-76649-7

Softcover reprint of the hardcover 1st edition 1993

Typesetting: FotoSatz Pfeifer GmbH, 8032 Gräfelfing
2119/3130-543210 – Printed on acid-free paper

Contributors

Eckhard Alt, M.D., I. Medizinische Klinik, Klinikum rechts der Isar, Technische Universität München, Ismaningerstr. 22, 8000 München 80

S. Serge Barold, M.D., Genesee Hospital, University of Rochester, School of Medicine and Dentistry, 224 Alexander Street, Rochester, New York 14607, USA

Tom Bennett, Ph.D., Medtronic Inc., Advanced Product Development, 7000 Central Ave., Minneapolis, MN 55432, USA

Wim Boute, Vitatron Medical B.V., Technical Division, Postfach 76, 6950 AB Dieren, The Netherlands

Johan Brandt, M.D., Dept. of Cardiothoracic Surgery, University Hospital, S-22 185 Lund, Sweden

Raul Chirife, M.D., Instituto de Cardiologia, Academia Nacional de Medicina de Buenos Aires, Cnel. Diaz 2423, 1425 Buenos Aires

Thomas Fahraeus, M.D., Dept. of Cardiothoracic Surgery, University Hospital, S-22 185 Lund, Sweden

Seymour Furman, M.D., Dept. of Cardiothoracic Surgery, Montefiore Hospital, 111 E. 210th Street, Bronx, New York 10467, USA

Pat Gordon, Ph.D., 494 Highgrove Road, Wayzata, MN 35391, USA

Jerry C. Griffin, M.D., University of California, Room 312 Moffitt Hospital, San Francisco, CA 94143, USA

John Helland, Ph.D., Pacesetter Systems INC., 12884 Bradley Ave., Sylmar, CA 91392, USA

Joel Kupersmith, M.D., Humana Hospital University, University of Louisville, 530 South Jackson Street, Louisville, Kentucky 40202, USA

Chu-Pak Lau, M.D., Division of Cardiology, University Dept. of Medicine, Queen Mary Hospital, Hong Kong

M. Lehmann, M.D., Klinikum der Albert-Ludwigs-Universität, Abt. Sport- und Leistungsmedizin, Hugstetterstr. 55, 7800 Freiburg

Harry G. Mond, M.D., Suite 14 Private Consulting Rooms, The Royal Melbourne Hospital, Victoria, 3050, Australia

Tibor A. Nappholz, Ph.D., Telectronics Pacing Systems, Research and Development, 7400 South Tuscon Way, Englewood, Colorado 80112, USA

Anthony F. Rickards, M.D., Royal Brompton and National Heart Hospital, Sydney Street, London SW 3 6NP, United Kingdom

Marten Rosenquist, M.D., Dept. of Medicine, Division of Cardiology, Karolinska Hospital, S-104 01 Stockholm, Sweden

Rodney W. Salo, Cardiac Pacemakers Inc., 4100 Hamline Ave. North, St. Paul, MN 55112-5798, USA

Massimo Santini, M.D., Largo di Vigna Stelluti, 12, I-00191 Roma

Hans Schüller, M.D., Dept. of Cardiothoracic Surgery, University Hospital, S-22 185 Lund, Sweden

Igor Singer, M.B., Humana Hospital University, University of Louisville, 530 South Jackson Street, Louisville, Kentucky 40202, USA

Karl Stangl, M.D., Bereich Medizin (Charité), Humboldt-Universität Berlin, Schumannstr. 20, 1040 Berlin

Contents

Preface

Treatment of patients with symptomatic bradycardia using pacemakers is one of the most successful therapeutic measures in modern cardiology. While pacing had already undergone a considerable evolution from its simple form of asynchronous pacing in the early 1960s to the dual-chamber demand pacing currently used, the enormous technical progress in microelectronics has recently opened up new possibilities: rate-adaptive cardiac pacing. While in former years cardiac pacing was predominantly used to prevent sudden cardiac death, syncopy or other symptoms concomitant with bradycardia at rest, cardiac pacing is evolving more and more towards being a therapy aimed at improving patients' quality of life and greatly increasing their capacity for physical exercise.

Since cardiac output and exercise capacity are closely linked to the variation of heart rate, and since a considerable percentage of pacemaker patients – 30-50% of all pacemaker patients are assumed to benefit from rate-adaptive pacing – show no or only limited chronotropic response to exercise, sensor parameters other than the natural sinus rate have to be used to determine the heart rate at which the patient should be paced under varying metabolic conditions. These new rate-adaptive systems vary the heart rate by means of one or several sensor parameters derived from a variety of body functions such as physical activity, ventilation, QT interval, intracardiac pressure or blood temperature, to name just some of them. Rate-adaptive pacing has gained more and more clinical importance within the last 5 years, and several hundreds of thousands of these systems have now been implanted worldwide.

This book is divided into four major parts, each comprising several chapters, that deal with the various clinical, functional, and technical issues in rate-adaptive pacing. The first part is devoted mainly to the basic hemodynamics of the paced heart, and the definition of chronotropic incompetence and the clinically important quest for indications for this innovative medical technology are also highlighted. The second part provides a concise description of the clinical and functional characteristics of the various sensors currently used for rate adaptation. It gives a clear and comprehensible insight into how the different systems function.

The third part is a guide to clinical and practical aspects of rate-adaptive pacing. It explains the correct follow-up, helps in understanding the electrocardiographic interpretation of the various new rate-adaptive systems, and defines their limitations, adverse effects, and possible interferences. Renowned scientists give competent answers to the important questions and demonstrate their meaning for clinical practice.

Finally, the fourth part is dedicated to future trends, new developments, and advanced concepts in the field of rate-adaptive pacing.

Leading authors from both sides of the Atlantic Ocean have contributed their expertise to make this book a comprehensive and clinically focused volume representing the state of the art in rate-adaptive pacing. We would like to express our gratitude to these authors for their excellent contributions and reviews.

The Editors

Foreword

It is a pleasure for me to be able to write a few words at the beginning of this book on rate-adaptive pacing. While several texts have been published recently that encompass a wide area of cardiac pacing, none has been devoted solely to a practical approach to indications, technique and management of rate-adaptive pacing. The text is intended as a practical delineation of how rate-adaptive pacemakers work and what functional, electrocardiographic and telemetric findings are associated with normal and abnormal functions. It is these analyses that help clarify the complexity of modern rate-adaptive cardiac pacing. A book that is written for the practising clinician, cardiology fellow, internist and clinical cardiologist is definitely needed, and the timely publication of this volume by Springer has delivered an up-to-date resource that will help the clinician make management decisions for patients in need of pacing. This book is a readable, accessible tutorial, responsive to the needs of the less experienced worker and valuable to the more experienced, in addition to being a significant contribution to the cardiac pacemaker literature. I recommend this book for all doctors taking care of patients with these problems.

Dr. Anthony F. Rickards, London, UK

The Evolution of Bradycardia Pacing

S. FURMAN*

There have been a series of definable streams in the evolution of clinical cardiac pacing since its introduction in 1952 by Zoll [1] using transcutaneous stimulation of the heart via high outputs through the intact chest wall. This technique was suitable for emergency use at the time of sudden asystole, but not for prolonged maintenance during continued bradycardia. It has been used for emergency purposes since that time and technologic evolution has again encouraged its revival in the recent past. Prolonged continuous transcutaneous pacing has been unsuccessful in stabilizing cardiac function and is not tolerated well by the patient.

The later direction of cardiac pacing was toward comfortable, continuous, and low-power stimulation. This was accomplished in two ways during 1957-1958. The first was the placement of direct myocardial wires when heart block had occurred during early open heart surgery [2]. These myocardial wires were connected to a portable battery-powered pulse generator which was not connected to the hospital power supply and would not stop pacing during a power outage, an event that actually occurred early on during the development of pacing. These myocardial wire leads, however, suffered a continuing increase in stimulation threshold until capture was lost, despite a progressive increase in pacemaker output. Continued investigation of a means of safe and prolonged stimulation demonstrated that transvenous, i.e. endocardial pacing of the right ventricle could be prolonged at a continuing low threshold. If either the cathode or both cathode and anode (bipolar) were within the ventricle, thrombus would not collect at the electrode. Virtually indefinite cardiac stimulation was possible [3]. During this time continued evaluation of myocardial electrodes determined, that stainless steel (as originally used) was unsuitable for prolonged stimulation and that platinum-iridium alloy in the myocardium was also associated with a prolonged stable threshold [4].

By 1959-1960 prolonged myocardial and endocardial stimulation by a battery-powered pacemaker, often on an outpatient basis, was demonstrated to be successful. In some designs battery replacement by the patient was possible, sometimes without assistance. Such external pulse generators, some connected by a radio-frequency (RF) [5, 6] link to an implanted receiver and the intracardiac lead system were subject to frequent damage, loss of contact, decoupling, and connector and lead breakage.

* Department of Cardiothoracic Surgery, Montefiore Medical Center, Bronx, New York, USA

The psychological burden associated with a patient carrying his/her "heart" exposed was substantial and gave further impetus to the need for a wholly implantable pulse generator.

A wholly implantable device implied a power source which could function for a prolonged period. Two efforts were made to have an RF link in which power source and pulse generator would be external. Both were unsuccessful because of difficulty with the integrity of the RF link and because of potential damage to the device. A wholly implantable, rechargeable device using nickel-cadmium batteries was introduced in 1958 and implanted using myocardial wires in a patient in his midthirties [7]. The first device failed within a day and the second model within 8 days. The patient remained without a pacemaker for 2 years until a wholly implantable, primary (mercury-zinc) cell device was developed. He then underwent implantation of the first of over 30 pulse generators and remains alive at beginning of 1992.

The mercury-zinc cell had been developed during the 1940s and had excellent characteristics of energy density, an output voltage of 1.35 V, and maintenance of constant voltage output until the end of service. This allowed an electronic circuit design which would maintain a constant stimulation rate from the time of manufacture until the end of battery life. A change in stimulation rate (some manufacturers designed a decrease and others an increase) signalled the end of the pacemaker's service. The first such device was introduced during 1960 [8]. The mercury-zinc cell, in a battery of four or five cells provided an output voltage of 5.2 or 6.5 V and was particularly suitable for the electrodes then in use. The life of such a pulse generator was, however, 18 months during the development of the pacemaker, and, at most, 36 months (on average) during the 1970s. As the average patient lived for 7 years after pacemaker implantation, several pulse generator replacements were required and costs for the individual patient remained relatively high compared to today. Since the earliest implanted pacemakers several directions have determined the state of cardiac pacing as it now exists.

Power Sources

The earliest power source for an implantable device was the rechargeable nickel-cadmium battery. It was, however, unsuitable for serveral reasons. One was that the device with a rechargeable battery had to be molded into plastic which rapidly equilibrated with the 100% moisture in the body and which caused short circuits and electronic deterioration. A second reason is that nickel-cadmium battery operation is distinctly temperature-dependent. While the battery operates at a usable level at normal ambient temperatures of 20°-25°C it's capacity and charge retention are far less satisfactory at 37°C. During the 1970s a new implantable rechargeable device using nickel-cadmium batteries was introduced, which it was predicted would function over a prolonged period [9]. It required weekly recharging for 1.5 h and had a high-failure rate. It was in clinical use for several years and then was displaced by primary cell devices, which even though requiring operative replacement were recognized as the most appropriate technology.

Because of the short life of mercury-zinc cell devices and the lack of availability of prolonged function devices, an effort was made to develop nuclear power source pacemakers. These were manufactured in the United States, France, and the Federal Republic of Germany. Two of the devices used plutonium (half-life 89 years) to power a thermal converter and had a projected pulse-generator longevity of 6 years (very long for that time), but which in actual use demonstrated a far greater longevity. Most of the devices implanted during 1972-1976 still remain functional during 1990. As the unites were implanted in relatively young people many patients remain alive.

Another power source was the isotope promethium (half-life 3.5 years), which, when in use gave a pulse generator an actual longevity of 5-6 years, which while prolonged at that time (early/mid 1970s) was soon overshadowed by newly introduced primary, nonnuclear cells [10]. While nuclear pacemakers have enjoyed prolonged low-level usage and reliability, the restrictions and reporting requirements associated with their use reduced enthusiasm. The weight of the pulse generator, which required extensive radiation shielding, made them heavier than primary-cell devices and the need, in each country of production, to move through a variety of governmental agencies for design approval made them electronically obsolete when compared to primary-cell units [11]. Few, if any, are now implanted.

During 1972 a new primary cell was introduced, made of a lithium anode and an iodine compound cathode. This cell had an immense capacity for a primary cell, 3 Ah. It was hermetically sealed and emitted no gas during the production of electricity (the nickel-cadmium and mercury-zinc cells did emit gas and required venting, i.e., a nonhermetic pacemaker). The cell could not produce large amounts of electricity because of high internal impedance, but was suitable for the operation of an electronic device which required lower amounts of current for prolonged periods [12]. This cell came into widespread use during 1974 and lithium-anode power sources soon became the standard [13]. A variety of cathodes were evaluated and five reached commercial use in implantable pacemakers. In addition to iodine, cupric sulfide, thionyl chloride, lead and silver chromate were all fabricated into pulse generators. Each eventually was found to be less suitable than lithium iodine and it alone powers all newly manufactured pacemakers worldwide.

All pulse generators are now hermetically sealed so that the incursion of body fluids has ended. The reliability of these devices is far better and more predictable than that of any early devices [14]. The longevity of the devices now depends up on the drain to which they are subjected and the size of the battery. Mercury-zinc batteries were virtually of a single size with a narrow range of capacity differences, but lithium-iodine batteries can be fabricated into a wide variety of sizes, each suitable for a specific use and intended pulse generator size and length of service. The first lithium battery pacemakers introduced were very large (weighing about 140 g) and operated for 10-15 years. More modern pacemakers have many more functions, weigh 20-30 g, and operate for 5-7 years.

Lead Systems

The first lead system was a pair of myocardial stainless-steel wires used with an external pulse generator to pace children who had developed complete heart block after the repair of congenital cardiac lesions. These wires developed extensive local reaction and progressively increasing thresholds [15]; they were clearly unsuitable for implantable devices which required a prolonged low and stable threshold. The second lead system available was an endocardial lead placed initially via the basilic vein (during 1958) and thereafter via the external jugular vein into the outflow tract of the right ventricle [16]. This lead too was initially attached to an external pulse generator which was originally line powered but later battery operated. It demonstrated stimulation threshold stability, a feature which had not previously existed. A group of patients were maintained for over a year with an external pulse generator and a transvenous lead [17].

The next lead design which was to be instrumental in the development of long-term myocardial, i.e. transthoracic, pacing included an electrode platform with two platinum-iridium pins which acted as the electrode and was attached to an external pulse generator. It too demonstrated stimulation threshold stability. Myocardial spring, i.e. flexible, electrodes were then introduced and, associated with the Chardack-Greatbatch implantable pulse-generator design, began the era of workable implanted pacing [18]. These spring electrodes remained available for several decades and many remain in service. In 1963 an endocardial unipolar lead system was introduced [19] and in 1965 a bipolar endocardial lead system [20]. Both lay in the right ventricular apex rather than the outflow tract and allowed prolonged endocardial stimulation which gradually displaced myocardial pacing, so that today few, if any, primary myocardial pacemaker implants are performed worldwide.

A later development in lead design involved the recognition that stimulation threshold was directly related to the size of the cathodal surface. Electrodes were then designed to have smaller cathodal surface areas and today, with the use of mesh and porous surfaces, a small area stimulates while a larger area senses the electrogram [21]. Much of the ability to reduce pulse-generator output and to correspondingly increase pulse-generator longevity has been based on improvements in electrode efficiency. As electrode size is directly related to the stimulation threshold and earlier electrode cathodes were almost ten times larger than at present, there has been a corresponding decrease in generator output needed to provide stable long-term stimulation. As programmability, i.e. the ability to change the output to correspond with the specific threshold achieved, low threshold can be readily translated into greater longevity. This change in electrode design has had a significant influence on present pulse-generator longevity, albeit little acknowledged.

Early leads fractured at an alarming rate, but the replacement of single metal wire coils with multifilar coils has immeasurably increased the durability and fracture resistance of the leads. Initial leads in Europe were insulated with polyethylene while in the United States silicone rubber was used. Silicone-rubber insulation tended to be thick and in bipolar lead systems two leads occupied too large a space within the venous system. In an effort to make leads smaller in diameter, a polyurethane material was introduced during 1979-1980. Different polyurethanes were used in different fabrications by various manufacturers. Most were distinctly better than older leads and have been durable over the past decade. One group of designs deteriorated while in situ causing significant pacing and clinical problems in a large portion of the 225 000 patients in whom they were implanted [22]. About 25% of these leads failed, though 5 years after implantation those that were to fail had already failed and those still functioning have been stable. [23]

Sensing Function

Despite all of the advancements enumerated above, there is one that can be considered to define modern cardiac pacing. That is the increasing ability of pacing systems to receive and interprete multiple channels of information. The earliest pacemakers did not respond to any incoming cardiac or extracardiac signals. The stimulation rate was set at manufacture, usually to be 60 or 70 beats per minute and only circuit failure or battery depletion could affect that rate. In the 1960s the need to provide sensitivity to atrial activity to restore the normal atrioventricular sequence, and to change rate with activity was accomplished and an atrial synchronous pacemaker was used clinically [24]. As the atrial lead then, and for many years, could only be implanted by thoracotomy, this system fell from use when endocardial pacing became dominant. A second and perhaps more important reason was that this pacing system sensed the atrium but not the ventricle, so that competitive ventricular stimulation could occur and produce ectopic rhythms of which the patient was aware and could occasionally cause ventricular tachycardia or fibrillation [25].

Sensitivity to atrial function allowed a physiologic response to activity, but did not meet the even greater need to be non-competitive with the chamber being paced. Ventricular sensitivity was introduced in 1968 with the introduction of the "demand" pacemaker which inhibited its output in the presence of a spontaneous ventricular event [26]. Another approach was that of triggering a ventricular stimulus in the presence of a spontaneous ventricular event, the ventricular-triggered (synchronous) mode of noncompetitive pacing. Pacing could now be performed in patients with complete and lesser degrees of heart block and rhythms, such as sick sinus syndrome [27] in which the pacemaker might be inhibited for prolonged periods, only stimulating when necessary. In 1970 it proved possible to restore the atrioventricular sequence in patients with sinus bradycardia by stimulating, not sensing atrial activity. In this instance the pacemaker could compete with atrial activity but only because it sensed ventricular activity and was noncompetitive with the ventricle [28]. However, only a single input channel was used for all of these mechanisms; atrial synchrony, ventricular synchrony, and atrioventricular sequential pacing. In 1977 circuits which could sense the atrium and also the ventricle were introduced and these dual-chamber pacemakers, either atrial synchronous or AV universal, have dominated since then. They provided the ability to track or pace the atrium and to stimulate or be inhibited by spontaneous or conducted ventricular activity.

In 1976 the first pacemaker capable of sensing a noncardiac function was developed; pH was evaluated to increase the stimulation rate in the presence of exercise which produced lactic acidosis. This reduced the pH and in this design increased the stimulation rate [29]. While the value of this approach did not seem immediately apparent, it was gradually realized that an increase in ventricular rate was the primary requirement for the increase in cardiac output during activity [30]. With this realization other sensors were introduced in the early 1980s and gradually achieved widespread popularity. These were the stimulus-T sensor, which responded to the abbreviation of the stimulus-T interval by increasing stimulation rate [31] , and the respiratory sensor, which measured the respiration rate and caused a corresponding increase in ventricular stimulation rate [32]. This was later followed by the activity sensor in which a piezo-electric crystal detected body activity and emitted small electrical signals to increase the pacemaker stimulation rate in a manner similar to that of the atrial synchronous pacemaker. All of these devices were ventricular inhibited as well as sensor driven. Two input channels were in use.

The next introduction was during the late 1980s with dual-chamber pacemakers capable of sensing and pacing the atrium and the ventricle coupled with sensors capable of driving the atrium and then the ventricle above the spontaneous atrial rate [33]. These devices had three channels of input, atrial, ventricular, and sensor and correspondingly far greater complexity and capability. The introduction of further sensitivity channels will increase the complexity and utility of these devices.

The bases of modern cardiac pacing can thus be summarized as:

1. The implantable device
2. Endocardial stimulation and sensing
3. Continued stimulation for many years
4. Progressive increase in the ability to sense multiple functions

References

1. Zoll PM (1952) Resuscitation of the heart in ventricular standstill by external electric stimulation. N Engl J Med 247:768-771
2. Weirich WL, Paneth M, Pott VL, Lillehei CW (1958) The treatment of complete heart block by the use of an artificial pacemaker and a myocardial electrode. Am J Cardiol 2:250
3. Lagergren H, Levander-Lindgren M (1984) Ten-year follow-up on 1000 patients with transvenous electrodes. PACE 7:1017-1020
4. Hunter SW, Roth NA, Bernardez D, Noble JLA (1959) A bipolar myocardial electrode for complete heart block. Lancet 1:506
5. Glenn WWL, Mauro A, Longo E, Lavietes PH, Mackay FJ (1959) Remote stimulation of the heart by radio-frequency transmission: clinical application to a patient with Stokes-Adams syndrome. N Engl J Med 261:948-951
6. Cammilli L, Pozzi R, Pizzichi G, DeSaint-Pierre G (1964) Radio-frequency pacemaker with receiver coil implanted on the heart. Ann NY Acad Sci 111:1007-1029
7. Elmqvist R, Senning R (1959) An implantable pacemaker for the heart. In Proceedings of the seventh international conference of Electrical Engineers. Iliffe, London, p 253
8. Chardack W, Gage AA, Greatbatch W (1961) Correction of complete heart block by self-contained and subcutaneously implanted pacemaker. J Thorac Cardiovasc Surg 42:814-830
9. Love JW, Lewis KB, Fischell RE, Schulman J (1974) Experimental testing of a permanent rechargeable cardiac pacemaker. Ann Thorac Surg 17: 152-156

10. Parsonnet V, Myers GH, Gilbert L et al. (1975) Clinical experience with nuclear pacemaker. Surgery 78:776
11. Parsonnet V (1977) Cardiac pacing and pacemakers: VII. Power sources for implantable pacemakers, part 2. Am Heart J 94:658:664
12. Greatbatch W (1975) The statistical reliability of lithium-iodine batteries. In: Schaldach M, Furman S (eds) Advances in pacemaker technology. Springer, Berlin, Heidelberg, New York, pp 345-355
13. Parsonnet V (1977) Cardiac pacing and pacemakers: VII. Power sources for implantable pacemakers, part 1. Am Heart J 94:517-528
14. Tyers GFO, Brownlee RR (1976) The non-hermetically sealed pacemaker myth. Or, Navy-Ribicoff 22,000-FDA-Weinberger O. J Thorac Cardiovasc Surg 71:253-254
15. Lillehei CW, Sellers RD, Bonnabeau RC Jr et al. (1963) Chronic postsurgical complete heart block. J Thorac Cardiovasc Surg 46:436-455
16. Furman S, Schwedel JB (1959) An intracardiac pacemaker for Stokes-Adams seizures. N Engl J Med 261:943-948
17. Siddons H (1978) Transvenous long-term pacing with an external pacemaker. What are the risks? PACE 1:163-165
18. Chardack WM, Gage AA, Schimert G, Thomson NB, Sanford CE, Greatbatch W (1963) Two years' clinical experience with the implantable pacemaker for complete heart block. Dis Chest 43:225-239
19. Lagergren H, Johansson L (1963) Intracardiac stimulation for complete heart block. Acta Chir Scand 125:562-566
20. Chardack WM, Federico AJ, Gage AA (1965) Clinical experience with an implanted pacemaker-catheter electrode system. Circulation 31-32:67
21. MacGregor DC, Wilson GJ, Lixfeld W, Pilliar RM, Bobyn JD, Silver MD, Smardon S, Miller SL (1979) The porous surfaced electrode: a new concept in pacemaker lead design. J Thorac Cardiavasc Surg 78:281-290
22. Hanson J (1984) Sixteen failures in a single model of bipolar polyurethane-insulated ventricular pacing lead. PACE 7:389-394
23. Stokes KB, Church T (1986) Ten-year experience with implanted polyurethane lead insulation. PACE 9:1160-1165
24. Nathan DA, Wu C, Keller W (1963) An implantable synchronous pacemaker for the long-term correction of complete heart block. Circulation 27:682
25. Bilitch M, Cosby RS, Cafferky EA (1967) Ventricular fibrillation and competitive pacing. N Engl J Med 276:598-604
26. Castellanos A, Lemberg L, Jude J, Mobbin-Uddin K, Berkovits B (1968) Implantable demand pacemaker. Br Heart J 30:29-33
27. Epstein S, Frieden J, Furman S (1968) Alternating supraventricular tachycardia and sinus bradycardia. NY State J Med 68:3066-3069
28. Harken DE (1971) Bifocal demand pacing. Chest 59:355-356
29. Cammilli L, Alcidi L, Papeschi G (1977) A new pacemaker autoregulating the rate of pacing in relation to metabolic needs. In: Watanabe Y (ed) Cardiac pacing. Proceedings of the 5th nternational symposium. Excerpta Medica, Amsterdam, pp 414-419
30. Karlof I (1975) Haemodynamic effect of atrial-triggered versus fixed-rate pacing at rest and during exercise in complete heart block. Acta Med Scand 197:195-206
31. Rickards AF, Donaldson RM, Thalen HJT (1983) The use of QT interval to determine pacing rate: early clinical experience. PACE 6:346-354
32. Rossi P, Prando MD, Magnani A, Aina F, Rognoni G, Occhetta E (1988) Physiological sensitivity of respiratory-dependent cardiac pacing: four-year follow-up. PACE 11:1267-1278
33. Hayes DL, Higano ST, Eisinger G (1989) Electrocardiographic manifestations of a dual-chamber, rate-modulated (DDDR) pacemaker. PACE 12:555-562

I. Basic Concepts

Hemodynamics of the Paced Heart

K. STANGL and E. ALT*

Basic Hemodynamic Considerations

Pacemaker-Specific Determinants

The hemodynamics of the pacemaker patient is subject not only to the general determinants of cardiac function, such as contractility of the myocardium, preload and afterload, but also to specific factors resulting from the nature of the patient's conduction defect and/or the particular pacing mode applied.

The physiological situation is characterized by the existence of exercise-adequate sinus rate control and ensured orthograde stimulus conduction and propagation, and thus an ensured physiological sequence between atrial and ventricular contraction. The degree of pathologically altered hemodynamics under pacemaker stimulation is expressed by the failure of one or both factors. The greater or lesser pathological adaptive mechanisms of the paced heart are not due solely to the underlying bradyarrhythmia, but are also affected substantially by the specific pacemaker system selected. The known hemodynamic problems of VVI pacing led to the development of so-called physiological systems. The term "physiological" refers to systems that restore atrioventricular (AV) synchrony. Physiological systems are thus the AV-synchronous pacing modes AAI, DVI, VAT, VDD and DDD, AAIR, and DDDR and DDIR (Table 1).

Specific determinants of the hemodynamics of the paced heart that result from conduction defect and pacing mode are: rate adaptation, AV synchrony, retrograde AV conduction, and AV interval in dual-chamber systems.

Rate Adaptation

Under physiological conditions the exercise-dependent variation in heart rate is the major mechanism in adapting cardiac output. The latter is composed of rate and stroke volume, whereby stroke volume can be increased during exercise by about 50%, but heart rate by approximately 250%. The exercise-induced increase in cardiac

* Humboldt-Universität Berlin, Bereich Medizin (Charité), 1040 Berlin, and First Medical Clinic, Technical University of Munich, 8000 Munich 80, FRG

Table I. AV synchrony and rate adaptation in various operating modes

Mode	AV Synchrony	Rate Adaptation
VVI	–	–
AAI	+	–
DVI	+	–
DDI	+	–
VAT, VDD, DDD	+	+
VVIR	–	+
AAIR	+	+
DDD(I)R	+	+

VVI, ventricular pacing, ventricular sensing, inhibited mode
AAI, atrial pacing, atrial sensing, inhibited mode
DVI, double pacing (atrial + ventricular), ventricular sensing, inhibited mode
DDI, double pacing, double sensing, inhibited mode
DDD, double pacing, double sensing, inhibited and triggered mode
R, rate adaptive (additional function)

output to four or five times the rest value is thus carried mainly by the heart rate component. In the case of chronotropic incompetence, cardiac output is modulated largely by stroke volume. This compensatory mechanism obviously presupposes an intact ventricular myocardium with the possibility of a variation in stroke volume. If this is impaired, or the stroke volume cannot compensate for the lack of rate increase, cardiac output will be compromised. The relationship between cardiac output and rate is thus crucially dependent upon the stroke volume component.

Controversely, the question of how an increase in heart rate affects cardiac output cannot be answered in general terms. What is initially crucial is the state of the myocardium: if the healthy myocardium, which is capable of changing stroke volume, is paced with increasing rates at rest, cardiac output will remain constant over a wide range of rates, only dropping after exceeding a critical limit at which the diastolic filling becomes limiting [156, 183, 184]. Under these hemodynamic conditions heart rate and cardiac output are almost independent variables within this range of rates. [11, 20, 33, 34, 57, 121, 156, 183] Cardiac output is effectively regulated by the two components: when the rate increases the decrease in stroke volume prevents an increase in circulation beyond the metabolic requirements under conditions of rest.

The myocardial situation is different when ventricular function is compromised. With insufficient stroke volume regulation one observes a proportionality between rate and cardiac output; rate becomes the sole determinant in an individually varying range [11, 156] with a shift of the critical rate beyond which cardiac output drops towards the left, i.e., to lower rates [11, 183, 184].

From the data shown, the importance of the two components (rate and stroke volume) for cardiac output can be summarized as follows: The importance of rate as the major factor for adaptation of cardiac output under rest and exercise conditions results from this component's greater ability to change under physiological conditions. It increases further under pathological conditions to the degree at which stroke volume is compromised or fixed in the case of an insufficient myocardium.

AV Synchrony

The term AV synchrony describes the physiological contraction sequence between the atria and ventricles which has short intervals under physiological conditions. Properly timed atrial contractions determine the atrial contribution to the ventricular stroke volume by influencing AV valve closure, end-diastolic ventricular volume, and the pressure in the atrium and ventricle. A disturbance in AV synchrony is of particular importance for the hemodynamics of the paced heart in two situations. It can initially be completely lost as a result of an AV dissociation in the case of an antegrade and retrograde AV block; the contraction sequence between the atrium and ventricle then follows a beat pattern. Secondly, it can lead to a reversal of the contraction sequence due to retrograde AV conduction under ventricular pacing. The atrial contraction then occurs in the ventricular ejection phase.

Atrial Contribution

A further relevant variable for the hemodynamics of the paced heart is the predetermined AV interval (AAI) or programmable AV interval (dual-chamber systems). The first of a series of systematic animal-experiment studies on the importance of atrial systole that are still being conducted today dates back to the beginning of this century. [4, 14, 20, 24, 26, 55, 56, 82, 106, 112, 113, 122, 162]. All in all, the results of the animal and human experiments can be summarized as follows.

Under physiological conditions the atrial contraction actively transports about 20% of the total inflowing blood volume during diastole into the ventricle and increases ventricular filling toward the end of diastole. What is far more important is that the atrial systole simultaneously increases the preextension of the myocardium of the ventricles which, according to Starling's law, is essential for the force and pressure development of the following contraction. This volume loading thus leads to a sufficiently high end-diastolic pressure in the ventricle for an optimal sarcomere length of the ventricular myocardium. The importance of the atrial contribution for the stroke volume of the ventricular myocardium is made clear by the working diagrams of the two different initial positions (Fig. 1).

In situations of low preextension, the atrial contraction leads to a rightward shift from the initial position into the optimal range of preextension. A lack of atrial contraction can cause a decrease in end-diastolic ventricular pressure and consequently an insufficient preextension of the ventricular myocardium. When there is no atrial contraction the prolonged diastolic filling time additionally prevents the presystolic closure of the AV valves [38, 69]; the valve closure takes place solely through the ventricular contraction which can lead to regurgitation at the AV valves in early systole. [1, 63, 107, 120, 122, 146, 154] The teleological sense of atrial contraction is that the end-diastolic pressure level can build up in the ventricle towards the end of diastole without correspondingly high atrial pressures having to exist during the entire cardiac cycle. The mean pressure in the pulmonary circulation can thus be kept low and pulmonary congestion prevented [24, 25, 105].

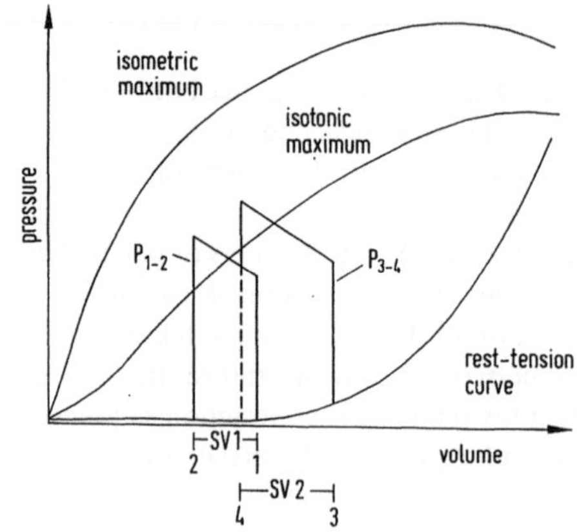

Fig. 1. Schematic representation of working diagrams and stroke volumes (*SV*) at different preextensions. *1*, the end-diastolic volume; *2*, the end-systolic volume at low preextension; *3*, the end-diastolic volume; *4*, the end-systolic volume at greater preextension. Lines *P 1-2* and *P 3-4* yield the particular stroke volumes

Rate vs Atrial Contribution

As stated above, the increase in cardiac output obtained during adaptation to exercise results firstly from the rate increase and the atrial contribution to stroke volume. The year-long discussion about the importance of the two components for the increase in cardiac output was reactivated by the development of atrial-independent, rate-adaptive, single-chamber systems and has been quite controversial over the past few years. In the studies investigating the importance of the two components for cardiac output [6, 10, 53, 85, 91, 110] the following test setup was selected with various slight modifications: predefined exercise protocols were conducted with the same patient in three different modes, namely VVI, an atrial-triggered pacing mode (VAT/VDD/DDD), and a rate-adaptive VVI mode (VVI-matched). VVI-matched means that the patients were paced with AV asynchrony at the rate they had reached under atrial-triggered pacing. With the same pacing rate in the ventricle this arrangement permits a direct intraindividual comparison between AV synchronous (VAT/VDD/DDD) and asynchronous (VVI-matched) pacing, and thus an estimation of atrial contribution. All studies indicated that the importance of the atrial contribution diminishes or disappears at increasing exercise levels [47, 48, 86, 103].

In the past few years similar effects have also been shown comparing DDD systems and rate-adaptive single-chamber ventricular systems (VVIR). In some studies the hemodynamics are compared, as in the above-described design, in the AV-synchronous DDD-mode and with asynchronous rate-adaptive pacing (VVIR) in patients with a third-degree AV block [30, 127, 143, 158, 168]. During exercise there was no difference in hemodynamics between the two pacing modes; in patients with additional sinual chronotropic incompetence VVIR pacing even proved to be superior [13].

Interestingly enough, the first comparisons between AV-synchronous, rate-adaptive, dual-chamber pacing (DDDR) and asynchronous VVIR pacing showed no differences in cardiac performance [180] in patients with total AV block during exercise, while a clear superiority of DDDR pacing over VVIR pacing can understandably (see below) be demonstrated in patients with retrograde conduction [77].

According to the data shown, the initial question as to the value of rate and atrial contribution in adapting cardiac output to exercise can presumably only be answered to the effect that the rate increase is of far greater importance [47, 48, 86, 87, 103]. In the individually high-load range the increase in cardiac output is carried almost solely by rate. These results appear to contradict the importance ov AV synchrony and atrial contribution for the hemodynamics of the paced heart as described above. The supposed contradictions result from the fact that the weighting of these factors changes during exercise with consecutively raised filling pressures. At a higher pressure level there are fundamental differences in the part played by atrial systole for ventricular filling and presystolic preextension of the ventricular myocardium. The atrial contribution to the ventricular stroke volume depends crucially on the mean atrial pressure. In patients with compromised myocardial pumping function and reduced compliance there is a corresponding pressure increase in the left atrium during exercise. Due to the existing pressure gradient between the atrium and the ventricle, the early diastolic filling of the ventricle is increased further; the filling takes place in a predominantly passive fashion. Under these conditions the atrial contraction takes place against the raised end-diastolic ventricular pressure which has already built up; its effect consequently decreases or disappears altogether [35, 93, 135]. At the same time, the effect of atrial contraction is determined by the mean pressure in the atrium itself: the efficiency of atrial contraction decreases to the point at which pathologically elevated pressures preextend the atrial myocardium beyond the optimal sarcomere length.

Summing up, one can conclude from the results of these studies that the atrial contribution is important in increasing cardiac output at rest and during moderate exercise, but this importance diminishes, or often can no longer be detected, upon increasing exercise with a corresponding increase in left ventricular filling pressures (Fig. 2).

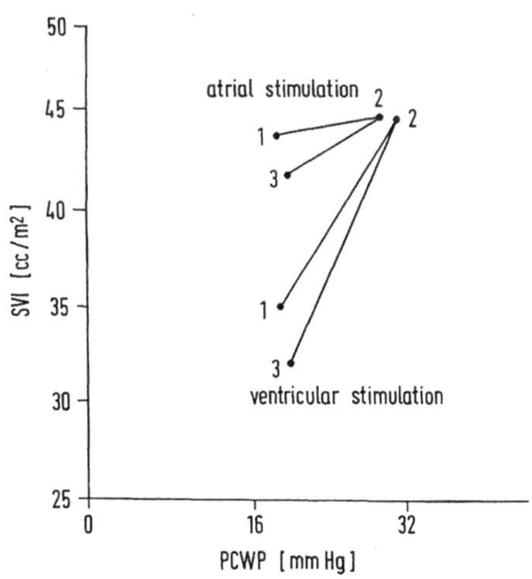

Fig. 2. Dependence of atrial contribution on filling pressure. The atrial contribution is calculated from the difference in points *1* and *2* between atrial pacing and ventricular pacing. (Modified from [67]).
PCWP, pulmonary capillary wedge pressure; *SVI*, stroke volume index

Retrograde AV Conduction

The hemodynamic situation deteriorates when there is a dissociation of atrial and ventricular action or a retrograde stimulation of the atria subsequent to ventricular pacing. AV dissociation is the result of a total AV block that is untreated or treated with a VVI system. Retrograde conduction results from ventricular pacing with retrograde atrial stimulation; it can also occur rarely in the case of an antegrade conduction block [31, 149]. In sick sinus syndrome its incidence is stated as being between 40% and 100% [64, 176, 186]. The clinical picture of this pacemaker-specific disturbance is summarized as pacemaker syndrome [5, 68, 125].

Several factors must be considered pathogenetic for the clinical picture of pacemaker syndrome. Contraction of the atria against the closed AV valves leads to an acute extension of the atria with the occurrence of cannon waves [83, 154]. These sudden pressure increases seem to be involved in triggering a reflex process with a drop in peripheral resistance [112, 113, 122] and cardiac output. [40, 114] Atrial contraction against the closed AV valves also leads to a reversal in the flow of blood with regurgitation into the pulmonary and systemic veins [44, 45, 112, 113, 122]. This consequently delays and compromises the rapid filling phase in early diastole, adversely affecting the filling of the corresponding ventricle. The hemodynamic situation is comparable with that in the case of mitral stenosis: the left atrial mean pressure is raised while the end-diastolic pressure in the left ventricle remains low.

In accordance with these findings, retrograde atrial activation is of central importance in pacemaker patients under VVI pacing (Fig. 3) [188]. Thus, patients without retrograde conduction showed no significant differences despite a higher rate under VVI pacing in comparison to the previously existing sinus bradycardia, while the cardiac index rose 19% under atrial pacing (AAI). By contrast, if there was retrograde atrial activation ventricular pacing led to a 14% drop in the cardiac index; these patients accordingly profited clearly more from AAI pacing with an increase of 42% over VVI pacing [164, 165, 191].

New aspects of the pathogenesis of pacemaker syndrome have been opened up by the study of atrial natriuretic peptide (ANP) in AV dissociation and retrograde conduction. The generally accepted secretion stimuli for this hormone, which is synthesized and liberated predominantly in the atria, are in particular chronically raised atrial pressures and/or the abrupt extension of the atria – factors that play a central part in pacemaker syndrome. The polypeptide acts on various target organs, but particularly its vasodilator effect appears interesting for the pathogenesis of pacemaker syndrome. On the basis of these previous findings, ANP liberation and chronic plasma levels in AV-synchronous and -asynchronous pacing modes were examined in two studies. As expected, in AV dissociation there was a higher release of the hormone at rest and during exercise of up to 200% (Fig. 4) [161, 177]. The value of acutely and chronically elevated ANP levels under nonphysiological pacing is not sufficiently clear at present, but the dilative effect of the peptide on the arteriolar musculature [22, 137] could be a connecting link between the observed drop in blood pressure and/or peripheral resistance in pacemaker syndrome.

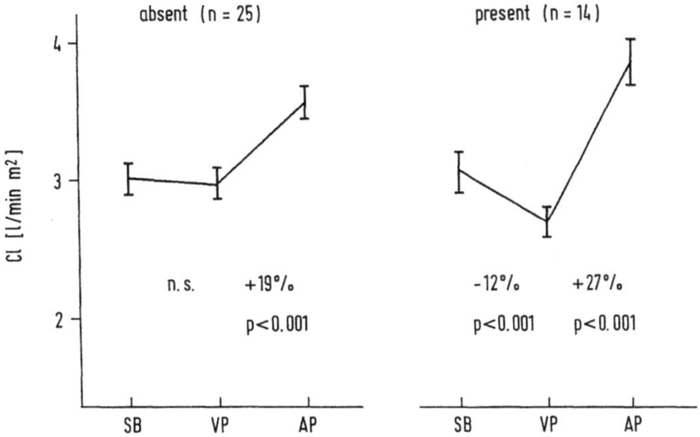

Fig. 3. Dependence of cardiac output on conduction conditions in various pacing modes. *Left*, cardiac index (*CI*) of patients with sick sinus syndrome without retrograde conduction with sinus bradycardia (*SB*), ventricular pacing (*VP*), and atrial pacing (*AP*). *Right*, cardiac indices with present retrograde conduction. (Modified from [188])

AV Interval

The use of AV-synchronous systems can restore AV synchrony and thus avoid the adverse effects of a reversal of the contraction sequence.

While the time interval between atrial and ventricular contraction is predetermined by the conduction time of the AV node and the intraventricular conduction system under atrial single-chamber pacing (AAI), the AV intervals are variable in dual-chamber systems. The question as to the optimal AV interval cannot be definitively answered at present; the literature contains some contradictory data ranging from 50 ms to 250 ms [8, 37, 46, 51, 62, 70, 71, 81, 88, 116, 118, 173, 179, 181]. The great variation may be partly due to methodological aspects, but there is certainly wide individual fluctuation between individual patients and examined populations, whereby differences in the patients' myocardial functions are an essential factor [145].

Indisputably, the AV intervals should become shorter as the rate increases, in accordance with the physiological situation [50, 104, 138, 139].

Hemodynamics Under Ventricular Single-Chamber Pacing (VVI)

Total AV-Block

Basic studies on the acute and long-term hemodynamic effects of VVI pacing date mainly back to the 1960s [2, 20, 59, 60, 78, 111, 147, 157]. Since at that time the indication was predominantly limited to total AV block, most studies deal with the hemodynamics of this conduction defect prior to and under VVI pacing.

There are clear differences with respect to hemodynamics and physical capability

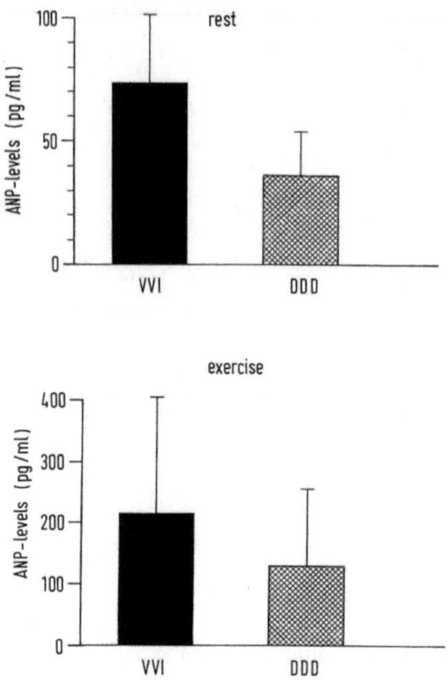

Fig. 4. Influence of AV synchrony on plasma levels of atrial natriuretic peptide (*ANP*) in patients with total AV block. Comparison between synchronous DDD pacing and asynchronous VVI pacing. (Modified from [161].)

between congenital and acquired forms of block. Patients with congenital AV block generally show approximately normal cardiac outputs at rest and during exercise; their capabilities are not restricted [79, 148]. This is due to the younger age and usually normal myocardial pump function of these patients, in contrast to the mainly elderly population with aquired AV conduction defects, and to the fact that patients with congenital AV block are capable of increasing their ventricular rate up to 100 beats/min during exercise, which is not normal but is hemodynamically sufficient [79].

By contrast, the aquired AV block situation is characterized by reduced cardiac outputs that manifest themselves with corresponding symptoms during exercise and even at rest [16, 111, 159].

VVI vs Intrinsic Rate

In most studies the cardiac output of the various populations is already lowered at rest, with cardiac indices between 1.9 l/m^2 per minute and 2.3 l/m^2 per minute [78, 147] or outputs between 2.8 l/min and 3.8 l/min [20, 60].

If the pacemaker rate of the heart is increased under conditions of rest in acute tests, there is an increase in cardiac output of between 21% and 57% [20, 59, 60, 78, 147, 156]. During exercise various studies show an increase in cardiac output of between 32% [49] and 50% [20] in acute tests under VVI pacing, in comparison to the spontaneous bradycardiac rhythm. Nevertheless, the cardiac output fails to reach normal values under VVI pacing even during exercise. Also, the pressure conditions often altered pathologically in symptomatic bradycardia remain largely unaffected by pacemaker therapy [111] . As a result of the reduced circulation the maximum oxygen uptake, as a measure of cardiac performance, is reduced [9, 129, 157] , being sometimes far below that of an age-appropriate and sex matched population [23, 150, 153].

Important aspects of cardiac energetics under VVI pacing were worked out in Baller's animal model [12] and in humans [89]. Under VVI pacing a 40% decrease in the efficiency of cardiac work and an increase of 22% [11] and 21% [89] in myocardial oxygen consumption were observed, in comparison to the AAI mode.

The hemodynamically favorable effect of the rate increase in acute tests is countered by long-term studies in which this initially observed increase in cardiac output was no longer reproducible [2, 111, 187].

Sick Sinus Syndrome

The hemodynamics ov VVI pacing in sick sinus syndrome is determined essentially by the basic rhythm and accompanying conduction conditions. What is crucial is whether there is retrograde AV conduction, so that the negative effects overlay the potential hemodynamic gain of the higher rates. Thus, under VVI pacing and retrograde conduction there was a drop in cardiac output, down to 25% below the spontaneous bradycardiac rhythm [164, 165, 188]. Even without retrograde conduction no hemodynamic improvement could be achieved under VVI pacing in comparison to the spontaneous rhythm [188]. No hemodynamic improvement can be achieved in patients with retrograde AV conduction under VVIR pacing either [77].

Bradyarrhythmia

The influence of VVI pacing on bradyarrhythmia (atrial fibrillation + slow ventricular response) is judged in different ways. No invasive data are available. While some authors report a clear improvement in cardiac performance and/or New York Heart Association (NYHA) classification [43, 108, 134] , the results of other studies are disappointing in regard to the progression of myocardial insufficiency or prognosis [19, 39, 75] .

However, a positive effect of VVI pacing must be seen in the extension of therapeutic possibilities to substances with positive inotropic and negative dromotropic action profiles.

Hemodynamics of Physiological Pacing Modes

Pacing modes are termed physiological when they restore the synchrony between the atrium and ventricle (Table 1) [65].

Fixed-Rate Atrial Single-Chamber Pacing (AAI) vs Intrinsic Rate

Atrial single-chamber pacing is the method of choice for sick sinus syndrome without a concomitant AV conduction defect. By restoring the normal AV sequence one can utilize the physiological contribution of atrial systole and avoid retrograde atrial stimulation. Under AAI pacing the cardiac outputs or cardiac indices are 13%-28% higher than with the spontaneous bradycardiac rhythm [18, 21, 70, 101, 164, 188], and 28%-45% higher compared to the hemodynamics under ventricular pacing [164, 188].

It is important that the acute hemodynamic effects described prove to be reproducible even after long periods of observation [18, 189].

Despite positive hemodynamic results, this pacing mode meets with considerable, presumably inappropriate, skepticism [167]. Looking through numerous studies on the development of life-threatening AV blocks one finds annual incidences below 1% in the majority of studies [142].

Fixed-Rate Sequential Pacing (DVI) vs Intrinsic Rate

DVI pacing was established as a further development of AAI pacing in order to make atrial pacing also possible for patients with AV conduction defects. However, it has become outdated through the development of DDD systems. Under DVI pacing there was an increase in cardiac output at rest with improvements in cardiac output of between 11% and 29% in comparison to the spontaneous rhythm [32, 36, 90, 115, 131, 133, 164, 174].

No data are available on hemodynamics during exercise.

Atrial-Triggered Pacing Modes (AT, VDD, DDD) vs VVI

Unlike AAI and DVI pacing, the atrial-triggered pacing modes VAT, VDD, and DDD not only preserve AV synchrony, but also open up the possibility of rate adaptation.

Since the early 1970s, the acute hemodynamic effects and cardiac performance of pacemaker patients under atrial-triggered pacing modes have been examined in comparison with VVI pacing in numerous studies. All studies, with one exception (sick sinus syndrome [18]), involve populations with high-degree AV blocks.

Under atrial-triggered modes there are improvements in hemodynamics at rest of between 10% and 43% over fixed-rate VVI pacing [18, 35, 41, 72, 84, 85, 93, 98, 116, 119, 126, 133, 140, 143, 163, 185, 189]. During exercise the atrial-triggered pacing modes proved superior with higher cardiac outputs of between 10% and 40%.

Several studies, furthermore, compare physical capabilities with various metabolic or physical variables as equivalents of cardiac performance under the two pacing modes. They find improvements in cardiopulmonary performance of between 9% and 43% [53, 91, 126, 128, 143, 166].

The increase in cardiac performance during exercise evidenced in all studies represents only one aspect of an improved hemodynamic situation. Another aspect is the influence of the pacing mode on left ventricular filling pressures, which are usually pathologically raised under VVI pacing. Five studies [84, 85, 119, 126, 143] examine this question additionally. Two studies can demonstrate a positive effect on hemodynamics whilst at rest under VAT pacing, with a 13% or 35% reduction in pulmonary capillary wedge pressure [84, 85]. On the other hand, there were no significant differences between the two pacing modes during exercise in any study. This result can be interpreted as being due to the fact that many pacemaker patients already have impaired myocardial compliance (e.g., in coronary heart disease, LV hypertrophy) that becomes apparent particularly during exercise; this can of course not be influenced by pacing.

In contrast to the merely temporary increase in cardiac output under VVI pacing [2, 111], a positive long-term effect is detectable under atrial-triggered pacing [18, 84, 128, 152, 166].

The effects of atrial-triggered pacing on hemodynamics and physical powers can be summarized as follows: In comparison to VVI pacing there is an increase in cardiac output of up to 10%-43% under physiological pacing at rest and between 10% and 40% during exercise. The resulting average improvement in physical powers is between 10% and 40%. Both effects show long-term behavior. Pathological pressure conditions under VVI pacing can only be influenced positively at rest.

Atrial-Independent Rate-Adaptive Pacing

Basic Considerations

Since the improvement in exercise hemodynamics under atrial-triggered pacing is carried largely by the rate, similar positive hemodynamic effects would also be expected from a pacing mode that does not use the sinoatrial rate as a control parameter, but is modulated by parameters varying in proportion to exercise. Such systems open up the possibility of adequate rate adaptation for patients with inadequate or no sinoatrial function. Since atrial-independent rate adaptation is no longer restricted to ventricular pacing (VVIR), but is now also possible as atrial single-chamber (AAIR) and dual-chamber pacing (DDDR, DDIR), it can be utilized for the three main indications, AV block, sick sinus syndrome, and absolute brady-arrhythmia, and constitutes a genuine expansion and improvement in pacemaker therapy for a great number of patients with chronotropic incompetence [190].

VVIR vs VVI

Hemodynamics at rest and during exercise under atrial-independent rate-adaptive pacing has been examined for several parameters since the early 1980s. In acute tests the increase in cardiac output during exercise is between 22% and 64% [3, 15, 27, 29, 76, 86, 117, 136, 140, 143, 178, 189] , more than comparable values under fixed-rate pacing.

There are also a large number of reports on improved performance and increased well-being under atrial-triggered pacing. Exercise protocols on the treadmill were used to test cardiac performance. Increases in performance were observed over a wide range of 13%-77% [17, 26, 28, 42, 52, 54, 80, 86, 92, 94, 96, 99, 100, 102, 123, 124, 130, 141, 155, 171, 192, 194].

Studies have been conducted on rate-adaptive pacing with physiological parameters other than activity. Improvements in cardiac performance of between 8% and 44% were found [7, 29, 58, 73, 74, 95, 97, 143, 144, 160, 172, 193, 194]. There are also reports of a normalization of performance in patients after His' bundle ablation under rate-adaptive VVI pacing [169], and of 24% lower plasma levels of ANP in comparison to the fixed-rate mode [170].

The question of the long-term effectiveness of rate-adaptive systems is dealt with in several studies, which show improved hemodynamics under VVIR pacing as a long-term effect [15, 28, 42, 103, 124].

AAIR vs AAI

The availability of atrial (AAIR [151]) and rate-adaptive dual-chamber systems (DDDR, DDIR) has resulted in a new therapeutic approach to patients with sick sinus syndrome.

The advantages of rate-adaptive AAI pacing (AAIR) over fixed-rate AAI pacing have already been shown in some studies [140, 141, 144]. The maximum oxygen uptake and treadmill distances under AAIR pacing were 18% and 20% higher, respectively, than in the fixed-rate AAI mode.

DDDR vs DDD

A comparison of the most recent pacing mode (DDDR) with DDD pacing in patients (some of whom have chronotropic incompetence) has already been dealt in two studies. DDDR proved superior with 11% [182] and an optimistic 67% [30]. Hemodynamic improvements under DDDR pacing also seem to have a long-term effect [109].

Summing up, the results demonstrate that similar hemodynamically favorable acute and long-term effects can be obtained under atrial-independent rate-adaptive pacing and under atrial-triggered pacing. If there is inadequate, or no sinoatrial rate adaptation this new pacing mode clearly improves the therapeutic possibilities.

References

1. Abinader EG, Goldhammer E, Hassan A (1987) The significance of properly timed ventricular systole on diastolic mitral regurgitation occuring in complete heart block. PACE 10:630
2. Adolph RJ, Homes JC, Fukusumi H (1968) Hemodynamik studies in patients with chronically implanted pacemakers. Am Heart J 76:829
3. Aguirre JM, Ruiz de Azuá E, Molinero E et al. (1987) Hemodynamic response to isotonic exercise of rate-responsive pacemaker Activitrax vs VVI. PACE 10:1205
4. Albani E, Amati PC, Destro A et al. (1983) Echocardiographic parameters in DDD AV-sequential paced patients. PACE 6:A-76
5. Alicandri C, Fouad FM, Tarazi RC et al. (1978) Three cases of hypotension and syncope with ventricular pacing: possible role of atrial reflexes. Am J Cardiol 42:137
6. Alt E, Wirtzfeld A, Klein G (1983) Hämodynamische Ergebnisse bei ventrikulärer und physiologischer Stimulation. Herz Kreislauf 2:31
7. Alt E, Völker R, Högl B et al. (1988) Kardiopulmonale Belastungstest unter frequenzvariabler Stimulation: Ein Vergleich von Activitrax- und Nova-MR-Schrittmachern zu VVI-/AAI-Simulation. Z Kardiol 77:456
8. Antonioli GE, Albani E, Amati PC et al. (1988) 2D and Doppler echocardiography in dual-chambered paced patients. PACE 11[Suppl):846
9. Astrand I, Landegren J (1965) The effect of varying rate on physical work capacity in patients with complete heart block. Acta Med Scand 177:657
10. Ausubel K, Steingart RM, Shimshi M et al. (1985) Maintenance of exercise stroke volume during ventricular versus atrial synchronous pacing: role of contractility. Circulation 72(5):1037
11. Baller D, Hoeft A, Korb H et al. (1981) Basic physiological studies on cardiac pacing with special references to the optimal mode and rate after cardiac surgery. Thorac Cardiovasc Surg 29:168
12. Baller D, Wolpers HG, Zipfel J et al. (1988) Comparison of the effects of right atrial, right ventricular apex and atrioventricular sequential pacing on myocardial oxygen consumption and cardiac efficiency: a laboratory investigation. PACE 11:394
13. Bathen J, Hegrenes L, Skjaerpe T (1983) Pulsed Doppler ultrasound for estimating blood flow in the aorta during cardiac pacing. PACE 6:A-87
14. Batey RL, Sweesy M, Scala M et al. (1990) Comparison of low-rate dual-chamber pacing to activity-responsive variable-ventricular pacing. PACE 13:646
15. Bellocci F, Montenero S, Scabbia E et al. (1988) Long-term follow-up of activity-sensing rate-responsive pacemaker. PACE 11[Suppl]:798
16. Benchimol A, Ellis J, Dimond G (1965) Hemodynamik consequences of atrial and ventricular pacing in patients with normal and abnormal hearts. Am J Med 39:911
17. Benditt AG, Mianulli M, Fetter J et al. (1987) Single-chamber cardiac pacing with activity-initiated chronotropic response: evaluation by cardiopulmonary exercise testing. Circulation 75:184
18. Bergbauer M, Sabin G (1983) Hämodynamische Langzeitresultate der bifokalen Schrittmacherstimulation. Dtsch Med Wochenschr 108:545
19. Bernstein V, Roem C, Peretz DI (1971) Permanent pacemakers: 8-year follow-up study. Incidence and management of congestive cardiac failure and performance. Ann Intern Med 74:361
20. Bevegard S, Johnsson B, Karlöf I et al. (1967) Effect of changes in ventricular rate and central pressures at rest and during exercise in patients with artificial pacemakers. Cardiovasc Res 1:21
21. Beyer J, Thorban S, Adt M et al. (1983) Physiological vs VVI pacing: Its effect on cardiac output with different left ventricular compliance. PACE 6:A-84
22. Bolli P, Müller FB, Linder L et al. (1987) The vasodilator potency of atrial natriuretic peptide in man. Circulation 75:221
23. Bolt W, Buchter A, Grosser KD (1971) Die Leistungsbreite bei Patienten mit Herzschrittmachern. Verh Dtsch Ges Inn Med 77:457

24. Braunwald E, Frahm CJ (1961) Studies on Starling's law of the heart. Observations on the hemodynamic functions of the left atrium in man. Circulation 14:633
25. Braunwald E, Sonnenblick EH, Ross J et al. (1967) An analysis of the cardiac response to exercise. Circ Res XX/I:44
26. Brofman P, Rossi P, Loures D et al. (1987) Rate-responsive pacemaker in Chagas' disease. PACE 10:1208
27. Buckingham T, Woodruff R, Pennington G et al. (1987) Hemodynamic effects of rate-responsive pacing in patients with left ventricular dysfunction measured by 2D and Doppler echocardiography. PACE 10/II:652, A90
28. Buetikofer J, Milstein S, Mianulli M et al. (1987) Sustained improvement in peak oxygen consumption with activity-initiated rate-variable pacing. PACE 10/II:652, A91
29. Camm AJ, Garratt CJ (1988) Rate-adaptive pacing guided by minute ventilation. In: Santini M, Pistolese M, Alliegro A (eds) Progress in clinical pacing. Excerpta Medica, Amsterdam, p 107
30. Capucci A, Caccin R, Boriani G et al. (1990) DDDR pacing modalities in patients with and without chronotropic incompetence compared to DDD and VVIR modes. PACE 13:1192
31. Castillo C, Samet P (1967) Retrograde conduction in complete heart block. Br Heart J 29:553
32. Chamberlain DA, Leinbach RC, Vassaux CE et al. (1970) Sequential atrioventricular pacing in heart block complicating acute myocardial infarction. N Engl J Med 282:577
33. Chan W, Kertes P, Mond H et al. (1983) The effects of altering heart rate on supine cardiac volumes at rest during ventricular-inhibited pacing. PACE 6:A-79
34. Contini C, Pauletti M, Moscarelli E et al. (1983) Evaluation of myocardial function in pacemaker (PM) patients (PTS) by means of a non-invasive Doppler technique. PACE 6:A-87
35. Costa R, Moreira LF, Martinelli F et al. (1988) Atrial synchronous pacing: a real benefit in cardiomyopathy? PACE 11[Suppl.]:816
36. Curtis JJ, Madigan NP, Withing RB et al. (1981) Clinical experience with permanent atrioventricular sequential pacing. Ann Thorac Surg 32:179
37. Curtis J, Walls J, Boley T et al. (1983) Importance of atrio-ventricular contraction interval on hemodynamics. PACE 6:A-83
38. Daubert JC, Roussel A, Langella B et al. (1983) Hemodynamic and echocardiographic consequences of ventriculo-atrial conduction (VAC) in man. PACE 6:A-78
39. Davidson DM, Braak CA, Preston TA et al. (1972) Permanent ventricular pacing. Effect on long-term survival, congestive heart failure, and subsequent myocardial infarction and stroke. Ann Intern Med 77:345
40. DiCarlo LA, Morady F, Krol R et al. (1987) Role of the atrium during ventricular pacing: hemodynamic consequences of atrio-ventricular and ventriculoatrial pacing in humans. PACE 10/128:438
41. DiCola VC, Stewart WJ, Harthorne JW et al. (1983) Doppler ultrasound measurement of cardiac output in patients with physiologic dual-chamber pacemakers. PACE 6:A-86
42. Djordjevic M, Stojanov P, Kocovic D et al. (1987) Comparative effects of rate-responsive activity pacing an VVI pacing on exercise capacity. In: Belhassen B, Feldmann S, Copperman Y (eds) Cardiac pacing and electrophysiology. R&L Creative Communications, Jerusalem, p 47
43. Dolder A, Halter J, Nager F (1975) Schrittmacherimplantation bei bradykarder Herzinsuffizienz. Dtsch Med Wochenschr 100:2070
44. Dreifus LS, Naito M, David D et al. (1983) Hemodynamic consequences of abnormal atrioventricular sequential pacing. PACE 6:81
45. Dreifus LS, Mitamura H, Rhauda A et al. (1986) Effects of AV-sequential versus asynchronous AV-pacing on pulmonary hemodynamics. PACE 9:171
46. Duval AM, Lellouche D, Dubois-Rande JL et al. (1988) Relationship between AV delay and left ventricular filling in VDD mode pacing. PACE 11[Suppl]:817
47. Edelstam C, Juhlia-Dannfeldt, Nordlander R et al. (1990) The hemodynamic importance of atrial systole – a function of the kinetic energy of blood flow? PACE 13:1194
48. Edelstam C, Hjemdahl P, Pehrsson et al. (1990) Is DDD pacing superior to VVI-R? Effects on myocardial sympathetic activity and oxygen consumption. PACE 13:1193
49. Eimer HH, Witte J (1974) Zur Leistungsbreite bei Patienten mit festfrequentem Herz-

Herzschrittmacher unter Berücksichtigung von Hämodynamik, arteriovenöser Sauerstoffdifferenz und Lungenfunktion. Z Kardiol 63:1099
50. Eisinger GE, Winston SA, McGaughey MD (1988) Rate-responsive AV-delay and its effect on upper rate limit performance in DDD pacemakers. PACE 11[Suppl]:815
51. Faerestrand S, Ohm OJ (1985) A time-related study of the hemodynamic benefit of atrioventricular synchronous pacing evaluated by Doppler echocardiography. PACE 8:838
52. Faerestrand S, Ohm OJ (1987) Activity-sensing rate-responsive ventricular pacing (VVI): relation between left ventricular dimensions and improvement in work capacity. PACE 10:1211
53. Fananapazir L, Srinivas V, Bennett DH (1983) Comparison of resting hemodynamic indices and exercise performance during atrial synchronized and asynchronous pacing. PACE 6:202
54. Fetter J, Mianulli M, Benditt DG (1987) Transcutaneous triggering of conventional implanted pulse-generators: a technique for predicting benefits of activity-initiated rate-variable pacing. PACE 10:432
55. Frank O (1895) Zur Dynamik des Herzmuskels. Z Biol (Munich) 32:371
56. Frank O (1901) Isometrie und Isotonie des Herzmuskels. Z Biol (Munich) 41:14
57. Fujiyama M, Furuta Y, Matsumura J et al. (1983) Reconsideration of heart rate (HR) -cardiac output (COP) curve and resting cardiac function in bradyarrhythmias. PACE 6:A-83
58. Gammage M, Schofield S, Pentecost B (1990) Benefit of rate-respnsive pacing compared with fixed-rate demand pacing using a single setting for rate-responsive mode in elderly patients. PACE 13:504
59. Gattenlöhner W, Schneider KW (1973) Schrittmachertherapie und Hämodynamik. Münch Med Wochenschr 115:2137
60. Gerhard W, Smekal P, Grosser KD (1976) Kreislaufdynamik bei totalem atrioventrikulären Block vor und nach Anwendung eines elektrischen Schrittmachers unter verschiedenen Frequenzen. Dtsch Med Wochenschr 34:1488
61. Gesell RA (1919) Cardiodynamics in heart block as affected by auricular systole, auricular fibrillation and stimulation of the vagus nerve. Am J Physiol 40:267
62. Gillespie WI, Greene DG, Karatzas NB et al. (1967) Effect of atrial systole on right ventricular stroke output in complete heart block. Br Med J 1:75
63. Gilmore J, Sarnoff SJ, Mitchell JH et al. (1963) Synchronicity of ventricular contraction: observations comparing hemodynamic effects of atrial and ventricular pacing. Br Heart J 25:299
64. Goldreyer BN, Bigger J (1970) Ventriculo-atrial conduction in man. Circulation 61:935
65. Goldreyer BN (1982) Physiological pacing: the role of AV synchrony. PACE 5:613
66. Greenberg P, Castellanet M, Messenger J et al. (1978) Coronary sinus pacing. Clinical follow-up. Circulation 57:98
67. Greenberg B, Chatterjee K, Parmley WW et al. (1979) The influence of left ventricular filling pressure on atrial contribution to cardiac output. Am Heart J 98:742
68. Haas JM, Strait GB (1974) Pacemaker-induced cardiovascular failure. Hemodynamic and angiographic observations. Am J Cardiol 33:295
69. Hamby RI, Aintablian A, Wisoff BG (1973) The role of atrial systole in valve closure. Chest 64:197
70. Hartzler GO, Maloney JD, Curtis JJ et al. (1977) Hemodynamic benefits of atrioventricular sequential pacing after cardiac surgery. Am J Cardiol 40:232
71. Haskell RJ, French WJ (1986) Optimum AV interval in dual-chamber pacemakers. PACE 9:670
72. Hayes DL, Furman S (1984) Stability of AV conduction in sick sinus syndrome patients with implanted atrial pacemakers. Am Heart J 107:644
73. Hedman A, Nordlander R (1988) Q-T-sensing rate-responsive pacing versus fixed-rate ventricular pacing – a controlled clinical study. PACE 11:506
74. Hedman A (1989) Long-term follow-up of patients treated with the Q-T interval-sensing rate-responsive pacemaker. J Intern Med 225:385
75. Hetzel MR, Ginks WR, Pickersgill AJ et al. (1978) Value of pacing in cardiac failure associated with chronic atrioventricular block. Br Heart J 40:864
76. Humen DP, Kostuk WJ, Klein GJ (1985) Activity-sensing, rate-responsive pacing: improvement in myocardial performance with exercise. PACE 8:52

77. Hummel J, Barr E, Hanich R et al. (1990) DDDR pacing is better tolerated than VVI in patients with sinus node disease. PACE 13:504
78. Humphries JO, Hinman EJ, Bernstein L et al. (1967) Effect of artificial pacing on cardiac and renal function. Circulation 36:717
79. Ikkos D, Hanson JS (1960) Response to exercise in congenital complete atrioventricular block. Circulation 12:583
80. Iwase M, Hatano K, Saito F et al. (1989) Evaluation by exercise Doppler echocardiography of maintenance of cardiac output during ventricular pacing with or without chronotropic response. Am J Cardiol 63:934
81. Janosik D, Pearson A, Redd R et al. (1987) The importance of atrioventricular delay fallback in optimizing cardiac output during physiologic pacing. PACE 10:410
82. Jochim K (1938) The contribution of the auricles to ventricular filling in complete heart block. Am J Physiol 122:639
83. Johnson AD, Laiken SL, Engler RL (1978) Hemodynamic compromise associated with ventriculoatrial conduction following transvenous pacemaker placement. Am J Med 65:75
84. Kappenberger L, Gloor HO, Babotai I et al. (1982) Hemodynamic effects of atrial synchronization in acute and long-term ventricular pacing. PACE 5:639
85. Karlöf I (1975) Haemodynamic effect of atrial-triggered versus fixed-rate pacing at rest and during exercises in complete heart block. Acta Med Scand 197:195
86. Kay GN, Bubien R (1988) Effect of His' bundle ablation and rate-responsive pacing on exercise capacity and quality of life in patients with atrial fibrillation. PACE 11:500
87. Kay GN, Bubien RS (1990) Paired exercise treadmill testing for comparison of pacing modes: the importance of randomized test sequence. PACE 13:534
88. Knapp K, Gmeiner R, Hammerle P et al. (1976) Der Einfluß der Vorhofkontraktion auf das Schlagvolumen bei Schrittmacherstimulation. Z Kardiol 65:783
89. Koretsune Y, Kodama K, Nanto S et al. (1983) The effect of pacing mode on external work and myocardial oxygen consumption. PACE 6:A-77
90. Kourkoulados C, Gialafos J, Paraskevas P et al. (1985) Assessment of left ventricular function in ventricular and AV pacing using systolic time intervals and thermodilution technique. In: Gomez FP (ed) Cardiac pacing, electrophysiology, tachyarrhythmias. Editorial Grouz, Madrid, p 610
91. Kristensson BE, Arnman K, Ryden L (1985) The hemodynamic importance of atrioventricular synchrony and rate increase at rest and during exercises. Eur Heart J 6:773
92. Ladusans E, Priestley K, Rosenthal E et al. (1987) Rate-responsive pacing improves effort capacity compared with VVI pacing in children with symptomatic bradycardia. PACE 10:1216
93. Lascault G, Bigonzi F, Lechat P et al. (1988) Efficacy of DDD pacing in dilated cardiomyopathy: assessment by pulsed Doppler echocardiography. Preliminary results. PACE 11[Suppl]:851
94. Lau C, Tse W, Camm AJ (1988) Clinical experience with Sensolog 703: a new activity-sensing rate-responsive pacemaker. PACE 11:1444
95. Lau C, Drysdale M, Ward D, Camm AJ (1988) Clinical experience of Meta: a minute ventilation-sensing rate-responsive pacemaker. PACE 11:507
96. Lau CP, Camm AJ (1988) Role of left ventricular function and Doppler-derived variables in predicting hemodynamic benefits of rate-responsive pacing. Am J Cardiol 62:906
97. Lau CP, Ward DE, Camm AJ (1989) Single-chamber cardiac pacing with two forms of respiration-controlled rate-responsive pacemaker. Chest 95:352
98. Laule M, Stangl K, Wirtzfeld A (1988) Adaptation to exercise: role of cardiac output, stroke volume and mixed venous oxygen saturation under atrial-triggered vs fixed-rate ventricular pacing. PACE 11[Suppl]:814
99. Lindemans FW, Rankin IA, Murtaugh R et al. (1986) Clinical experience with an activity-sensing pacemaker. PACE 9/II:978
100. Lipkin DP, Buller N, Frenneaux M et al. (1987) Randomized crossover trial of rate-responsive Activitrax and conventional rate-ventricular pacing. Br Heart J 58:613
101. Liu P, Burns RL, Weisel RD et al. (1983) Comprehensive evaluation of left ventricular function during physiological pacing. PACE 6:A-77
102. Manz M, Pfitzner P, Lüderitz B (1987) Rate-responsive pacing after His' bundle ablation and for sick sinus syndrome. PACE 10:1219

103. McMeekin JD, Lautner D, Hanson S et al. (1990) Importance of heart-rate response during exercise in patients using atrioventricular synchronous and ventricular pacemakers. PACE 13:59
104. Mehta D, Gilmour S, Lau C et al. (1987) Optimal atrioventricular interval in patients with dual-chamber pacemakers. PACE 10:437
105. Mitchell JH, Gilmore JP, Sarnoff SJ (1962) The transport function of the atrium. Am J Cardiol 9:237
106. Mitchell JH, Gupta DN, Payne RM (1965) Influence of atrial systole on effective ventricular stroke volume. Circ Res 17:11
107. Moreira LFP, Costa R, Fernandes PMP et al. (1985) Reevaluation of the role of atrial systole in the closure of atrioventricular valves. In: Gomez FP (ed) Cardiac pacing, electrophysiology, tachyarrhythmias. Editorial Grouz, Madrid, p 554
108. Müller OF, Bellet S (1961) Treatment of intractable heart failure in the presence of complete atrioventricular heart block by the use of the internal cardiac pacemaker. N Engl J Med 265:769
109. Mugica J, Henry L, Attuel P et al. (1990) Long-term inprovement of patients' behaviour with rate-modulated pacemakers. PACE 13:1205
110. Munteanu J, Wirtzfeld A, Stangl K et al. (1985) Is the hemodynamic benefit of VDD pacing due to AV synchrony or to rate responsiveness? In: Gomez FP (ed) Cardiac pacing, electrophysiology, tachyarrhythmias. Editorial Grouz, Madrid, p 893
111. Nager F, Bühlmann A, Schaub F (1966) Klinische und hämodynamische Befunde beim totalen AV-Block nach Implantation elektrischer Schrittmacher. Helv Med Acta 33:240
112. Naito M, Dreifus LS, Mardelli TJ et al. (1980) Echocardiographic features of atrioventricular and ventriculoatrial conduction. Am J Cardiol 46:625
113. Naito M, David D, Michelson EL et al. (1980) Pulmonary venous regurgitation: a major factor adversely affecting hemodynamics ventriculoatrial pacing. PACE 3:381
114. Narahara KA, Blettel ML (1983) Effect of rate on left ventricular volumes and ejection fraction during chronic ventricular pacing. Circulation 67/2:323
115. Nishimura RA, Gersh BJ, Vlietstra RE et al. (1982) Hemodynamics and symptomatic consequences of ventricular pacing. PACE 5:903
116. Nitsch J, Seiderer M, Büll U et al. (1983) Auswirkungen unterschiedlicher Schrittmacherstimulation auf linksventrikuläre Volumendaten-Untersuchungen mit der Radionukleid-Ventrikulographie. Z Kardiol 72:718
117. Nobile A, Montenero S, Scabbia E et al. (1987) Long-term follow-up of activity-sensing rate-responsive pacemaker. PACE 10:1223
118. Noll B, Krappe J, Goeke B (1988) Beeinflussung des atrialen natriuretischen Faktors durch die AV-Überleitungszeit bei Schrittmacherträgern. Dtsch Med Wochenschr 113:1994
119. Nordlander R, Pehrsson SK, Aström et al. (1987) Myocardial demands of atrial-triggered versus fixed-rate ventricular pacing in patients with complete heart block. PACE 10:1154
120. Norman R, West RO, Burggraf GW (1986) Echocardiographic assessment of tricuspid regurgitation during ventricular demand pacing. PACE 9:290
121. O'Connor AMJ, Arentzen CE, Anderson RW et al. (1988) Contribution of atrioventricular synchrony to left ventricular systolic function in a closed-chest canine model of complete heart block: implications for single-chamber rate-variable cardiac pacing. PACE 11:404
122. Ogawa S, Dreifus L, Shenoy PN et al. (1978) Hemodynamic consequences of atrioventricular and ventriculoatrial pacing. PACE 1:8
123. Page E, Wolf JE, Billette A et al. (1988) The usefulness of a noninvasive method to predict the benefits of rate-responsive pacing in patients with complete atrioventricular block previously implanted in VVI mode. PACE 11[Suppl]:850
124. Pasquier J, Adamec R, Velebit V et al. (1986) Amelioration à long terme des performances à l'effort des porteurs du stimulateur cardiaque à frequence asservie à l'activite physique. Schweiz Med Wochenschr 116:1604
125. Patel AK, Yap VU, Thomsen JH (1977) Adverse effects of right ventricular pacing in a patient with aortic stenosis. Hemodynamic documentation and management. Chest 72:103
126. Pehrsson SK, Aström H (1983) Left ventricular function after long-term treatment with ventricular-inhibited compared to atrial-triggered ventricular pacing. Acta Med Scand 214:295

127. Pehrsson SK, Hedman A, Hjemdahl P et al. (1987) Myocardial oxygen uptake and sympathetic activity – a comparison between fixed-rate ventricular pacing (VVI), atrial synchronous (VAT) and rate-responsive QT-sensing (TX) pacing. PACE 10:1224
128. Perrins EJ, Morley ChA, Chan SL et al. (1983) Randomized controlled trial of physiological and ventricular pacing. Br Heart J 50:112
129. Petzold D, Haan D, Sill V (1970) Langzeitelektrokardiographie und Spiroergometrie bei Schrittmacher-Patienten. Intensivmed 7:39
130. Pipilis A, Bucknall C, Sowton E (1988) Sensolog – one year on. PACE 11[Suppl]:804
131. Raza ST, Lajos TZ, Lewin AN et al. (1983) Hemodynamic advantages of AV-sequential (DVI) pacing. Further enhancement by optimizing cardiac function. PACE 6:A-80
132. Rediker DE, Eagle KA, Homma S et al. (1988) Clinical and hemodynamic comparison of VVI versus DDD pacing in patients with DDD pacemakers. Am J Cardiol 61:323
133. Reiter MJ, Hindman MC (1982) Hemodynamic effects of acute atrioventricular pacing in patients with left ventricular dysfunction. Am J Cardiol 49:687
134. Rettig G, Schieffer H, Doenecke P et al. (1975) Langzeitprognose bei Schrittmacherpatienten. Herz Kreislauf 10:497
135. Reynolds DW, Wilson MF, Burow RD et al. (1983) Hemodynamic evaluation of atrioventricular sequential versus ventricular pacing in patients with normal and poor ventricular function at variable heart rates and posture. PACE 6:A-80
136. Rickards AF, Donaldson RM, Thalen HJT (1983) The use of QT interval to determine pacing rate: early clinical experience. PACE II/6:346
137. Richards AM, Nicholls MG, Ikram H, Webster MW et al. (1985) Renal, hemodynamic, and hormonal effects of human alpha atrial natriuretic peptide in healthy volunteers. Lancet 1:545
138. Ritter P, Daubert C, Mabo Ph et al. (1987) Improvement of the hemodynamic benefit of dual-chamber pacing by a rate-adapted AV delay. PACE 10/II:734
139. Ritter P, Daubert C, Mabo P et al. (1989) Haemodynamic benefit of a rate-adapted AV-delay in dual-chamber pacing. Eur Heart J 10:637
140. Rognoni G, Occhetta E, Prando MD et al. (1986) Benefits of rate-responsive ventricular pacing with or without atrioventricular synchrony in patients with advanced or complete AV block. In: Santini M, Pistolese M, Alliegro A (eds) Progress in cardiac pacing. Excerpta Medica, Amsterdam, p 20
141. Rosenquist M, Ahren C, Nordlander R et al. (1988) Atrial rate-responsive pacing-effect on exercise capacity. PACE 11:514
142. Rosenquist M, Obel IWB (1989) Atrial pacing and the risk for AV-block: is there a time to change in attitude? PACE 12:97
143. Rossi P, Rognoni G, Occhetta E et al. (1985) Respiration-dependent ventricular pacing compared with fixed-ventricular and atrial-ventricular synchronous pacing: aerobic and hemodynamic variables. J Am Coll Cardiol 6:646
144. Rossi P, Prando DM, Magnani A et al. (1988) Physiological sensitivity of respiratory-dependent cardiac pacing: four-year follow-up. PACE 11:1267
145. Ryden L, Karlsson Ö, Kristensson BE (1988) The importance of different atrioventricular intervals for exercise capacity. PACE 11:1051
146. Sakai M, Ueda K, Ohkawa S et al. (1983) Echocardiographic and pathologic studies on tricuspid regurgitation induced by transvenous right ventricular pacing. PACE 6:A-75
147. Samet Ph, Bernstein WH, Bernstein WH et al. (1964) Effect of alteration in ventricular rate on cardiac output in complete heart block. Am J Cardiol 14:477
148. Scarpelli EM, Rudolph AM (1964) The hemodynamics of congenital heart block. Prog Cardiovasc Dis 6:327
149. Scherf D, Cohen J, Orphanus RP (1964) Retrograde activation of the atria in atrioventricular block. Am J Cardiol 13:219
150. Schmid P, Klein WW, Hard H et al. (1969) Körperliche Belastbarkeit von Herzschrittmacherträgern. Z Kariol 68:763
151. Schüller H, Brandt J, Fahraeus T et al. (1990) Feasibility of rate-adaptive atrial pacing: clinical results in 44 patients. PACE 13:1209
152. Sedney MI, Weijers E, van der Wall EE et al. (1989) Short-term and long-term changes of left ventricular volumes during rate-adaptive and single-rate pacing. PACE 12:1863

153. Sidney KH, Shephard RJ (1977) Maximum and submaximum exercise tests in men and women in the seventh, eighth, and ninth decades of life. J Appl Physiol 43:280
154. Skinner NS, Mitchell J, Wallace AT et al. (1963) Hemodynamic effects of altering the time of atrial systole. Am J Physiol 205:499
155. Smedgard P, Kristensson BE, Kruse I et al. (1987) Rate-responsive pacing by means of activity-sensing versus single-rate ventricular pacing: a double-blind cross-over study. PACE 10/I:902
156. Sowton E (1964) Hemodynamic studies in patients with artificial pacemakers. Br Heart J 26:737
157. Sowton E (1967) The relationship between maximal oxygen uptake and heart rate in patients with artificial pacemakers. Cardiologia 50:15
158. Spencer WH, Goodman DA, Hargis J et al. (1987) Comparison of exercise performance in three rate-responsive pacing modes. PACE 10:1229
159. Stack MF, Rader B, Sobol BJ et al. (1958) Cardiovascular hemodynamic functions in complete heart block and the effect of isopropylnorepinephrine. Circulation 17:526
160. Stangl K, Wirtzfeld A, Göbl G et al. (1986) Rate control with an external SO_2 closed-loop system. PACE 9:992/II
161. Stangl K, Weil J, Seitz K et al. (1988) Influence of AV synchrony on the plasma levels of atrial natriuretic peptide (ANP) in patients with total AV block. PACE 11:1176
162. Starling EH (1915) The lineacre lecture on the law of the heart. Longmans, Cambridge
163. Stewart WJ, Dicola VC, Harthorne JW et al. (1984) Doppler ultrasound measurement of cardiac output in patients with physiological pacemakers. Effects of left ventricular function and retrograde ventriculoatrial conduction. Am J Cardiol 54:308
164. Sutton R, Citron P (1979) Electrophysiological and hemodynamic basis for application of new pacemaker technology in sick sinus syndrome and atrioventricular block. Br Heart J 41:600
165. Sutton R, Perrins EJ, Citron P (1980) Physiological cardiac pacing. PACE 3:207
166. Sutton R, Perrins EJ, Morley C et al. (1983) Sustained improvement in exercise tolerance following physiological cardiac pacing. Eur Heart J 4:781
167. Sutton R, Kenny RA (1986) The natural history of sick sinus syndrome. PACE 9/II:1110
168. Swift PC, Cowell LC, Woolard KV (1987) A comparison of the exercise response to DDD and activity-response ventricular pacing. PACE 10/II:751
169. Trappe HJ, Klein H, Frank G et al. (1988) Rate-responsive pacing as compared to fixed-rate VVI pacing in patients after ablation of the atrioventricular conduction system. Eur Heart J 9:642
170. Travill CM, Varadas P, Ingram A et al. (1988) Benefits of VVIR over VVI: Atrial natriuretic peptide (ANP) – a new quantitative assessment? PACE 11 [Suppl]:860
171. Treese N, Hungfleisch S, Rhein S et al. (1988) Cardiopulmonary exercise: a new approach for control of rate-responsive pacing. PACE 11[Suppl]:847
172. Treese N, Stegmaier A, Slamer P et al. (1990) Rate-responsive pacing improves the oxygen uptake work rate ratio. PACE 13:1213
173. Tscheliessnigg KG, Stenzl W, Dacar D et al. (1985) Hemodynamic importance of a constant AV delay. In: Gomez FP (ed) Cardiac pacing, electrophysiology, tachyarrhythmias. Editorial Grouz, Madrid, p 572
174. Unger G, Biolonozyk C, Leonhartsberger H et al. (1983) Influence of pacing mode on parameters of left ventricular function (LVF) measured by Tc-nucleid-ventriculography (TcN). PACE 6:A-80
175. Van Erckelens F, Sigmund M, Reupke C et al. (1990) exercise responsiveness of cardiopulmonary function under rate-adaptive pacing: Q-T interval vs minute ventilation for regulation. PACE 13:1193
176. Van Mechelen R, Hagemeijer F, de Boer H et al. (1983) Atrioventricular and ventriculo-atrial conduction in patients with symptomatic sinus node dysfunction. PACE 6:13
177. Vardas P, Williams M, Travill C et al. (1987) Atrial natriuretic peptide in complete atrioventricular block, untreated and after DDD and VVI pacing. In: Belhassen B, Feldmann S, Copperman Y (eds) Cardiac pacing and electrophysiology. R&L Creative Communications, Jerusalem, p 261
178. Velimirovic YD, Djordjevic M, Kocovic D et al. (1988) Metabolic and hemodynamic assessments of rate-responsive pacing: a comparative study. PACE 11[Suppl]:851
179. Videen JS, Huang SK, Bazgan ID et al. (1986) Hemodynamic comparison of ventricular

pacing, atrioventricular sequential pacing and atrial synchronous ventricular pacing using radionuclide ventriculography. Am J Cardiol 57:1305
180. Vogt P, Goy JJ; Kuhn M et al. (1988) Single-versus dual-chamber rate-responsive pacing: comparison by cardiopulmonary exercise testing. PACE 11[Suppl]:797
181. v. Bibra H, Busch U, Wirtzfeld A (1984) Hemodynamic effects of short AV intervals in DDD pacemaker patients. Circulation 70:408
182. Weinhold C, Fülle P, Steinbeck G (1990) Hemodynamic investigation in patients with dual-chamber rate-responsive pacemakers under exercise. PACE 13:1214
183. Wessale JL, Geddes LA, Fearnot NE et al. (1988) Cardiac output versus pacing rate at rest and with exercise in dogs with AV block. PACE 11:575
184. Wessale JL, Voelz MB, Geddes LA (1990) Stroke volume and the three phase cardiac output rate relationship with ventricular pacing. PACE 13:673
185. Westermann KW (1972) Hämodynamische Untersuchungen bei Schrittmacherträgern während AV-Block, starrfrequenter und vorhofgesteuerter Stimulation. Intensivmed 9:360
186. Westveer DC, Stewart JR, Goodfleish R et al. (1984) Prevalence and significance of ventriculo-atrial conduction. PACE 7:184
187. Winters WL, Tyson RR, Barrera F et al. (1965) Cardiac pacemaking. Physiological studies. Ann Intern Med 62:220
188. Wirtzfeld A, Himmler FC, Präuer HW et al. (1979) Atrial and ventricular pacing in patients with the sick sinus syndrome. In: Meere CM (ed) Cardiac pacing. Proceedings of the VIth world symposion on cardiac pacing, Montreal
189. Wirtzfeld A, Himmler FC, Blömer H (1981) Klinische Gesichtspunkte der Schrittmachertherapie bradykarder Herzrhythmusstörungen. Verh Dtsch Ges Kreislaufforsch 47:98
190. Wirtzfeld A, Schmidt G, Himmler FC et al. (1987) Physiological pacing: present status and future developments. PACE 10:41
191. Witte J, Dressler L, Schröder G (1979) 10 years of experience with permanent atrial electrodes. In: Meere CM (ed) Cardiac pacing. Proceedings of the VIth world symposion on cardiac pacing, Montreal
192. Zegelman M, Cieslinsky G, Kreuzer J et al. (1987) 140 times body activity directed pacing – nonphysiological sensor with satisfying clinical results? PACE 10:1234
72/5:1037
194. Ziljstra F, Polak PE, Tanis CJ et al. (1987) Comparison of two pacing modes of rate-responsive pacing. In: Belhassen B, Feldmann S, Copperman Y (eds) Cardiac pacing and electrophysiology. R&L Creative Communications, Jerusalem, p 133

Chronotropic Incompetence and Natural History of Sick Sinus Syndrome

M. SANTINI[1], G. ANSALONE[2], G. CACCIATORE[2], and B. MAGRIS[1]

Introduction

Chronotropic incompetence can be defined as an inadequate heart-rate increase to a given level of exercise. In particular a peak heart rate as below the double-standard deviation of the mean peak exercise heart rate defined for normal subjects is considered as inadequate.

Maximal exercise heart rate declines progressively with age [1]. It is therefore difficult to distinguish the true effects of aging from those due to physical deconditioning or unrecognized cardiac disease. A sedentary lifestyle is frequently observed in elderly subjects, and clinically undetected significant coronary heart disease may be present in more than 25% of persons older than 45 years of age [2, 3].

Kostis et al. [4] studying 101 subjects with normal hearts have shown that during maximal exercise stress test older subjects achieve lower maximal exercise heart rates, have a lower exercise tolerance, show a steeper increase in heart rate with exercise, and a slower decline in heart rate after exercise. Such behaviour may be due to changes induced by the aging of intrinsic pacemaker cells, to decreases in cardiovascular responsiveness to autonomic changes, and to a decrease in adrenergic receptor sensitivity.

Chronotropic incompetence, however, may be due not only to physiological changes, but also to coronary heart disease and to sinus node disease.

Chronotropic Incompetence in Coronary Artery Disease

It has been shown that chronotropic incompetence may be an indicator of coronary artery disease, even in the absence of manifest and significant sinus node disease. Bruce et al. [5] showed that peak heart rates for patients with coronary artery disease were lower than those of normal subjects at maximal exercise. Ellestad and Wan [6] studying a population of patients with and without chronotropic incompetence

[1] Pacemaker Center, S. Camillo Hospital, Rome, Italy
[2] Cardiology Center, C. Forlanini Hospital, Rome, Italy

observed, during the follow-up, an increased incidence of coronary events in the group with chronotropic incompetence. Finally, Chin et al. [7] found an increased prevalence of coronary artery disease at angiography in patients who showed chronotropic incompetence during exercise when compared to patients with normal heart-rate response.

Chronotropic incompetence, in some instances, may be the only exercise marker of coronary artery disease. Wiens et al. [8] studying 312 patients submitted to coronary angiography divided the study population into two subgroups, with and without significant coronary obstructions and with and without chronotropic incompetence. Of the 312 Patients, 18 (6%) showed chronotropic incompetence and coronary artery disease was present in 16 of them (93%).

The possible causes of chronotropic incompetence in coronary artery disease are still controversial. In some instances beta-blocking therapy may be responsible, while in others exercise training may reduce the maximal exercise heart-rate response [9, 10]. It has been postulated that sinus node disease might coexist with coronary artery disease and might be caused by coronary artery disease itself. In contrast with this view are the data of Wiens et al. [8] who showed that only 12% of patients with chronotropic incompetence had obstructions near the sinus node artery. Furthermore, Chin et al. [7] observed a normal sinus node recovery time in 23 patients with chronotropic incompetence and Shaw et al. [11] found in post-mortem angiography of 25 patients with sinus node disease a sinus node artery stenosis greater than 50% in only seven subjects.

An abnormal left ventricular function has also been advocated as a possible cause of chronotropic incompetence in patients with coronary artery disease. However, ejection fraction of patients with and without chronotropic incompetence does not show any significant difference [8].

Chronotropic Incompetence in Patients with Sinus Node Disease

Sinus node disease undoubtedly encompasses the vast majority of patients in which chronotropic incompetence is observed (Figs. 1-3). Macieira-Coelho et al. [12] studied 40 patients with sick sinus syndrome (SSS) using a maximal graded bicycle exercise test and found a maximal heart rate below the one predicted according to age in 80% of them. In 55% of patients the exercise stress test was stopped because of the appearance of clinical symptoms. It should also be emphasized that although patients with sinus node disease may achieve peak heart rates comparable to those of control subjects (Fig. 1)., the temporal course of heart-rate acceleration may be markedly abnormal [7, 13]. Graded exercise testing may therefore be very helpful in the differentiation of those patients with resting bradycardia, but essentially normal exercise heart-rate responses (physically well-trained individuals, subjects with marked predominance of parasympathetic tone at rest), from patients with more severe degrees of chronotropic incompetence (Fig. 2 [7, 8]).

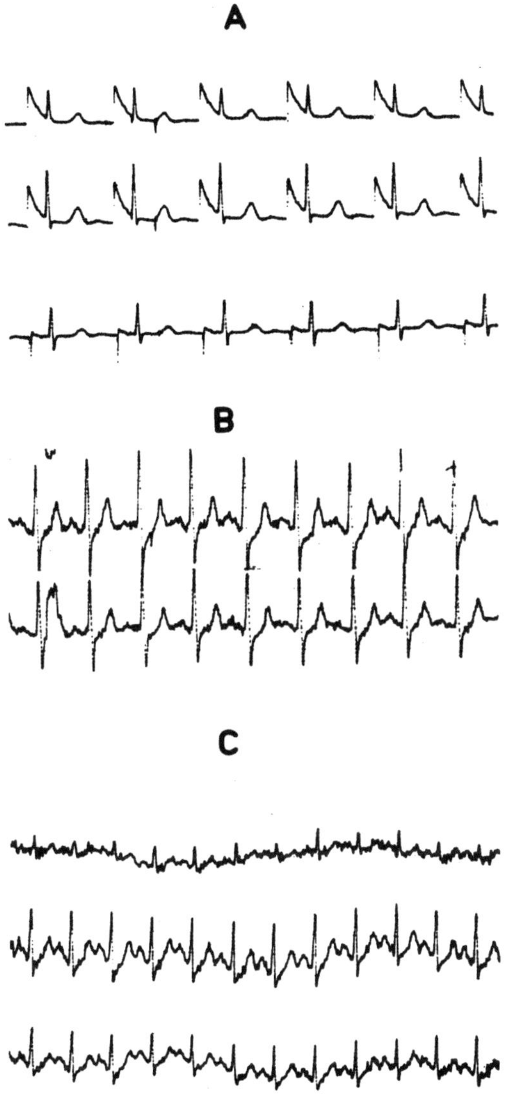

Fig. 1. A-C. Stress test in AAI-paced SSS patients: normal increase in heart rate. *A* AAI pacing at rest at 70 beats per minute. *B, C* During the stress test the sinus rate progressively increases reaching values almost similar to normal people

Administration of atropine may also be used to differentiate extrinsic from intrinsic sinus node disease, but it cannot help in selecting people with chronotropic incompetence. In Abbot's series [14], in fact, the administration of atropine to patients with sinus bradycardia resulted in a significant increase in resting heart rate, so that preexercise heart rate was similar to that of control subjects. Such a response indicated that hypervagotonia was present in patients with sinus node disease who received the medication, but there was no difference between peak rates achieved with and without atropine.

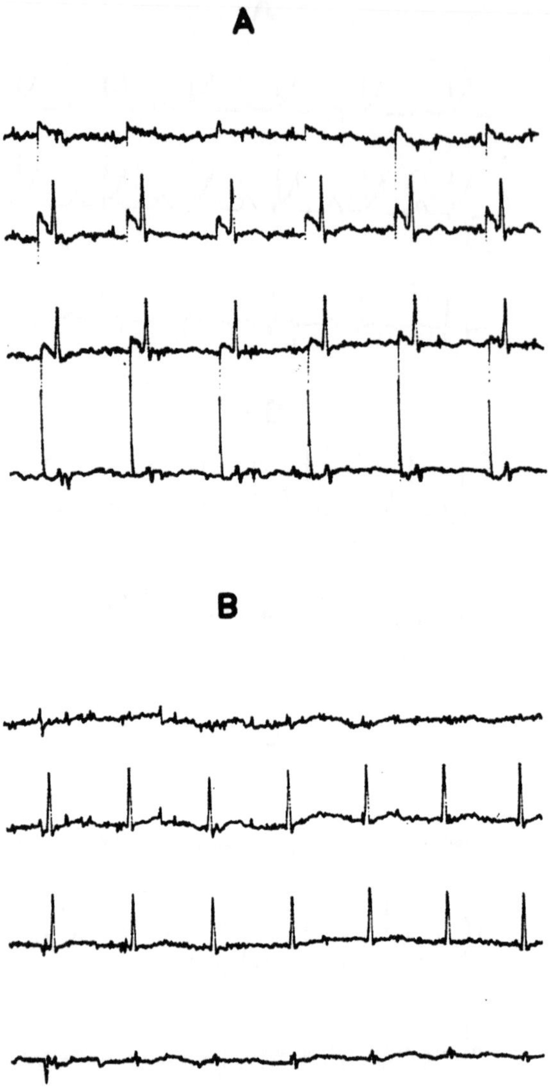

Fig. 2. A, B. Stress test in an AAI-paced SSS patient: poor response of heart rate. *A* AAI pacing at rest at 70 beats per minute. *B* At the maximum level of the stress test only a junctional rhythm with a rate of nearly 80 beats per minute can be observed

It may be difficult to identify chronotropic incompetence using only a single exercise stress test because in the same patient the sinus node response to exercise may vary from day to day [15], resulting in different findings according to the time of day.

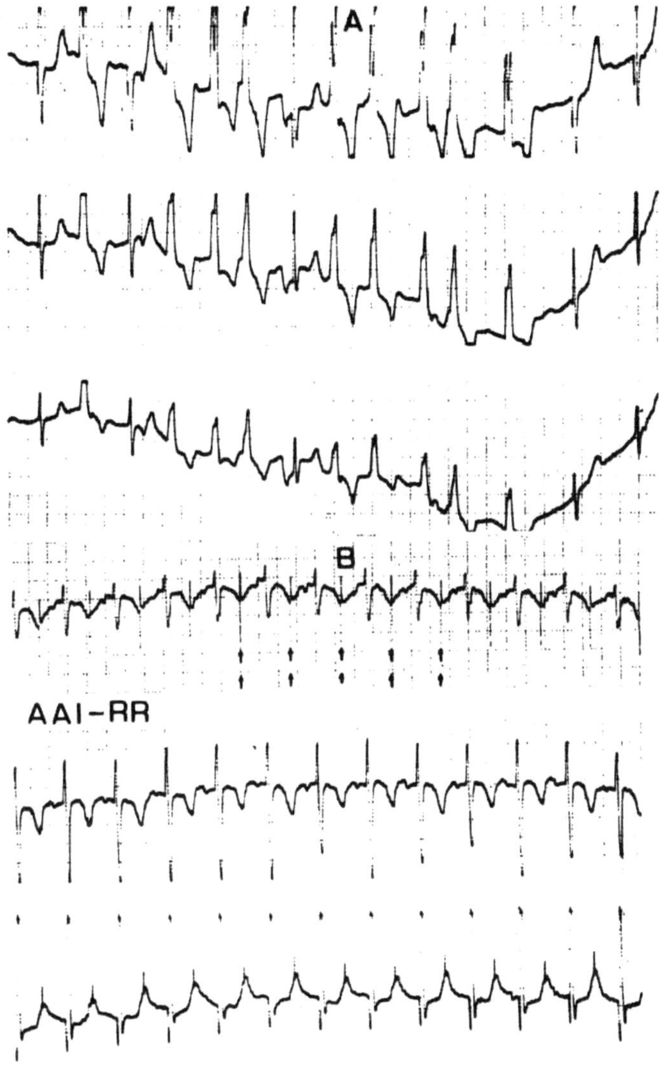

Fig. 3. A, B Antiarrhythmic benefits of AAI rate-responsive pacing. *A* Stress test during AAI pacing at a fixed rate of 70 beats per minute. The pacemaker is inhibited by the spontaneous rhythm which is disturbed by frequent and repetitive ventricular ectopic beats. *B* Stress test in the same patients during AAI rate-responsive mode. The pacing rate reaches 150 beats per minute and no arrhythmia can be observed

Benefits of Rate-Responsive Physiological Pacing in Patients with Sinus Node Disease and Chronotropic Incompetence

Because of the high incidence of chronotropic incompetence in SSS patients, AAI (atrial pacing, atrial sensing, inhibited mode) and DDD (double pacing, double sensing, d for inhibited and triggering mode) pacing modes appropriate for patients with sinus node dysfunction and symptomatic bradycardia have substantially increased with the advent of rate-adaptive pacing systems using on-line sensors capable of determining an appropriate pacing rate independent of native atrial activity. At present, the large clinical use of these devices permits the evaluation of their possible hemodynamic and antiarrhythmic benefits.

In SSS patients with chronotropic incompetence, DDDR (rate-adaptive) pacing has been shown to improve exercise performance, providing a greater exercise duration than observed during DDD pacing at fixed heart rate (Fig. 3).

Capucci et al. [16], estimated that the exercise duration in SSS patients with chronotropic incompetence was 6.7 min during DDD pacing at fixed heart rate and 11.2 min during DDDR pacing mode ($p < 0.01$).

Higano et al. [17] demonstrated that DDDR pacing minimizes sympathetic stimulation (lower atrial natriuretic factor, ANF, and norepinephrine levels) during exercise over both DDD and VVI (ventricular pacing, ventricular sensing, inhibited mode) pacing. ANF release during exercise is lower in DDDR pacing mode compared to VVIR (rate-adaptive VVI) pacing, even in patients without retrograde ventriculo-atrial conduction, providing clear-cut evidence of more physiologic cardiac activity during DDDR [18].

AV delay may significantly influence both the cardiac output and the increase in cardiovascular sympathetic nervous system activity during exercise [19]. Theodorakis et al. [20] showed that adrenergic activity is lower during exercise in DDD with shorter AV delay (100 ms) than in DDD with 150 ms AV interval, or VVI pacing mode. Finally, DDDR pacing mode has not shown any deleterious arrhythmogenic effect when compared to DDD pacing mode in the same subjects [21, 22, 23].

The same hemodynamic benefits documented with DDDR pacing have also been reported in SSS patients affected by chronotropic incompetence during AAIR (rate-adaptive AAI) pacing mode. Pouillot et al. [24] reported in their SSS patients a maximal exercise duration of 9.7 ± 4 min during AAI pacing and of 12.1 ± 5 min during AAIR pacing mode. Our results [25] show that exercise tolerance in eight patients subjected to ergometric stress test was better during AAIR pacing mode than during AAI pacing mode (8 min versus 5 min respectively, < 0.02). These results agree with the findings of Pouillot et al [24].

AV conduction is not negatively influenced by heart-rate increase if the pacemaker is adequately programmed. In our series [25], as well as in Edelstam et al. [26] and Schuller et al. series [27] , during a follow-up of over 2 years no problem was observed with AV conduction during exercise.

Regarding the slope of heart-rate increase, if the pacemaker is not adequately programmed or the patient does not have a good AV conduction in basal conditions, we can observe the emergence of AV block during the initial phase of the ergometric test, when sympathetic acitivity has still scarcely been augmented and paced heart rate is strongly increased.

If AV interval is greatly delayed, we can observe the same hemodynamic damage as that induced by retroconduction during VVI stimulation. Two cases of pacemaker syndrome induced by AAIR-pacing mode were described by Pouillot et al. [28].

Thus, AAIR pacing mode can be largely utilized in SSS patients with chronotropic incompetence in the presence of good AV conduction (Fig. 3). At the present time, infact, many studies have shown that the AV conduction in SSS subjects with a high Wenckebach threshold (120-140 min) at the time of pacemaker implant does not decline during a 5-year follow-up period [29, 30, 31].

In our series of 135 AAI-paced SSS patients, with a Wenckebach threshold less than 140 min at the time of implantation, we could observe during the follow-up of over 5 years a significant deterioration in AV conduction in only seven cases (5%) [30]. In six of them, AV-conduction deterioration was due to the dromotropic negative effect of pharmacological treatment (verapamil, digitalis, etc. [30]).

Prevention of Atrial Flutter or Atrial Fibrillation by Physiological Pacing

It is well-known that VVI pacing mode has a well-defined arrhythmogenic effect in SSS patients, inducing chronic atrial fibrillation in a high percentage of them [29, 30, 31]. Physiological pacing, on the contrary, showed a remarkable antiarrhythmic effect both alone or if associated with drug therapy [30]. In AAI-paced patients recurrences of supraventricular arrhythmias in the absence of drug therapy range from 9% [32] to 13% [33], 25% [34], and 45% [35].

Worthy of note are the data of Lemke et al. [35], who reported a high prevalence of arrhythmia recurrences (45%), related to AAI-paced patients examined with 24 h Holter monitoring.

It is well-known, that arrhythmia recurrences after pacemaker implantation are more frequent in those patients suffering from preimplant atrial fibrillation than in those who experienced only sinus bradycardia before pacemaker implantation (24%-35% versus 4%-8.4%, respectively [36, 37]). It could also be speculated that a higher atrial pacing rate could induce recurrences of atrial fibrillation more frequently than a lower atrial pacing rate. In fact, in a group of physiologically paced patients Galley et al. [36] documented a higher prevalence of atrial fibrillation recurrences after pacemaker implantation at an atrial rate pacing of >80/min (31%) than at an atrial pacing rate of < 80/min (9.4%, $p < 0.05$).

Moreover, in our experience [30] the presence of an atrioventricular conduction defect associated with SSS does not seem to influence the prevalence of arrhythmia recurrences after pacemaker implantation, and does not reflect any greater anatomic damage of the atria in these patients than in those with SSS and without an associated conduction disturbance.

Prevention of Congestive Heart Failure by Atrial Pacing

Atrial pacing can successfully decrease heart failure in patients with SSS compared to VVI pacing. Rosenquist et al. [29] showed in their series of permanently paced SSS patients a heart failure rate of 7% in the AAI group versus 15% in the VVI group in the first 2 years of follow-up. After 4 years of follow-up 23% of AAI patients showed signs of heart failure versus 37% of VVI patients.

Thromboembolic Incidence During the First Year Postimplant

Thromboembolisms are much more frequent in SSS patients treated by means of VVI pacing (12.3%) than in those atrially paced (1.6%, $p < 0.001$) [31]. In VVI-paced SSS patients thromboembolic phenomena are observed more frequently in those who have atrial fibrillation (23%) than in those with sinus rhythm (68%) [31]. Double-chamber pacing pacemakers also seem to be a pacing modality which prevent thromboembolisms. Sasaki et al. [38] report no incidence of thromboembolisms in their SSS patients paced in DDI and DDD modalities. Anticoagulation is advisable in SSS patients treated by VVI pacing in order to reduce embolism. Sasaki et al. [38] showed an 8% incidence of thromboembolisms in the VVI-paced SSS patients who were on anticoagulants versus 31% in those without anticoagulation.

Decrease in Cardiac and Stroke Mortality by Physiological Pacing in SSS Patients

In our series of SSS patients cardiac mortality was found to be higher in the VVI group (14%) than in the AAI group (3%), ($p < 0.001$) [30]. This difference remained significant in patients older than 70 years ($p < 0.001$) in whom cardiac mortality was 4% in the AAI mode and 15% in the VVI group. In patients younger than 70 years no significant difference in cardiac mortality was found between the VVI and AAI groups. There were no statistical differences in cardiac mortality between the AAI and the DDD group when analyzed regardless of age, or separately according to age (over and under 70 years).

Stroke mortality was higher in the VVI group (8%) compared to that in the AAI group (2%) and the DDD group (2.5%), but only the difference between AAI and VVI is significant ($p < 0.01$). In terms of both pacing mode and age, stroke mortality remained higher in the VVI group (17%) than in the AAI (3%, $p < 0.001$) and DDD (3%) groups (difference not significant), but only for patients older than 70 years.

Conclusions

In spite of our knowledge today about the development and diagnosis of SSS, there are still some questions which need to be answered:

1. Which group of SSS patients can benefit from anticoagulation? Should we treat only VVI-paced patients with atrial fibrillation with anticoagulants, or all VVI patients, or whom else?
2. What is the real benefit of AAIR and DDDR pacing with regard to functional capacity and survival in large numbers of SSS patients?

3. Can an AAIR-DDDR increase in pacing rate be arrhythmogenic in patients with brady-tachy syndrome?
4. Should we treat all patients physiologically paced for brady-tachy syndrome with antiarrhythmic drugs immediately after pacing instauration, or should we wait for the first postimplant recurrence of the arrhythmia before prescribing drugs?

We still need several large trials to answer these questions.

References

1. Sheffield LT, Maloof JA, Sawyer JA, Roitman D (1978) Maximal heart rate and treadmill performance of healthy women in relation to age. Circulation 57:79
2. Gerstenblith G, Lakatta EG, Weisfeldt ML (1976) Age changes in myocardial function and exercise response. Prog Cardiovasc Dis 19:1
3. Raven PB, Mitchel J (1980) The effect of aging on the cardiovascular response to dynamic and static exercise. Aging 12:269
4. Kostis BJ, Moreyra AE, Amendo MT, Di Pietro J, Cosgrove N, Kuo PT (1982) The effect of age on heart rate free of heart disease. Circulation 65:141
5. Bruce RA, Fisher LD, Cooper MN, Gey GO (1974) Separation of effects of cardiovascular disease and age on ventricular function with maximal exercise. Am J Cardiol 34:757
6. Ellestad MHJ, Wan MKC (1975) Predictive implication of stress testing. Follow-up of 2700 subjects after maximum treadmill stress testing. Circulation 51:363
7. Chin CF, Messinger JC, Greenberg PS, Ellestad MH (1979) Chronotropic incompetence in exercise testing. Clin Cardiol 2:12
8. Wiens RD, Lafia P, Carey MM, Evans RG, Kennedy HL (1984) Chronotropic incompetence in clinical exercise testing. Am J Cardiol 54:74
9. Bruce RA, Kulsuma F, Hosmer D (1973) Maximal oxygen intake and nomographic assessment of functional aerobic impairment in cardiovascular. Am Heart J 85:546
10. Schever J, Tipton CM (1977) Cardiovascular adaptation to physical training. Annu Rev Physiol 29:221
11. Shaw DB, Linker NJ, Heaver PA, Evans I (1987) Chronic sinoatrial disorder (sick sinus syndrome) – a possible result of cardiac ischemia. Br Heart J 58:598
12. Macieira-Coelho E, Silva E, Alves MG, Machado HB (1989) Postexercise electrocardiographic and clinical changes in patients with sick sinus syndrome. J Electrocardiol 22:139
13. Benditt DG, Milstein S, Gornick CC et al. (1987) Sensor-triggered rate-variable cardiac pacing: current technologies and clinical implications. Ann Intern Med 107:714
14. Abbott JA, Hirschfeld DS, Kunkel FW et al. (1977) Graded exercise testing in patients with sinus node dysfunction. Am J Med 62:330
15. Benditt DG, Buetikofer J, Fetter J et al. (1988) Variability of sinoatrial rate-responsive during exercise testing in sinus node dysfunction. PACE 11:798 (abstr)
16. Capucci A, Cazzin R, Zardo F, Boriani G, Zanuttini D, Piccolo E (1990) DDDR – pacing modalities in patients with and without chronotropic incompetence compared to DDD and VVIR modes. PACE 13:1192 (abstr)
17. Higano S, Hayes D, Christiansen J (1990) Metabolic effects of atrioventricular synchrony during low levels of exercise. Rev Eur Technol Biomed 12/3:28 (abstr)
18. Blanc JJ, Mansourati J, Ritter P, Nitzsche R, Genet L, Morin JF (1990) Atrial natriuretic factor (ANF) release during exercise in patients successively paced in DDD and VVIR "like" mode. Rev Eur Technol Biomed 12/3:28 (abstr)
19. Vogt P, Goy JJ, Schlaepfer J, Fromer M, Kappenberger L (1990) Haemodynamic consequences of atrioventricular delay in DDDR pacing. Rev Eur Technol Biomed 12/3:58 (abstr)
20. Theodorakis G, Kremastinos D, Markianos M, Livanis E, Archodakis C, Karavolias G, Toutouzas P (1990) The c-AMP and ANP levels in VVI and DDD pacing with different AV delays during daily activity and exercise. Rev Eur Technol Biomed 12/3:29 (abstr)

21. Spencer W, Markowitz T, Alagona P (1990) Rate augmentation and atrial arrhythmias in DDDR pacing. PACE 13:1211 (abstr)
22. Sutton R, Travill C, Fitzpatrick A, Ahmed R, Gibbs S, Guneri S, Ingram A (1990) DDDR pacing in severe chronotropic incompetence. Rev Eur Technol Biomed 12/3:56 (abstr)
23. Stangl K, Seitz K, Wirtzfeld A, Alt E, Laule M (1990) Differences in prognosis and incidence of atrial arrhythmias between AAI and VVI pacing in patients with sick sinus syndrome. Rev Eur Technol Biomed12/3:93 (abstr)
24. Pouillot C, Mabo P, Clement C, Druelles P, Lelong B, Paillard F (1990) Sinus node disease with atrial chronotropic incompetence: AAIR or DDDR pacing? Rev Eur Technol Biomed 12/3:56 (abstr)
25. Santini M, Messina G, Alexidou G, Ceci V, Macali L, Porto MP (1986) Rate-responsive atrial pacing: selection of candidates. In: Santini M, Pistolese M, Alliegro A (eds) Progress in clinical pacing. Excerpta Medica, Amsterdam, pp 5-19
26. Edelstam C, Nordlander R, Wallgren E, Rosenquist M (1990) AAIR pacing and exercise–what happens to AV conduction? PACE 13:1193
27. Schuller H, Brandt J, Fahraeus T, Ogawa T (1990) Feasibility of rate-adaptive atrial pacing: clinical results in 44 patients. PACE 13:1209
28. Pouillot C, Mabo P, Cazeau S, Le Breton H (1990) A potential limitation for AAIR pacing: the frequent lack of adaptation of the PR interval to heart rate. Rev Eur Technol Biomed 12/3:90 (abstr)
29. Rosenquist M, Brandt J, Schuller H (1988) Long-term pacing in sinus node disease: effects of stimulation mode on cardiovascular morbidity and mortality. Am Heart J 116:16-22
30. Santini M, Alexidou G, Ansalone G, Cacciatore G, Cini R, Turitto G (1990) Relation of prognosis in sick sinus syndrome to age, conduction defects, and modes of permanent cardiac pacing. Am J Cardiol 65:729
31. Sutton R, Kenny RA (1986) The natural history of sick sinus syndrome. PACE 9:1110-1114
32. Jordaens L, Robbens E, Van Wassenhove E, Clement DL (1989) Incidence of arrhythmias after atrial or dual-chamber pacemaker implantation. Eur Heart J 10:102-107
34. Kerr CR, Frank G, Tyers O, Vorderbrugge S (1989) Atrial pacing: safety and efficacy. PACE 12:1049-1054
35. Lemke B, Holtman BJ, Selbach H, Barmejer J (1989) The atrial pacemaker: retrospective analysis of complications and life expectancy in patients with sinus node dysfunction. Int J Cardiol 22:185-193
36. Galley D, Elharrar C, Ammor M, Scheffer J, Codjia R, Tirkawi R, Pavy O, Delporte B (1990) Is chronic atrial pacing protective against atrial fibrillation (AF)? Rev Eur Technol Biomed 12/3:92 (abstr)
37. Benditt DG, Mianulli M, Buetikofer J, Milstein S (1990) Prior arrhythmia history is the major determinant of postimplant atrial tachyarrhythmias in DDDR pacemaker patients. Rev Eur Technol Biomed 12/3:95 (abstr)
38. Sasaki Y, Shimotori M, Akahane K, Yonekura H, Hirano K, Endoh R, Koike S, Kawa S, Furuta A, Homma T (1988) Long-term follow-up of patients with sick sinus syndrome: a comparison of clinical aspects among unpaced, ventricular inhibited, and physiologically paced groups. PACE 11:1575-1583

The Impact of Exercise Metabolism; Catecholamine Levels and Individual Fitness

M. LEHMANN*

The Importance of the Sympathetic System for Adaptation to Stress

The importance of the sympathetic system for adaptation to stress, such as orthostasis and physical exertion becomes especially clear in patients with an insufficient sympathetic system, that is with patients suffering from PRIMARY ORTHOSTATIC HYPOTENSION [30, 31]. This disease is probably attributable to a genetically caused degeneration of sympathetic neurones and the adrenal cortex; in the advanced stage, there are only marginal concentrations of the neurotransmitters and hormones dopamine, noradrenaline, and adrenaline in the plasma [30, 31]. The renal elimination of catecholamines in 24 h, as an indication of total conversion, also decreases to marginal values [30, 31]. In the advanced stage, these patients can hardly right themselves from a horizontal position without immediate circulatory collapse, resulting from a decrease in arterial pressure to values no longer measurable without an essential increase in heart rate [30, 31]. At rest and in the supine position, inconspicuous cardiac dimensions and function parameters are found [30,31]. As a result of deficient sympathetic drive, however, no adjustment in cardiac function to physical exertion is possible, that is, the cardiac output can only be slightly increased at rest; the Frank-Starling mechanism is meaningless. Even during physical exertion in the supine position, there is a decrease in pressure, again without an increase in heart rate [30, 31]. Physical inactivity leads to a loss of training in the skeletal muscles; this means that the aerobic work capacity of the skeletal musculature, determined amongst other things by the number and size of mitochondria, is clearly reduced. Even during mild ergometric exertion in the supine position, corresponding to about 1-1.5 w/kg body weight, there is a clear increase in the lactate level in the blood to values of about 8 mmol/l (Fig. 1), which indicates a marked limitation in the oxidative mitochondrial capacity.

To compensate, there is a higher proportion of anaerobic glycolysis in the energy supply, recognizable by the increase in the lactate level.

* Medical University Hospital Freiburg, Department of Sport and Performance Medicine, 7800 Freiburg, FRG

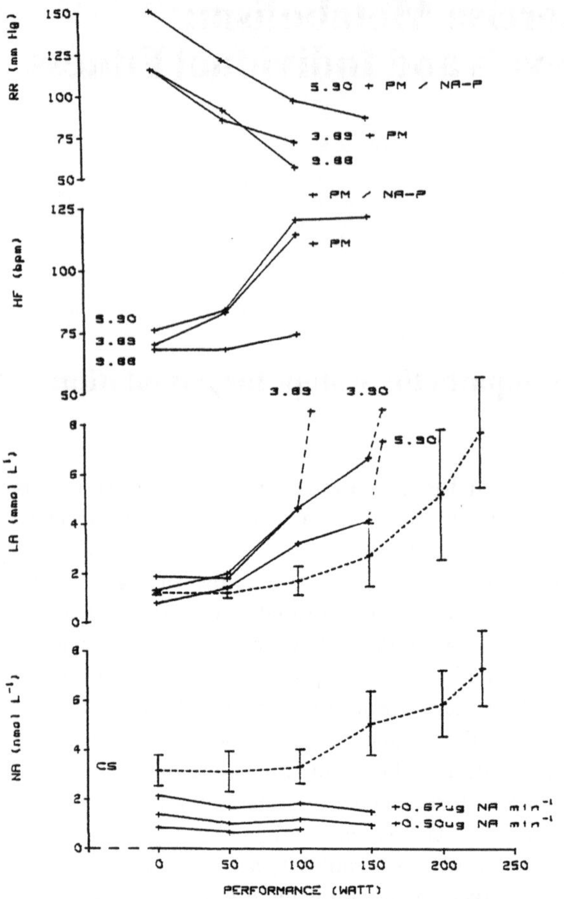

Fig. 1. Noradrenaline (*NA*) and lactate (*LA*) levels in a patient suffering from primary orthostatic hypotension (primary sympathetic insufficiency) (——) and in healthy control subjects (– – –) at rest and during graded ergometric supine exercise. Also heart rate responses (*HF*) and behaviour of mean arterial blood pressure (*RR*) of the patient in September 1988 (baseline examination), in March 1989 (with rate-responsing pacing system), and in May 1990 (with pacing system, *PM*, and microdosing noradrenaline pump, *NA-P*)

This example also demonstrates that the sympathetic activity in activating phosphorylase (glycogenolysis) and anaerobic glycolysis can only be of secondary importance in everyday stress. Clearly elevated noradrenaline and adrenaline levels are assumed to be necessary only at the maximum glycolytic flux rate [17]. Sympathetic insufficiency thus acts primarily on the cardiovascular system in this disease.

An increase in cardiac output by a rate-responsive pacing system of about 2 l/min during mild physical exercise cannot decisively improve the exercise capacity or energy metabolism (greater oxygen supply); this is only possible when noradrenaline can be administered subcutaneously at the same time via a programmable micropump (Fig. 1).

Behavior of Sympathetic Activity and Energy Metabolism During Physical Exercise

The appropriate textbooks can be consulted with respect to the configuration and function of the sympathetic system; the required brevity does not permit repetition at this point. Questions about energy metabolism can also only be considered to a limited extent for the same reason.

The sympathetic activity can be evaluated on the basis of, amongst other things, its influence on the organism, for example, based on increases in blood pressure and heart rate. Due to the complex regulation of these parameters, however, such a method remains problematical. Usually, the evaluation of sympathetic activity is now based on an analysis of plasma and urinary catecholamines [11, 20-29, 45]. The positive correlation between the response of the heart to sympathetic stimulation and the release of endogenous catecholamines into the coronary sinus of the dog [49] may be of basic importance. Of more importance is the positive correlation between sympathetic activity in sympathetic fibres of the peroneus communis in humans, recorded by means of microelectrodes, and the venous noradrenaline concentration of the corresponding extremity [47]. That is, the determination of the catecholamine levels permit sufficient evaluation of sympathetic activity [40]. There are differences in noradrenaline concentration in samples of arterial, venous and coronary venous blood drawn simultaneously, but positive correlations between the samples of various vascular areas [7, 33], especially during exercise [7]. The evaluation of the noradrenaline level in arterial blood is considered to be particularly favourable [1, 45], since the concentration in venous blood may be changed considerably following its passage through the organs, both by additional release and by elimination. The requirement can be met by determining the noradrenaline levels in earlobe capillary blood [1, 29].

The plasma catecholamine level, that is the noradrenaline concentration, is determined by release and spillover on the one hand and by plasma clearance on the other. The plasma half-life in healthy individuals is about 2–3 min at rest; it does not change decisively even during physical exercise [12, 33]. That means changes in the plasma catecholamine level in healthy individuals during physical exercise can be primarily explained by changes in release. During incremental exercise (Figs. 2, 3 [27]) the sympathetic system probably becomes important for the adaptation of cardiac output and energy metabolism, starting at the half- to submaximum exercise intensity, that is, with plasma catecholamine levels of at least 5–6 nmol/l present [45]. However, the sensitivity of the organism is increased during physical exercise [6] and the influence of antagonists, such as the vagus, is reduced [10], so that a physiological importance can be assumed even at lower levels during physical exercise. The sensitivity to catecholamines in the presence of disease, such as PRIMARY ORTHOSTATIC HYPOTENSION can also be increased to ten times the normal level [30, 31], or markedly reduced in the presence of chronic cardiac disease [4, 5].

In general, it can thus be concluded that a reduction in vagal activity and an increase in venous return is more important than an increase in sympathetic activity in healthy

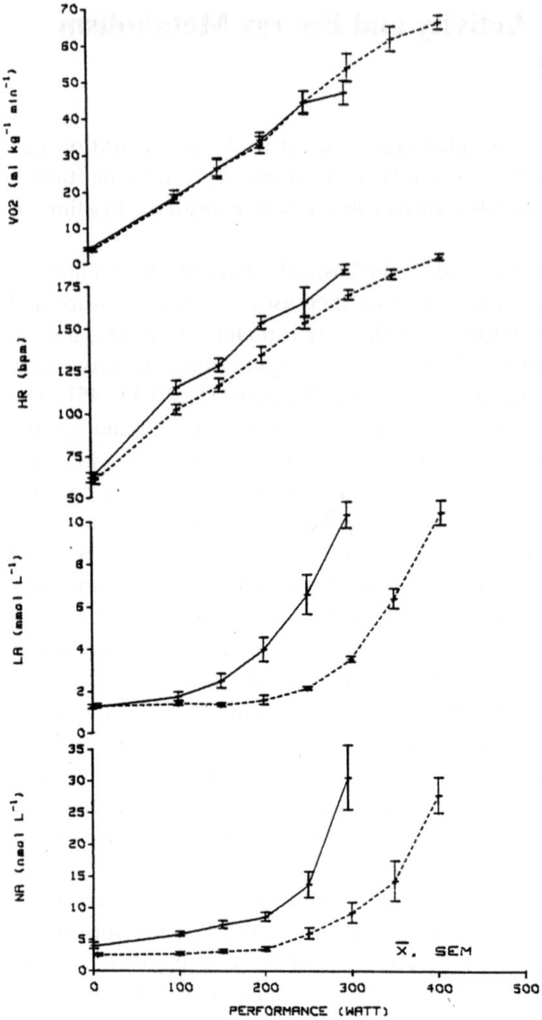

Fig. 2. Behaviour of free plasma noradrenaline (*NA*), lactate levels (*LA*), heart rate responses (*HR*) and oxygen uptake capacity (VO_2max) in endurance trained cyclists (– – –) and untrained control subjects (——)

individuals during everyday exertion. An increase in sympathetic activity seems to be necessary only during submaximum to maximum physical exercise. The latter applies as well to energy metabolism.

The Influence of Physical Training on Sympathetic Activity

Physical training of an endurance type probably results initially in an increase in vagal activity [38], followed by a reduction in sympathetic drive or the sympathetic activity [13, 24–26, 32, 39, 48]. This is called the vegetative adaptation of the

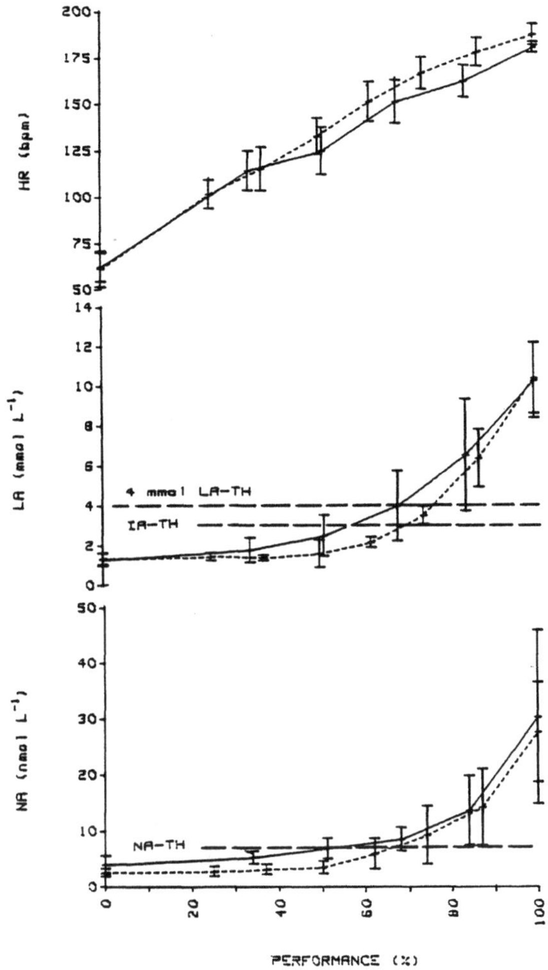

Fig. 3. Noradrenaline (*NA*), lactate levels (*LA*) and heart rate responses (*HR*) of the trained (– – –) and untrained (——) subjects in relation to relative workload. The 4 mmol lactate threshold (*LA-TH*), the individual anaerobic threshold of the trained athletes (*IA-TH*) and the assumed noradrenaline threshold (*NA-TH*) are marked additionally

organism. The reason for this vegetative adaptation is the economization of cardiovascular activity with a reduction in the myocardial oxygen requirement [15, 44]. The maximum cardiac output, and thus the maximum cardiac work capacity, can only be increased by reducing the heart rate and increasing the cardiac stroke volume at the same absolute exercise level.

Physiological cardiac hypertrophy is an additional factor in high-performance endurance sports [41]. This vegetative adaptation can probably be controlled very decisively by, e.g., a training-related improvement in the aerobic performance capacity of the skeletal muscles [18, 46]. The minimum training is about 30 – 60 min endurance training three times per week over 3–4 weeks with an intensity of 60%–70% of the maximum oxygen uptake capacity [32], until a reduction in plasma catecholamines becomes apparent. The plasma clearance shows no training dependency in healthy individuals [34, 35], that means that the reduction in the plasma catecholamine level

(Fig. 2) is based primarily on a reduction in release. In relation to the relative exercise intensity, trained and untrained healthy subjects show comparable plasma catecholamine levels and lactate concentrations (Fig. 3). The so-called 4-mmol lactate threshold [36], which separates a workload with a mostly aerobic energy supply from one with an aerobic-anaerobic energy supply, is at about 70%–80% of the maximum performance capacity (Fig. 3). As discussed earlier, it can be assumed that no essential increase in sympathetic activity occurs in healthy individuals during exercise up to 50% of maximum performance, or that only sub-threshold plasma levels are present [45]. The reduction in the plasma catecholamine level and thus the sympathetic activity in endurance-trained subjects is, however, followed by an increase in the sensitivity to catecholamines based on an increase in beta-adrenoreceptors [3, 6, 25]. The anticipated elevated sensitivity of the sinus node to beta-adrenergic stimuli is, however, masked by a concurrent elevation in vagotony in trained individuals.

In sub-threshold training stimulation, that is training which is too little in scope and too low in intensity, no vegetative adaptation and no marked improvement in endurance performance capacity and maximum cardiopulmonary capacity can be expected [14].

This also applies to too great a training scope with overexertion of the athlete [34, 35]. Under these conditions, a further increase in the noradrenaline plasma level at the same submaximum exercise level must be expected [34, 35]. Thus, training at an optimal level rather than training per se is decisive.

The Influence of Age on Endurance Performance Capacity, Cardiopulmonary Capacity, and the Sympathetic System

A reduction in endurance performance capacity and maximum cardiopulmonary capacity of about 30%–50% must be expected between 30 and 70 years of age [16]. This is the result, in addition to aging which cannot be influenced, of a lack of training of the skeletal muscles. As a result, the endurance performance capacity of older people can be favourably influenced by training (i.a. [16]). The age-related reduction in endurance performance and maximum cardiopulmonary capacity is accompanied by a clear increase in plasma catecholamine levels at the same exercise level (Fig. 4) [19, 22, 23, 42]. A markedly higher lactate level is found as an expression of the reduced oxidative capacity of the skeletal muscles (Fig. 4). In relation to the relative intensity of exercise, the differences seem to just about equal out, but a clear difference remains in the noradrenaline levels, which cannot be explained by the reduction in performance [28]. In relation to the relative exercise and age, higher noradrenaline levels are in part the result of an age-dependent decrease in plasma clearance [11] and also in part the result of the reduction in sensitivity to catecholamines in aging [19, 42], from which a somewhat higher compensatory release can be expected. This agrees with the positive relationship between the 24 h noradrenaline excretion and age [23].

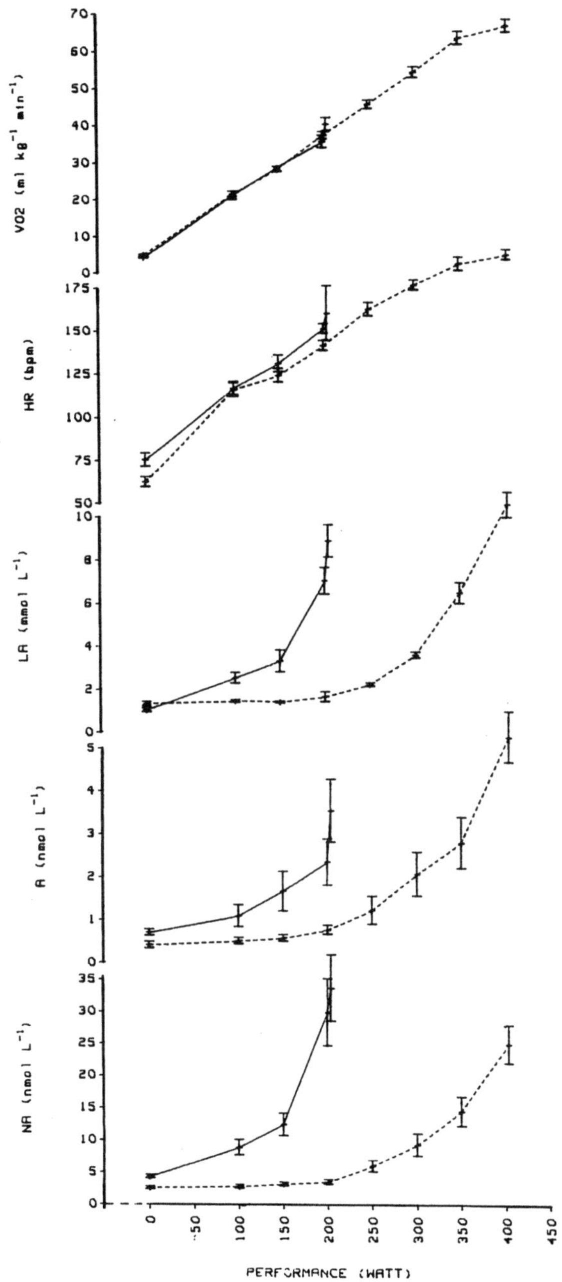

Fig. 4. Behaviour of noradrenaline (*NA*), adrenaline (*A*), lactate levels (*LA*), heart rate responses (*HR*) and oxygen uptake capacity ($VO_2\,max$) in trained older (66.2 ± 6.1 years of age) (——) and younger (25.5 ± 3 years of age) (– – –) cyclists

The Relationship Between Cardiac Function and Sympathetic Activity

A disease-related reduction in cardiac function is usually accompanied by a compensatory increase in sympathetic activity, recognizable by elevated plasma catecholamine levels and catecholamine excretions [4, 7, 9, 20, 21, 28, 33, 37] Impaired vagal activity can also be demonstrated [8]. In chronic sympathetic hyperstimulation, there is a decrease in sensitivity to beta-adrenergic stimulation, which is ascribed to a decrease in the density of beta-adrenoreceptors [2, 5]. In the late stages of heart failure, depletion of the sympathetic system must be expected as a result of overexertion and damage [33].

The increase in sympathetic activity, which can be observed in cardiac patients and which cannot usually be considered favourable since it results in increased stress to the heart without improving cardiac function, is in no way ascribably solely to a reduction in cardiac function; rather the heart disease leads to an increasing training deficit of the skeletal muscles, which in healthy subjects is also accompanied by a clearly excessive sympathetic activity [13, 24–26, 32, 39, 48]. This, one might say, unnecessary proportion of the increase in sympathetic activity can be clearly reduced by specific physical therapy [9, 26].

This means that even in patients with reduced cardiac function, specific physical therapy can produce an improvement in the working economy of the heart [9, 26, 32], even in the final stage of the disease [43]. During short-term physical therapy in patients following heart surgery, with daily training over about 4 weeks, intermittent training is probably superior to continuous training [38, 43]. To what extent this also applies to long-term physical therapy for cardiac patients remains open.

According to current opinion, sympathetic activity in cardiac patients is controlled by a complex mechanism increasing pressure during diastole in the low-pressure system (expansion receptors), to which the left atrium and left ventricle belong; moreover, decreasing cardiac output (a reduction in the oxygen supply in essential organs) and arterial pressure (baroreceptors). In addition, there is the decrease in aerobic working capacity of the inactivated skeletal muscles as discussed.

Summary

The sympathetic system regulates the cardiovascular and metabolic adaptation to physical exercise, if the exercise intensity exceeds 50%–70% of the maximum exercise capacity in healthy subjects. The free-plasma catecholamine levels may be seen as indicators of the sympathetic activity because there are positive correlations between the neuronal sympathetic activity and the plasma catecholamine concentrations. Adequate endurance training causes an economization of cardiovascular and metabolic adaptation to exercise, based on a decrease in sympathetic activity at identical absolute workloads and an increase in vagal tone. However, the plasma catecholamine concentrations are quite similar in trained and untrained subjects when related to the relative workload. Aging goes along with a clear increase in plasma noradrenaline levels at the same absolute workload and to a lesser extent also to the relative intensity of exercise, which may be explained by a lack of skeletal muscle training, a decrease in plasma clearance of catecholamines, and a reduction in sensitivity to catecholamines from which a somewhat higher compensatory release can be expected. A reduction in cardiac function and a consecutive training deficit of the skeletal muscles are seen to be two main factors of an increased sympathetic activity in cardiac patients, which cannot be considered favourable with respect to cardiac load and myocardial oxygen consumption. That part of excess sympathetic activity in cardiac patients which is caused by training deficit can be also reduced by training, that is by physical therapy.

References

1. Baumgartner H, Wiedermann CJ, Hörtnagel H, Mühlberger V (1985) Plasma catecholamines in arterial and capillary blood. Naunyn Schmiedebergs Arch Pharmacol 328:461-463
2. Baumann G, Riess G (1982) Verhalten kardialer β-Rezeptoren bei akutem Myokardialinfarkt und chronischem Herzversagen. Mögliche Rolle von H2-Rezeptor-Agonisten. Herz Kreislauf 14:169
3. Bieger W, Zittel R, Zappe H, Weicker H (1982) Einfluß körperlicher Aktivität auf Katecholamin-Rezeptoraktivität. Dtsch Z Sportmed 33:249
4. Braunwald E (1965) The control of ventricular function in man. Br Heart J 27:1
5. Bristow MR, Ginsburg R, Minobe W (1982) Decreased catecholamine sensitivity and ß-adrenergic receptor density in failing human hearts. N Engl J Med 307:205
6. Brodde OE, Daul A, O'Hara N (1984) ß-adrenoceptor changes in human lymphocytes induced by dynamic exercise. Naunyn Schmiedebergs Arch Pharmacol 325:190-192
7. Dominiak P, Schulz W, Delius W, Kober G, Grobecker H (1981) Catecholamines in patients with coronary heart disease. In: Delius W, Gerlach E, Grobecker H, Kübler W (eds) Catecholamines and the heart. Springer, Berlin Heidelberg New York, pp 223-233
8. Eckberg DL, Drabinsky M, Braunwald E (1971) Defective cardiac parasympathetic control in patients with heart disease. N Engl J Med 258:877
9. Ehsani AA, Heath GW, Martin III WH, Hagberg JM, Holloszy JO (1984) Effect of intensive exercise training on plasma catecholamines in coronary patients. J Appl Physiol 57:154-159
10. Ekblom B, Kilbom A, Soltysiak A (1973) Physical training, bradycardia and autonomic nervous system, Scand J Clin Lab Invest 32:251
11. Esler M, Jennings G, Korner P, Willet I, Dudley F, Hasking G, Anderson W, Lamberg G (1988) Assessment of human sympathetic nervous system activity from measurement of norepinephrine turnover. Hypertension 11:3-20
12. Hagberg JM, Hickson RC, McLane JA, Ehsani AA, Winder WW (1979) Disappearance of norepinephrine from the circulation following strenuous exercise. J Appl Physiol 47:1311-1314
13. Hartley LH, Mason JW, Hogan PR, Jones LG, Kotchen TA, Mougey EH, Wherry FE (1972) Multiple hormonal responses to graded exercise in relation to physical training. J Appl Physiol 33:602-606
14. Henritze J, Weltman A, Schurrer RL, Barlow K (1985) Effects of training at and above the lactate threshold on the lactate threshold and maximal oxygen uptake. Eur J Appl Physiol 54:84-88
15. Heiss HW, Barmeyer J, Wink K, Huber G, Breiter J, Keul J (1975) Durchblutung und Substratumsatz des gesunden menschlichen Herzens in Abhängigkeit von Trainingszustand. Verh Dtsch Ges Kreislaufforsch 41:247
16. Hollmann W, Liesen H, Rost R, Heck H, Satomi J (1985) Präventive Kardiologie. Bewegungsmangel und körperliches Training aus epidemiologischer und experimenteller Sicht. Z Kardiol 74:46-54

17. Jakovlev NN, Viru AA (1985) Adrenergic regulation of adaptation to muscular activity. Int J Sports Med 6:255-265
18. Kniffki KD, Mense S, Schmidt RF (1981) Muscle receptors with fine afferent fibers which may evoke circulatory reflexes. Circ Res 48 [Suppl I]:25-31
19. Lake CR, Ziegler MG, Coleman D, Kopin IJ (1977) Age-adjusted plasma norepinephrine levels are similar in normotensive and hypertensive subjects. N Engl J Med 4:208-209
20. Lehmann M, Dickhuth HH, Franke T, Huber G, Keul J (1983) Simultane Bestimmung von zentraler Hämodynamik und Plasmakatecholaminen bei Trainierten, Untrainierten und Patienten mit Kontraktionsstörung des Herzens in Ruhe und während Körperarbeit. Z Kardiol 72:561-568
21. Lehmann M, Rühle K, Schmid P, Klein H, Matthys K, Keul J (1983) Hämodynamik, Plasmakatecholaminverhalten und ß-Adrenorezeptorendichte bei Trainierten, Untrainierten und Herzinsuffizienten. Z Kardiol 72:529-536
22. Lehmann M, Schmid P, Keul J (1984) Age- and exercise-related sympathetic activity in untrained volunteers, trained athletes and patients with impaired left ventricular contractility. Eur Heart J 5 [Suppl E]:1-7
23. Lehmann M, Keul J (1986) Urinary excretion of free noradrenaline and adrenaline related to age, sex and hypertension in 265 individuals. Eur J Appl Physiol 55:14-18
24. Lehmann M, Keul J (1986) Free plasma catecholamines, heart rates, lactate levels and oxygen uptake in competition weight lifters, cyclists and untrained control subjects. Int J Sports Med 7:18-21
25. Lehmann M, Dickhuth HH, Schmid P, Porzig H, Keul J (1984) Plasma catecholamines, ß-adrenergic receptors, and isoproterenol sensitivity in endurance trained and non-endurance trained volunteers. Eur J Appl Physiol52:362-369
26. Lehmann M (1988) Sympatho-vagal changes induced by physical training in cardiac patients. Eur Heart J 9 [Suppl F]:55-62
27. Lehmann M, Keul J, Korsten-Reck U, Fischer H (1981) Einfluß der Ergometerarbeit im Liegen und Sitzen auf Plasmakatecholamine, metabolische Substrate, Sauerstoffaufnahme und Herzfrequenz. Klin Wochenschr 59:1237-1242
28. Lehmann M, Keul J (1986) Age-associated changes of exercise-induced plasma catecholamine responses. Eur J Appl Physiol 55:302-306
29. Lehmann M, Keul J (1985) Capillary-venous differences of free plasma catecholamines at rest and during graded exercise. Eur J Appl Physiol 54:502-505
30. Lehmann M, Gastmann U, Tauber R, Weiler C, Pilot R, Hirsch FH, Auch-Schwelk W, Keul J (1986) Katecholaminverhalten, Adrenorezeptorendichte an intakten Zellen und Katecholamin-Empfindlichkeit bei einer Patientin mit primärer orthostatischer Hypotonie. Klin Wochenschr 64:1249-1254
31. Lehmann M, Hirsch FH, Auch-Schwelk W, Alnor J, Ochs A, Gastmann U, Keul J (1986) Primäre orthostatische Hypotonie. Ein Fallbericht. Z. Kardiol 75:117-121
32. Lehmann M (1989) Trainierbarkeit des Herz-Kreislauf-Systems bei Gesunden und Herzkranken. In: Hopf R, Kaltenbach M (eds) Bewegungstherapie für Herzkranke. PMI, Frankfurt, pp 27-38
33. Lehmann M, Hasenfuß G, Samek L, Eastman U (1990) Catecholamine metabolism in heart failure patients and healthy control subjects. Drug Res 40:1310
34. Lehmann M, Dickhuth HH, Lazar W, Thum M, Keul J (1990) Four-week training / overtraining study in middle- and long-distance runners. Dtsch Z Sportmed 41:112-124
35. Lehmann M (1990) Performance diagnostic relevance of catecholamine determinations. Dtsch Z Sportmed 41:124-129
36. Mader A, Liesen H, Heck H, Philippi H, Rost R, Schürch P, Hollmann W (1976) Zur Beurteilung der sportartspezifischen Ausdauerleistungsfähigkeit im Labor. Sportarzt Sportmed 27:80, 199
37. Mäurer W, Tschada R, Manthey J, Ablasser A, Kübler W (1981) Catecholamines in patients with heart failure. In: Delius W, Gerlach E, Grobecker H, Kübler W (eds) Catecholamines and the heart. Springer, Berlin Heidelberg New York, pp 236-245
38. Meyer K, Lehmann M, Keul J, Weidemann H (1990) Effects of interval – vs continuous exercise training on physical performance, cardiac work, metabolism and catecholamines after coronary bypass surgery. European Society of Cardiology, Brussels, p 42

39. Péronnet F, Cléroux J, Perrault H, Cousineau D, dChamplain J, Nadeau R (1981) Plasma norepinephrine response to exercise before and after training in humans. J Appl Physiol 51:812-815
40. Da Prada M, Zürcher G (1976) Simultaneous radioenzymatic determination of plasma and tissue adrenaline, noradrenaline and dopamine within the fentomole range. Life Sci 19:1161-1174
41. Reindell H (1987) Das Sportherz, geschichtliche Entwicklung und neue Aspekte. In: Rost R, Webering F (eds) Kardiologie im Sport. Deutscher Ärzte-Verlag, Cologne, p 109
42. Roth GS (1980) Changes in hormone action during aging. Glucocorticoid regulation of adipocyte glucose metabolism and catecholamine regulation of myocardial contractility. Proc Soc Exp Biol Med 165:188-178
43. Samek L, Hauf GF, Roskamm H (1990) Exercise training in patients with impaired left ventricular function. European Society of Cardiology, Brussels, p 48
44. Sarnoff SJ, Braunwald E, Welch CH Jr, Case RB, Stansby WN, Marcruz R (1958) Hemodynamic determination of oxygen consumption of the heart with special reference to the tension-time-index. Am J Physiol 12:148-158
45. Silverberg AB, Shah SD, Haymond MW, Cryer PE (1978) Norepinephrine: Hormone and neurotransmitter in man. Am J Physiol 234:E252-256
46. Trap-Jensen J, Christensen NJ, Clausen JP, Rasmussen B, Klausen K (1973) Arterial noradrenaline and circulatory adjustment to strenuous exercise with trained and non-trained muscle groups. In: Seliger V (ed) Physical fitness. Karlova University Press, Prague, pp 414-418
47. Wallin BG (1981) Relationship between sympathetic outflow to muscles, heart rate and plasma norepinephrine in man. In: Delius W, Gerlach E, Grobecker H, Kübler W (eds) Catecholamines and the heart. Springer, Berlin Heidelberg New York, pp 11-17
48. Winder WW, Hickson RC, Hagberg JM, Ehsani AA, McLane JA (1979) Training-induced changes in hormonal and metabolic response to submaximal exercise. J Appl Physiol 46:766-771
49. Yamaguchi N, de Champlain J, Nadeau R (1975) Correlation between the response of the heart to sympathetic stimulation and the release of endogenous catecholamines into the coronary sinus of the dog. Circ Res 36:662-668

General Characteristics of Sensors Used in Rate-Adaptive Pacing: The Ideal Sensor-Open- and Closed-Loop Concept

A.F. RICKARDS[1] and W. BOUTE[2]

Since their introduction, rate-adaptive pacemakers have rapidly gained acceptance by the medical community. Automatic adaptation of the pacing rate to the momentary metabolic needs of the individual patient significantly improved the patient's exercise tolerance. As this was recognized several sensors were investigated as to their ability to indicate the required pacing rate. Table I gives an overview of sensors that are either available or are under review.

Table I. Sensors currently available or under investigation

Sensor signal	Sensor	Status
Mechanical:		
Body activity	Piezo crystal	Available
	Accelerometer	Available
Temperature	Thermistor	Available
ECG:		
QT interval	Unipolar lead	Available
Depolarization gradient	Bipolar lead	Investigation
Impedance:		
Respiration rate	Auxiliary lead	Available
Minute ventilation	Bipolar lead	Available
Stroke volume	Multipolar lead	Investigation
Pre-ejection interval	Multipolar lead	Investigation
Other:		
dp/dt	Pressure sensor	Investigation
O_2 saturation	Light-emitting diode and opto sensor	Investigation

Early difficulties with rate-adaptive pacemakers involved both the sensor and the algorithm. Several manufacturers introduced second and third generation devices, in which improvements were made in sensor performance and/or the algorithm, i.e. the conversion from sensor signal into pacing rate.

[1] Royal Brompton and National Heart Hospital, Sydney Street, London SW 3 6NP, UK
[2] Vitatron Medical B.V., Technical Division, Postfach 76, 6950 AB Dieren, The Netherlands

Sensor Description

Acitivity. Activity-sensing pacemakers use a piezo crystal bonded to the inside of the pacemaker casing. Physical activity normally produces pressure waves which travel through the body and cause micro deflections of the piezo crystal, which in turn transforms these into an electrical signal. These electrical signals will change, in amplitude and/or frequency, depending on the type of physical activity.

The processing of the piezo signal is simple: only signals that exceed a programmable threshold are used to drive a counter process which in turn affects the pacing rate. Later generations have more advanced algorithms in order to obtain a pacing-rate increase that is more proportional to the level of exercise. These devices also take the energy of the piezo signal into account by the integration of the piezo crystal signal. Sensor artefacts may occur if mechanical vibrations that are not a result of physical activity affect the body. On the other hand, the piezo sensor does not respond to, e.g. isometric exercise and emotional stress.

Body activity can also be sensed via an accelerometer which of course has characteristics that differ from those of the piezo-crystal sensor and therefore the performance of such a pacing system is reported to be somewhat more specific to body exercise, especially if only filtered parts of the signal are used to control the pacing rate.

Temperature. Temperature is known to vary with physical activity. However, sensing of the venous blood temperature requires a specialized pacing lead that incorporates a thermistor. This makes such devices unsuitable for pacemaker replacements and one is committed to the future use of this type of rate-adaptive pacemaker once the lead has been implanted.

Clinical tests revealed another phenomenon: as soon as exercise starts the temperature will first decrease. This is known as the "dip". Highly sophisticated algorithms were developed which could recognize the dip and use it for an initial rate increase. However, the acceptance of temperature as a reliable sensor is hampered, mainly due to system complexity and the necessity for a special lead. For the future it might regain clinical importance in combination with an activity sensor.

QT Interval. The QT interval was one of the first sensors that became commercially available. The QT interval reacts to both physical and emotional stress. These pacemakers measure the interval between the stimulus and the maximum downslope of the evoked T wave. Shortening of this interval causes the pacing rate to increase and vice versa. First generation QT interval-sensing pacemakers were hampered by poor detection of the evoked T wave and/or nonexercise-related pacing-rate variations. The latest generation, however, has largely solved both problems. However, the measurement of QT interval is feasible only with paced, not with sensed cardiac beats.

Depolarization Gradient. Another electrocardiographic-related sensor is the depolarization gradient, which is defined as the area of the evoked R wave. The depolarization gradient decreases with stress and increases when the heart rate increases, thereby providing the means of using a closed-loop type algorithm. Limited investigations have shown encouraging results. This sensor only works with stimulated, not with intrinsic heart beats, as well.

Respiration. Respiration rate-sensing pacemakers have been used since the early 1980s. The basic principle of sensing the respiration rate is based on Ohm's law: the pacemaker emits small, constant current pulses and measures the subsequent pulse voltage which then reflects the impedance. When the sensing dipole is placed over (part of) the respiratory system, the impedance changes are largely related to respiration. The use of an auxiliary lead for respiratory rate-sensing has limited its acceptance.

Minute Ventilation. Later generations of respiratory parameter-sensing pacemakers did not only measure the respiration rate but also took into account the depth of breathing which then results in measuring the minute ventilation which is greatly proportional to the level of stress.

Pre-ejection Interval and Stroke Volume. Impedance measurement techniques can also be applied to the heart itself when the sensing dipole is situated in the heart. This enables the sensing of stroke volume and/or the pre-ejection interval. Clinical testing of these concepts have shown encouraging results. At this moment a drawback of this system is that it has to use a multi-polar lead.

Others. Other investigations include advanced sensors for sensing the right ventricular pressure and oxygen saturation. The need for a special pacing lead and the absence of long-term data on the stability and reliability slow the introduction of such systems.

The Ideal Sensor. The ideal sensor continuously provides the pacemaker with information on the exact required heart rate, thereby meeting the momentary metabolic needs of the patient.

Open- and Closed-Loop Concepts

A crucial part of all rate-adaptive pacemakers is the algorithm which translates changes in the sensor signal into changes in pacing rate. The sensor signal indicates whether the pacing rate should increase or decrease. The important question for the algorithm is by how much the pacing rate should be changed. The answer to this question greatly depends upon the type of sensor used.

All rate-adaptive pacemakers using the sensors as listed in Table I are capable of indicating the correct heart rate. However, for some sensors this will involve many reprogramming procedures and exercise tests, mainly because these sensors require the physicians judgement as to whether the pacing rate adaptation is adequate or not. If not, the physician needs to reprogramme the device and repeat the test and judgement procedures.

Other sensors are able to provide the pacemaker with additional information, namely whether the pacing rate has reached or exceeded the required heart rate. Now the judgement has been built into the sensor signal.

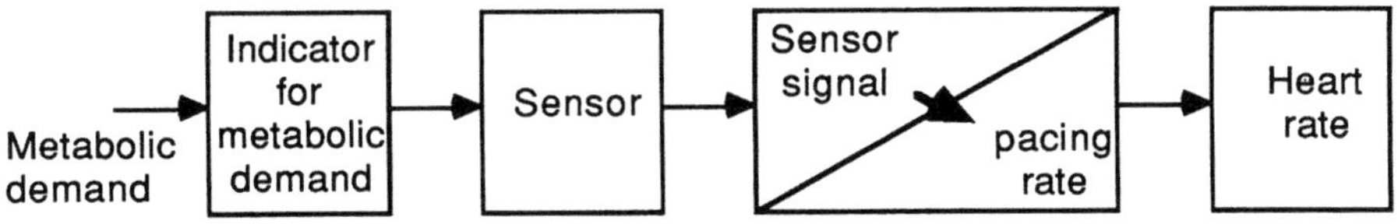

Fig. 1. An open-loop system

Both systems require different algorithms, known as open- and closed-loop systems, respectively.

Open-Loop Systems. An open-loop system is basically a one-way system (Fig. 1). The sensor delivers an electrical signal to the algorithm and the algorithm transforms changes in the sensor signal into changes in pacing rate. The most important factor in this process is how much the pacing rate should change when the sensor signal is changing by one unit.

In open-loop systems this factor, known as rate-response curve or slope, has to be programmed by the physician. However, defining the correct value for this factor is often difficult. The main reason is because most sensors only have an indirect relationship to the pacing rate. Take, for example, temperature. It is known that temperature rises when patients exercise and vice versa. However, the temperature increase that should produce a 25 ppm pacing rate increase differs from patient to patient and is not easy to measure in each individual patient. Therefore often the "trial and error" method is used to programme the correct rate-response factor. Depending on the results from Holter monitoring and/or exercise stress tests the physician decides to change the rate-adaptive parameters. The more experience the physician has with a particular sensor the easier and quicker he may find the correct rate-adaptive parameter settings.

Closed-Loop Systems. In closed-loop systems the sensor has a more direct relationship with the pacing rate. Now the sensor signal is influenced by both metabolic demand and by the momentary pacing rate. A basic requirement for closed-loop systems is that both influences have an inverse effect on the sensor signal, e.g. if metabolic demand increases the sensor signal will increase, and if the pacing rate increases the sensor signal will decrease.

The algorithm of closed-loop systems is normally designed to maintain a constant sensor signal level: the reference value. If we take the example as mentioned above, the sensor signal will increase if the patient starts exercising. Because the sensor signal has increased the pacemaker will respond by increasing the pacing rate. This increase in pacing rate, however, will decrease the sensor signal and the algorithm will continue to increase the pacing rate until the sensor signal has reached its reference value. Only when the sensor signal is equal to the reference value will the pacing rate be stable and this point is regarded as being the optimal pacing rate. The critical parameter in closed-loop systems is the reference value. If the reference value is incorrect the result will be a continuously incorrect rate response (Fig. 2).

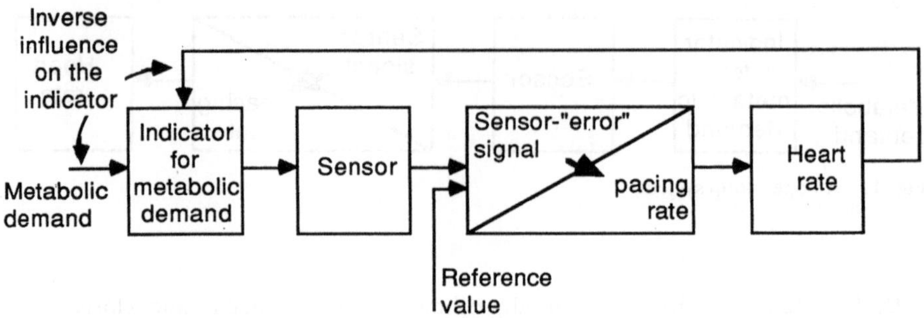

Fig. 2. A closed-loop system

The QT interval has a little bit of both. The QT interval is influenced by both metabolic demand and by heart rate, however, both have the same and not an inverse effect on the QT interval. An increase in metabolic demand and an increase in pacing rate will both shorten the QT interval. As such the QT interval is not a suitable sensor for closed-loop type algorithms.

However, the fact that heart rate does influence the QT interval, or in other words the rate dependency of the QT interval, provides the pacemaker with important information, namely it determines the maximal value of the rate-response factor as described under open-loop systems. Since the rate dependency of the QT interval can easily be measured it provides significant assistance in programming QT interval-sensing pacemakers. The latest generation of QT interval-sensing pacemakers automatically measure this every day and set the rate-responsive parameters accordingly. Sensor parameters that feature a true negative feedback (an increase in heart rate or pacing rate causes a decrease in the specific sensor signal) are oxygen saturation, stroke volume, pre-ejection interval, pacer depolarization integral, and also partly temperature. These parameters could be used in so-called closed-loop systems in the future if intelligent algorithms are capable of handling the sensor signal accordingly.

Conclusion

Several sensors have proven to be suitable for indicating the required heart rate. On the other hand several authors report poor sensor performance under certain circumstances, e.g. the sensor is influenced by factors other than physical exercise or emotional stress.

Advanced sensors such as oxygen saturation seem to have fewer problems, however, the need for a specialized pacing lead and the unknown long-term stability and reliability slow the introduction of such systems.

Therefore in the medium term, combinations of sensors are the way to go. Sensor combinations should be chosen that combine the strong points of each individual sensor while the weak points of one sensor should be covered by the other, and vice versa. In particular body activity seems to be one of the two sensor parameters in any combination due to its easy realisation and clear indication of start and end of physical exercise.

Indications for Implanting Rate-Adaptive Cardiac Pacemakers

E. ALT, M. MATULA, and M. HEINZ[1]

Introduction

Pacemaker therapy has developed into one of the most successful treatment methods in the field of cardiology. Initially implanted mainly to prevent Adams-Stokes attacks and to decrease the mortality of life-threatening bradycardias, pacemakers are increasingly implanted today for hemodynamic reasons, i.e. to improve the quality of life. The purpose is often not only to alleviate congestive heart failure at rest but also to enhance physical performance by improving cardiac output on exertion [1]. Other aims of rate-adaptive pacing are to provide an adequate rate response for different forms and levels of exercise, a rate adaptation under changing metabolic or circulatory conditions not due to exercise, a rate adaptation in terms of biorhythmics, a rate reaction in the case of emotional responses and to prevent the occurrence of especially atrial rhythm disorders.

An increase in cardiac output during exercise depends much more clearly on an increase in heart rate than on an increase in stroke volume (Fig. 1) [2]. This holds true for pacemaker patients even more than for normal people.

Numerous studies in the past have verified the importance of rate variation for improving exercise capacity and have found a strong correlation between the increase in work capacity and the increase in heart rate [3, 4]. A study conducted by our working group on two different patient populations with physiological pacemakers (AAI, atrial pacing, atrial sensing, inhibited; and DDD, double pacing, double sensing, inhibited and triggered) has also demonstrated that not only atrioventricular synchronization, but also adequate rate variation are decisive factors for a feeling of well-being. In both patient groups, those with sick sinus syndrome and limited subjective rate variation, and those with a complete AV block, the implantation of a physiological pacemaker (AAI for sick sinus syndrome and DDD for AV block) was able to restore the AV synchronization. But physical performance was much more favorable in the group with DDD pacemakers with an AV block and preserved normal sinus rate regulation than in the group with sick sinus syndrome and limited rate variation (Table I) [5].

The patient's well-being is affected not only by the maximum attainable heart rate, but also by the rate variation at submaximum stress levels. We were able to show that

[1] First Medical Clinic, Technical University of Munich, 8000 Munich 80, FRG

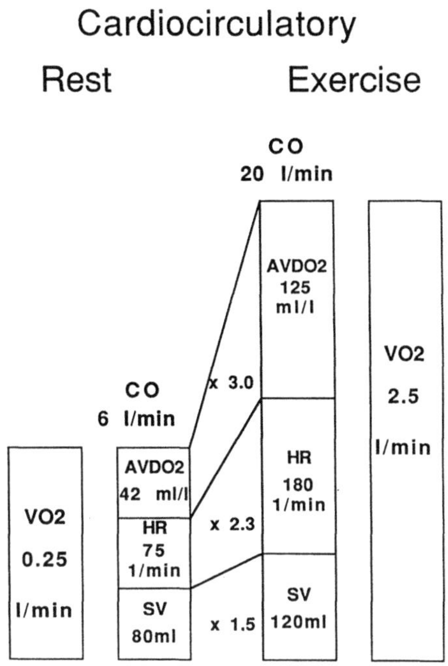

Fig. 1. The increase in cardiac output (CO) from about 6 l/min at rest to about 20 l/min under exercise conditions is achieved in healthy persons by three mechanisms: an increase in the arteriovenous oxygen difference ($AVDO_2$) by a factor of 3, an increase in heart rate (*HR*) by a factor of 2.3, and an increase in stroke volume (*SV*) by 1.5. One can see that an increase in heart rate during exercise is one of the essential mechanisms for increasing cardiac output from 6 to 20 l/min and oxygen uptake (VO_2) from 0.25 l/min at rest to 2.5 l/min under maximum exercise conditions.

Table 1. Improvement in New York Heart Association (NYHA) classification before and after pacemaker implantation

	AAI		DDD	
	Pre (%)	Post (%)	Pre (%)	Post (%)
NYHA I	27	48	0	86
NYHA II	33	43	36	14
NYHA III	20	7	29	0
NYHA IV	20	0	36	0

Functional results before (Pre) and after (Post) implantation of a physiological system (either AAI or DDD). Both patient groups (those with atrial [AAI] and those with dual chamber [DDD] pacemakers) showed atrioventricular synchronization after implantation of the physiological pacemaker system. Whereas the patient group with AAI pacemakers for sick sinus syndrome were limited in their sinus rate increase to an average of 104 bpm, the patients with DDD systems showed normal rate regulation during exercise. The functional pre- and postoperative results in terms of the NYHA classification differ accordingly [5]. There was a significant better improvement in NYHA functional classification in patients with DDD pacemakers compared to those with AAI pacemakers ($p < 0.05$) following pacemakers implantation reflecting the importance of not only AV synchrony but also of adequate rate adaptation.

adequate rate adaptation has a favorable effect on metabolic parameters not only at maximum stress levels (Fig. 2a), but even at submaximum stress levels (Fig. 2b) [6]. This agrees with findings by other authors [7, 8].

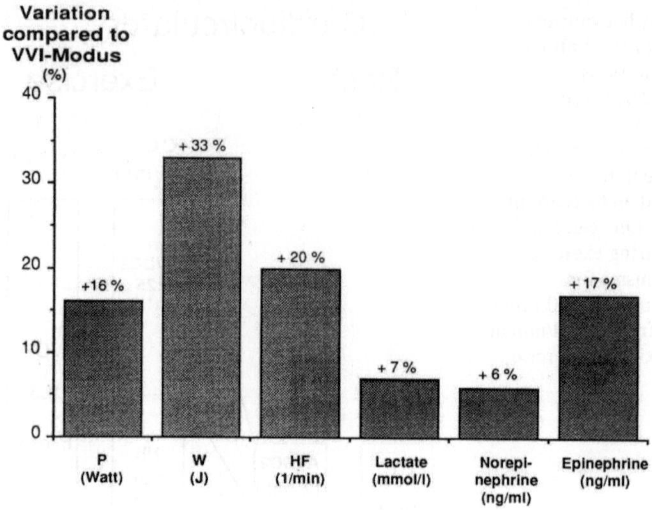

Fig. 2a. Effect of rate-adaptive pacing maximum performance (*P*), work (*W*), maximum heart rate (*HF*), serum lactate value, norepinephrine, and epinephrine levels in comparison to VVI pacing.

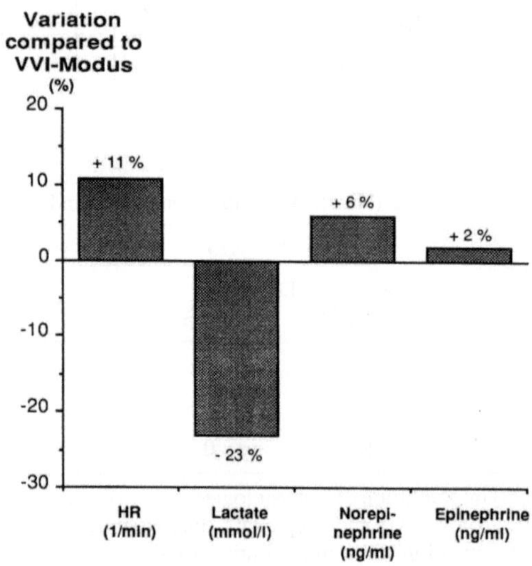

Fig. 2b. Influence of rate-adaptive pacing in comparison to VVI pacing at a fixed 50-watt exercise level with respect to heart rate (*HR*), serum lactate, norepinephrine, and epinephrine levels. The 23% lower lactate value at the same exercise level could also be interpreted as a better aerobic capacity under everyday stresses in the rate-adaptive mode [6]

Adequate and Inadequate Heart Rate Behavior in the Individual Patient

While the favorable influence of rate-adaptive pacing is confirmed for all patients with manifest chronotropic incompetence [8], the question of chronotropic competence or incompetence is not easy to assess in the individual patient. The simplest way of gauging rate behavior might be to measure the maximum heart rate reached at the maximum stress level. One can use, as an approximate guideline, the heart rate attained by a patient group with normal sinus node function, AV block and correctly functioning dual-chamber pacemaker systems (Fig. 3). The maximum rates found in everyday life are generally reached while the patient climbs stairs, as can be determined by means of a 24 h Holter ECG.

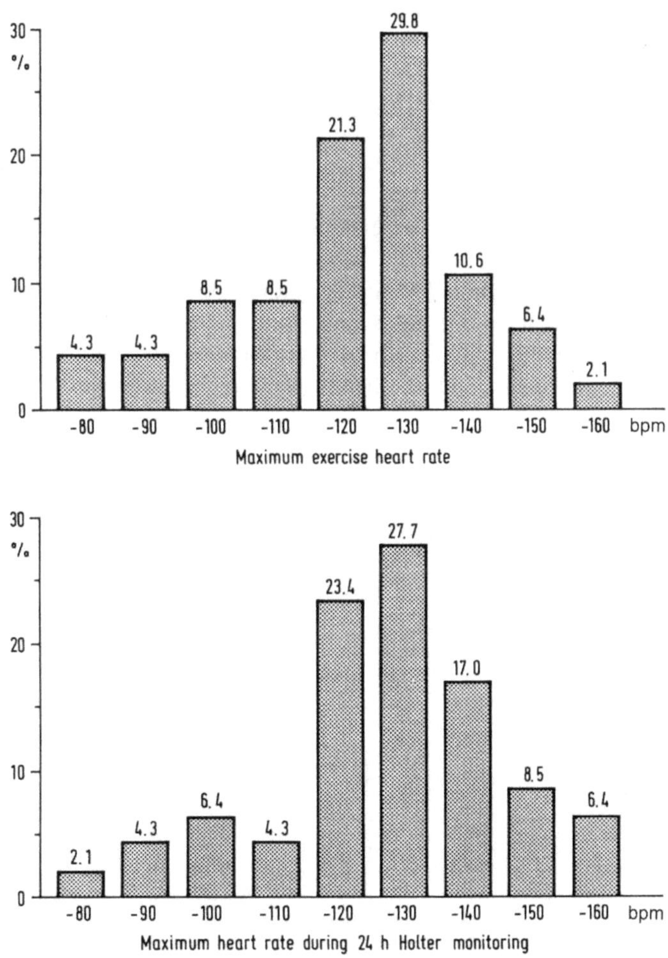

Fig. 3. Histogram of the heart rates reached in 94 patients with implanted DDD pacemaker systems in a normal pacemaker patient population. When climbing stairs, (*top*) 21% of the patients reached rates up to 120 bpm, just under 30% reached values up to 130 bpm, while as many as 19% showed values of more than 130 bpm when climbing stairs. The distribution is similar when one evaluates the 24 h Holter ECGs (*bottom*). Here, the percentage of patients who reach rates of more than 120 bpm in everyday life is, about 60%. Since these patients are average pacemaker patients with all their accompanying diseases, these rate values can also be used as indications of the possible heart-rate values to be attained under rate-adaptive pacing.

Our studies showed that more than half of all patients (60%) with normal sinus function and dual-chamber systems reach maximum rates of more than 120 bpm in everyday life [9]. These values can serve as guidelines for the rate response of sensor-driven pacemakers.

Heart Rate Reserve

A criterion for determining adequate heart rates under stress conditions is generally seen to be the maximum attained rate of 220 bpm minus age. Incompetence is termed chronotropic when 80% of the rate reserve is not attained [10]. In this connection, the heart-rate reserve is defined as the possible difference between the resting heart rate and the predicted maximum heart rate (220 bpm minus age). A 70-year-old patient with a resting heart rate of 60 bpm would have a rate reserve of 220 bpm minus 70 bpm equaling 150 bpm, minus 60 bpm at rest, resulting in a rate reserve of 90 bpm. Eighty percent of this rate reserve is 72 bpm. Thus, a maximum rate upon exertion of 132 bpm or more would be considered normal; maximum rates below this level would be judged to be chronotropically incompetent [10].

Rate Profile in Pacemakers Patients with VVI Systems

However, this distinction may be inadequate in individual cases; one must always take account of the patient's overall state of health. In a study [11] at our clinic on 107 pacemaker patients who were within the range of normal pacemaker indications and average age, and who had implanted nonrate-adaptive VVI systems, an average

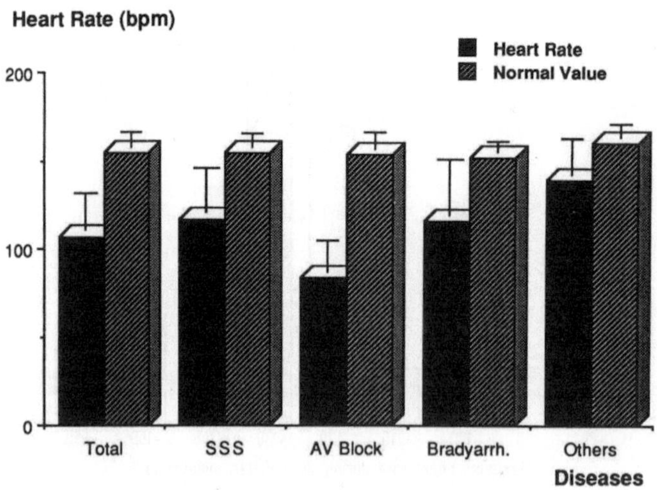

Fig. 4a. Heart rate reached by 107 patients supplied with VVI pacemaker systems and subjected to maximum treadmill exercise. The greatest difference between expected maximum heart rate (220 bpm – age) and measured heart rate is found in the patients with an AV block. *SSS*, sick sinus syndrome; *bradyarrh*, bradyarrhythmia

Fig. 4b. The maximum performance reached at the heart rates in Fig. 4a

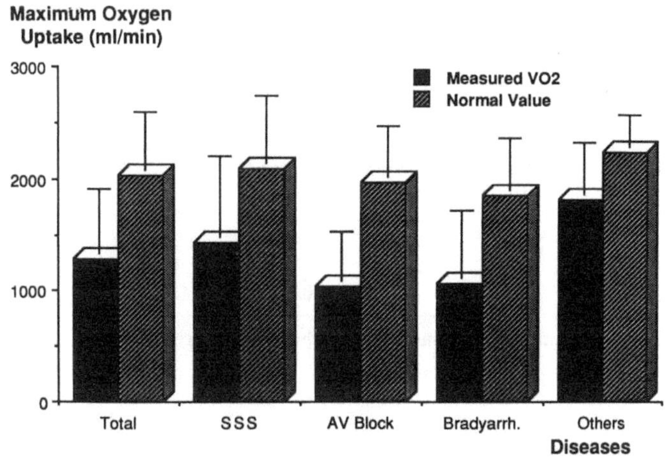

maximum rate of 107.5 ± 23 bpm upon maximum exercise was found for the patients altogether. Patients with sick sinus syndrome reached a maximum rate of 117 bpm, a clearly higher level than those with an AV block who reached only 84 bpm. Patients with bradyarrhythmia showed an average maximum rate of 116 bpm (Fig. 4a). Patients who had received pacemakers for other indications, such as hypersensitive carotid sinus syndrome or intermittent AV block, attained an average maximum heart rate of 139.6 bpm, reflecting a less-compromised chronotropic rate regulation. The maximum work capacity attained corresponds to the heart rates in the individual groups (Fig. 4b).

Inquiring into the reasons leading to the discontinuation of stress tests in this study, we found physical exhaustion in 32% of cases, tiring of muscles in 10%, shortness of breath in 26%, dizziness in 10%, angina pectoris in 17%, and a peripheral circulatory disturbance in 5% (Table 2). It is often difficult to judge in a given case whether the particular complaints are related to an unsatisfactory increase in heart rate and thus in cardiac output, or whether they are due to previous general diseases in the largely elderly patient group. Taking all aspects into account, we assumed that a rate increase would have been clinically advantageous in about half the patients examined. Patients with a complete AV block and normal sinus node function who would have been ideally treated with a DDD system were not taken into account.

Beneficiaries of Rate Adaptive Systems

Other studies have arrived at similar figures. MacBride et al. [12] found in their patient population that 41% would have profited from a rate-adaptive pacemaker, the distrubution being 12% for AAI-R, 16% for VVI-R, and 13% for DDD-R. Simonsen [13] also found in his studies that 40% of patients reached a heart rate of less than 110 bpm upon maximum stress and must therefore be considered potential

Table 2. Reasons for discontinuing exercise tests on 107 patients supplied with conventional nonrate-adaptive VVI systems

	No./%	Physical exhaustion No./%	Muscular fatigue No./%	Dyspnea No./%	Dizziness No./%	Stenocardia No./%	Claudication joint pain No./%
Total	107/100	35/32.7	11/10.3	28/26.2	10/9.3	18/16.8	5/4.7
SSS	50/100	17/34.0	6/12.0	9/18.0	7/14.0	9/18.0	2/4.0
AV Block	37/100	8/21.6	5/13.5	12/32.4	2/5.4	7/18.9	3/8.1
Bradyarrh.	12/100	4/33.3	0/0.0	6/50.0	0/0.0	2/16.7	0/0.0
Others	8/100	6/75.0	0/0.0	1/12.5	1/12.5	0/0.0	0/0.0

SSS = sick sinus syndrome. Bradyarrh. = bradyarrhythmia

beneficiaries of a rate-adaptive system. By contrast, Prior's study found that his group of 24 relatively young patients reached an average maximum heart rate of 137 bpm, or 87% of the predicted maximum rate; these patients would therefore not have benefited from an additional chronotropic sensor [14].

A differentiated examination of the clinical benefit of rate-adaptive pacemakers is provided by Corbelli et al [15]. They base their decision of whether a rate-adaptive system is of clinical benefit not only on the maximum heart rate attained, but also on the course of heart rate over the entire increasing stress period. Different rate patterns are shown here. In one group there is a fast initial rate increase during the first level of stress, but virtually no further increase at higher stress levels. A second heart rate pattern also frequently found shows a continuous rate increase at increasing stress levels, but the particular rate values are always altogether too low. The third pattern involves virtually no rate increase at the onset of stress, but a sudden drastic increase as stress becomes longer and greater, so that an almost normal maximum heart rate is attained by the end of stress. For these patients it is therefore unsuitable to focus on maximum heart rate to judge the clinical benefit of a rate-adaptive system. The unsatisfactory rate increase at low-stress levels should be taken into account here, since it can lead to an increase in blood and tissue lactate concentrations, although the maximum heart rate reached at maximum stress levels can be nearly normal (Fig. 2b) [8]. Furthermore, one should also consider the heart-rate response after the end of exercise when judging chronotropic behavior; too rapid a drop in heart rate, particularly after great effort, can be manifested by clinical complaints such as dizziness and a drop in blood pressure.

Assessment of Chronotropic Incompetence

The assessment of chronotropic incompetence is basically just as multifaceted and subject to different influences as the assessment of sinus node recovery time is as a parameter for normal or disturbed sinus node function. Since the sinus node reacts to numerous sympathetic and vagal influences, the heart-rate reaction varies during the course of the day. For example, Sulke et al. [17] found that a sinus node can function normally, or nearly so, in the morning, while the maximum heart rates attained in the afternoon can be in the pathological range of under 100 bpm.

In order to gauge chronotropic incompetence of the sinus node and thus the indication for rate-adaptive pacemaker therapy, one should answer the following questions:

1. What is the maximum heart rate attained at maximum exercise, or the rate reserve at a particular submaximum stress level?
2. How does the heart rate behave during light, moderate, and heavy physical activity?
3. What is the patient's biological state as a whole?
4. Do complicating factors exist, such as disorders of the locomotor system or the peripheral circulation, or has the patient not recovered well from a stroke?
5. Can a possible increase in cardiac output based on an increase in heart rate be turned into an improved quality of life?
6. Is an additional treatment of tachyarrhythmias necessary? Particularly in patients with brady-tachy syndrome, there is often an indication for pacemaker therapy due to necessary drug treatment for tachyarrhythmias, which strengthens a previously existing tendency toward bradycardia and makes it in need of treatment.
7. What is the biological age and the expected course of bradyarrhythmia?

These questions all vary in importance depending on the individual patient. For an elderly patient who does not make any great demands on his physical fitness a maximum achievable heart rate of 110 bpm might be sufficient, while a numerically older, but biologically younger patient might be limited in his quality of life by a maximum heart rate of 110 bpm due to his higher expectations in terms of exercise capacity.

With regard to the progression of sinus node dysfunction over the years, the studies by Seitz et al. [18] on 110 patients showed that the maximum heart rate achieved upon maximum exercise decreased from 115±21 bpm, at the time of implantation, to 93±7 bpm in the course of an average 52-month period.

In general, a negative correlation has been found between sinus node recovery time at rest and the maximum heart rate attained during stress [11]. This aspect should also influence the decision in favor of a rate-adaptive system, especially for younger patients already showing clearly pathological sinus node recovery times (> 2.0 s), even if the intrinsic heart rate upon maximum exercise was still sufficient at the time of implantation.

Rate Adaptive Pacing in Patients with Coronary Heart Disease

There has been no agreement up to now about the extent to which a concomitant coronary heart disease influences the decision whether to use a rate-adaptive system. There is no doubt that heart rate plays a major part in determining myocardial oxygen consumption since it forms the so-called double product together with peripheral resistance. One of the ways of treating coronary heart disease accordingly consists in limiting the rate increase during stress by corresponding drugs, e.g., beta blockers.

Patients with coronary heart disease should certainly have a less-steep increase in heart rate during exercise than healthy people. However, if the rate reserve is limited too strongly this can result in an inadequate increase in end-diagnostic filling pressure, which can lead to an increase in myocardial oxygen consumption. Studies on healthy volunteers have shown that an increase in cardiac output effected by an increase in stroke volume is much more economical than an increase in cardiac output due to rate increase [19]. But these findings cannot be readily applied to coronary patients, since an increase in end-diastolic filling pressure leads primarily to an increase in stroke volume in a healthy person with a normal contractility reserve, whereas in coronary patients with compromised contractility, an increase in filling pressure beyond a given point leads to a drop in stroke volume and thus to a further deterioration of the myocardial oxygen supply.

Thus, a study conducted by de Cock at al. [20] has shown that pacemaker patients with coronary heart disease and reduced myocardial function also benefit from rate-adaptive pacing. The increase in heart rate only causes a dramatic deterioration in an existing latent myocardial ischemia in exceptional cases. We ourselves observed the negative effect of an individually excessive increase in heart rate during exercise in a patient with very high grade coronary stenosis, who experienced a dramatic drop in central venous oxygen saturation, reflecting a considerable worsening of cardiac output. It must thus be expected that so-called closed-loop systems, which also optimize the pacing rate in terms of maximum myocardial effectiveness, will set the optimal heart rate for the particular case in the future. Parameters suitable for such closed-loop control include, e.g., stroke volume and oxygen saturation in the right ventricle. The principle of closed-loop pacing will overcome the current limitations of slopes that link sensor signals and pacing rate in a fixed and predetermined manner.

But, in general, coronary heart disease is not a contraindication for the implantation of a rate-adaptive pacemaker. In a given case it may be necessary to adapt the slope of the rate increase during exercise to the coronary status and to select a somewhat lower upper rate limit.

The percentage of pacemaker patients who can benefit from a rate-adaptive system at the time of implantation is assumed to be around 30% in most reports. Those who consider the group of potential beneficiaries of rate-adaptive pacing to be very small, or even nonexistent [21] are exceptional, as are those who assume that more than 90% of pacemaker patients would profit from rate-adaptive pacing. Our data, which involve a reasonable estimation of the clinical benefit, effort, cost and risks associated with rate-adaptive pacing, confirm that at least 30% would be suitable at present for rate-adaptive pacing (Fig. 5), and are supported by the figures from other centers [22].

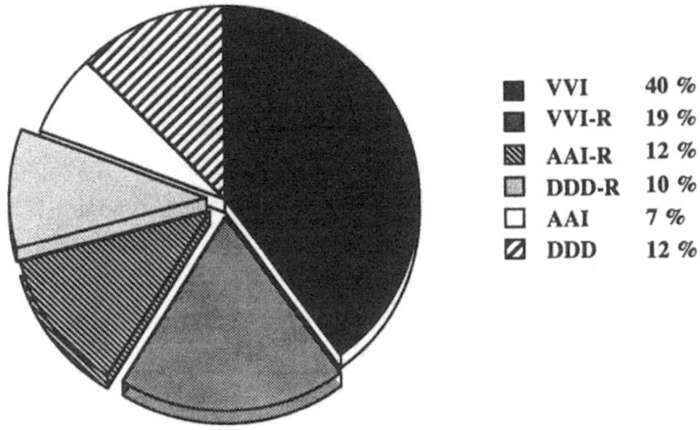

Fig. 5. Distribution of the various pacing modes in our patient population

Criteria for Selecting a Rate-Adaptive Pacemaker System for Patients with Sick Sinus Syndrome

Sick sinus syndrome is characterized by a great number of clinical features. Along with a constant sinus bradycardia there may be sinus arrhythmia with alternating foci. The clinical picture includes sinoatrial blockages, sinus arrest, and prolonged preautomatic pauses, as well as an abnormal response to carotid pressure and vagal stimuli. Patients with sick sinus syndrome frequently have not only bradycardia, but also intermittent tachycardias often requiring antiarrhythmic therapy, which further reduces the pulse in slow phases and therefore necessitates the implantation of a pacemaker system. A reduced response to atropine may indicate a damaged sinoatrial node, as may an inadequate rate increase during exercise. One must remember that the sinoatrial node shows great dependence on both sympathetic and vagal stimuli and can thus reflect circadian and emotional changes in the vegetative basic tonus.

When selecting the pacemaker system for patients with sick sinus syndrome one should focus on whether an adequate rate response exists. The criteria for adequate or inadequate rate response were shown above and should be oriented toward the picture of the total personality, the patient's expectation of his physical fitness, and his mobility. One will generally regard an exercise-induced rate increase to values of 110 to 130 bpm as an adequate rate response and lower values as inadequate. Two factors are of essential importance in selecting the pacemaker system for patients with sick sinus syndrome, and these have often been insufficiently heeded in the past.

Occurrence of Atrial Fibrillation

One point relates to the question of the occurrence of atrial fibrillation under various pacemaker systems and the second to the consequences of the occurrence of atrial fibrillation, such as cardiac insufficiency and thromboembolic events. In the past the most important goal in treating sick sinus syndrome was often only to raise the rate as such. However, numerous studies show the hemodynamic deterioration under ventricular pacing in patients with sick sinus syndrome in comparison to their spontaneous rhythm. This applies particularly to patients with retrograde conduction. One study [23] has shown that when the pacemaker provides the command variable for rate, the occurrence of atrial fibrillation was 28.5% in the second year after implantation of a VVI (ventricular pacing, ventricular sensing, inhibited) system in patients with sick sinus syndrome, while the proportion of patients with atrial fibrillation was only 3.4% after 2 years in the patient group supplied with AAI pacemakers for sick sinus syndrome. The corresponding figures after 4 years were 47% atrial fibrillation in the VVI group as compared to 6.7% for the patients with AAI pacemakers. In this study by Rosenquist et al. [23] the two patient groups (VVI and AAI pacemakers) were comparable in terms of electrophysiological and demographic parameters. Other surveys [24] also show that the frequency of atrial fibrillation was 22.3% in the group with VVI pacemakers as compared to 3.8% in the group with AAI pacemakers within a control period of 33 months.

Thromboembolic Events

The occurrence of atrial fibrillation is increasingly regarded as a cause for thromboembolic events. Whereas idiopathic atrial fibrillation without a rheumatic abnormality used to be considered a rather harmless disease of old age, there has recently been increasing clinical evidence that atrial fibrillation not induced by cardiac abnormalities (so-called nonrheumatic atrial fibrillation) involves a clearly higher rate of thromboembolisms. In 1978 the Framingham study already described a four times higher risk of thromboembolic events in patients with chronic nonrheumatic atrial fibrillation, including patients with coronary heart disease and cardiac insufficiency, in comparison to the normal population [25, 26]. Atrial fibrillation furthermore increases the risk of silent cerebral infarctions in comparison to sinus rhythm [27].

A recent publication by Petersen in *Lancet* [32] has accordingly shown that thromboembolic complications under anticoagulation with coumarin occurred in only five patients out of a group of 1007 patients with chronic nonrheumatic atrial fibrillation. In the patient group taking 75 mg aspirin a day, 20 patients suffered thromboembolic events, and in the group taking the placebo 21 thromboembolic events occurred. Thus, not only the frequency of thromboembolic events, but also the mortality rate due to embolic complications were significantly lower in the patient group taking coumarin, than in the groups taking aspirin and placebo, between which there were no significant differences. Further studies, some of which have not yet been concluded, such as the SPAF (Stroke Prevention in Patients with Atrial Fibrillation) study, [33], confirm the significant influence of anticoagulation therapy on the reduction in thromboembolic events (18 strokes in 459 patients without anticoagulation versus only 5 strokes in 477 patients under anticoagulation). Interestingly enough, the anticoagulation was conducted as low-dose coumarin therapy. The goal was to prolong the prothrombin time to 1.2–1.5 times (comparable with European Quick's values of 30%–50%).

Different frequencies of thromboembolic complications are also described for pacemaker patients, i.e., for patients with VVI pacemakers and atrial fibrillation in comparison to patients with AAI pacemakers. The figures from five nonrandomized studies involving 321 patients with AAI pacemakers and 532 patients with VVI pacemakers, show a significant difference with respect to systemic embolisms of 13% in the VVI mode versus 1.6% in the AAI mode [24].

The study by Rosenquist, who followed up 168 patients, found a higher number of strokes in the patient group with VVI pacemakers (13% in the VVI group versus 4.5% in the AAI group) after 2 years [24]. Whereas the risk of a stroke was not linked significantly with the occurrence of chronic atrial fibrillation in this group (19% versus 12%), there was a significantly higher proportion of patients with strokes in the group which had shown atrial tachyarrhythmias preoperatively (20% versus 7.1%, $p < 0.05$) [18, 28].

Cardiac Insufficiency

The same holds true for the development of congestive heart failure after implantation of a VVI pacemaker system in comparison with an AAI pacemaker system in patients with sick sinus syndrome. Rosenquist's study found that after 2 years 23% versus 7% and after 4 years 37% versus 15% of patients in the VVI group versus the AAI group developed signs of cardiac insufficiency and required treatment [24]. Both the loss of AV synchronization and retrograde atrioventricular conduction with VVI pacing lead to the development of cardiac insufficiency and to a clear reduction in contractility. Furthermore, the myocardial oxygen balance also worsens in patients with coronary heart disease, since the unfavorable VVI pacing leads to a relativ increase in myocardial oxygen consumption [29]. This is not altered by the implantation of a VVI-R system, since the ergonomically less favorable contraction of the ventricle cannot be compensated for by rate adaptation during exercise after the disappearance of atrioventricular synchronization [30].

Further indications of the unfavorable effect of VVI and VVI-R pacemakers on sick sinus syndrome are found in the studies by Vardas et al. [37] and Hull et al. [38]. These authors describe a significant increase in atrial natriuretic peptide and in plasma katecholamines in patients with sick sinus syndrome under VVI pacing, which is explained by the loss of AV synchronization.

Suppression of Atrial Arrhythmias

A further important aspect when selecting a rate-adaptive pacemaker system for patients with sick sinus syndrome is the suppression of atrial arrhythmias. Kato et al. [31] examined the frequency of supraventricular extrasystoles and atrial fibrillation and flutter in 28 patients with sick sinus syndrome. The patient group with VVI pacemakers showed a mean hourly frequency of supraventricular extrasystoles of 220 in the 24 h ECG, while patients with AAI pacemakers showed 12.9. The number of supraventricular extrasystoles was significantly lower in the patient group with AAI-R pacemakers (1.2 per h). This significant difference between the two groups of AAI and AAI-R is not surprising, considering the pathophysiological foundations of the origin of extrasystoles. A mechanical extension alone can lead to the occurrence of extrasystoles in the animal model. In pacemaker patients an inadequate rate increase during exercise leads to a greater extension of the atrium due to a stronger increase in the filling pressures. In addition, the shorter duration of diastole with AAI-R presumably has a favorable effect on the suppression of supraventricular extrasystoles in terms of an overdrive suppression phenomenon.

AAI Pacing and the Risk of AV Block

On the question of the optimal therapy for sick sinus syndrome, regardless of the question of rate adaptation, experts have different views depending on their personal estimations. There is a group of physicians who fundamentally consider it too uncertain to implant an atrial pacemaker system (AAI) alone, on the grounds that the danger of an AV block exists in principle in the course of time. These colleagues additionally implant a ventricular lead along with an atrial lead for reasons of safety. Another group assumes that the occurrence of an AV block can be ruled out with sufficient certainty, due to certain clinical criteria in patients with sick sinus syndrome and that the implantation of an atrial pacemaker system must be preferred after weighing up the benefits and risks. A recent study [35] examines the risk of an AV block occurring in patients with sick sinus syndrome with reference to an extensive survey of the literature covering 1876 patients in 28 different studies. It arrives at an annual incidence of 0.6% for the development of an additional AV block, and states that the occurrence of an AV block must be expected in altogether 2.1% of cases as the mean value from all studies. As far as we know, there is no indication in the literature that a patient was vitally threatened or died due to the sudden occurrence of a deep-seated AV block after the implantation of an atrial pacemaker system. AV blockages which occur in the course of time in patients with sick sinus syndrome and primarily normal AV function are thus generally of the Wenckebach type, and therefore allow sufficient time for implanting an additional ventricular lead if necessary.

The relatively low probability (0.6% a year) of the occurrence of AV blockages should be balanced against the complications that can occur with dual-chamber systems (DDD and DDD-R). These include reentry tachycardias, difficulties of venous access with the second lead, difficulties in removing the leads in case of infection, larger dual-chamber aggregates in comparison with single-chamber systems, higher prices, and complicated follow-ups with DDD and DDD-R systems in comparison to AAI and AAI-R pacemakers. After comparing the benefits and risks we, like the Working Group on Cardiac Pacing of the German Cardiac Society, are of the view that the implantation of an atrial pacemaker in patients with sick sinus syndrome and primarily normal AV node function is clearly the more advantageous method. There is really no sensible reason for withholding an atrial pacemaker system with or without rate adaptation from a patient with sick sinus syndrome if the AV node function is normal at the time of implantation and the probability of an AV block occurring later is low as described below.

Assessment of AV Node Function

The decision whether to use an AAI-R or a DDD-R system must be made contingent upon the behavior of the AV node. We assume that, depending on the age of the patient and in accordance with the basic vegetative tonus, a 1:1 conduction of 110–130 bpm provides a sufficient guarantee that no AV block will occur later, if 1) no severe coronary heart disease exists additionally and 2) a cardiomyopathy can likewise be excluded. It is known that the stimulus conduction system is often involved in a degenerative process in patients with cardiomyopathy. To be on the safe side one should exclude patients with bundle-branch block from implantation of an AAI atrial pacemaker system. A further criterion should be that no AV blockages are detectable in the long-term ECG and no AV blockages must occur upon carotid pressure, particularly upon pressure on the left carotid bifurcation. If these criteria are heeded the implantation of an atrial pacemaker system should be the remedy of choice.

If long term stable AV conduction is not ensured adequately, particularly in patients requiring treatment with class I or III antiarrhythmic drugs, one should additionally implant a second ventricular lead for safety reasons. In this case a dual-chamber system is suitable. Only in exceptional cases, if there are technical difficulties in placing the atrial lead, if the atria are fibrotic or very large and thus insufficient P waves (smaller than 1.5 mV) or inacceptably high stimulus threshold values (above 1.5 Volt at 0.5 ms) are attainable, one may resort to implanting a VVI-R system. Patients in whom frequent atrial tachyarrhythmias and considerably enlarged atria make it improbable for a normal sinus rhythm to exist on a long-term basis should also be supplied with a VVI-R system. However, with these patients one must assume that chronic atrial fibrillation or atrial flutter will arise within a short time after implantation. This occurs relatively quickly, particularly in cases in which a retrograde ventriculoatrial conduction exists. Apart from such exceptions the implantation of a VVI-R system in patients with sick sinus syndrome is regarded as obsolete nowadays and should therefore be rejected [36].

Doubts have been expressed in the past about whether a prolonged interval between the spike and the QRS complex might not lead to indirect Wenckebach's signs and thus to the occurrence of a pacemaker syndrome in patients with rate-adaptive atrial pacemakers. These views were based on the fact that a relative increase in the AV interval or the spike-QRS interval was observed upon a rate increase at rest without a corresponding sympathetic tone in the patient. However, recent studies [39] show that the same heart rate involves a substantially shorter stimulation-QRS interval during exercise than is the case with an artificial rate increase at rest. This is due to the improved AV conduction under sympathicotonic drive. One therefore need not expect the occurrence of cannon waves with rate-adaptive atrial pacemakers during physical stress which were implanted with regard to the abovementioned safety provisions during physical stress of primarily normal AV conductivity.

Therapy with Rate-Adaptive Pacemakers in Patients with Bradyarrhythmia (Atrial Fibrillation and Slow Ventricular Response)

Patients who require a pacemaker for bradyarrhythmia have not only chronic atrial fibrillation but also clearly reduced conductive properties in the AV node. Atrial fibrillation in otherwise healthy persons with normal sympathetic and vagal tone on the AV node leads to resting rates of between 110 and 130 bpm. Patients with normal AV conductive properties must accordingly be slowed down with conduction-inhibiting drugs if atrial fibrillation occurs. One generally uses digitalis, calcium antagonists, and beta blockers for this purpose.

Patients with bradyarrhythmia who require a pacemaker are accordingly impaired not only in the normal atrial automaticity but also in the conduction conditions in the AV node. The latter are often associated with structural changes in the heart. The patient group with bradyarrhythmia and cardiac pacemakers accordingly have the worst prognosis for survival of all pacemaker patients [40]. Pacemaker therapy is also chosen for these patients in only 14% of cases due to syncope in the anamnesis; in 86% the goal of pacemaker therapy is to improve an existing cardiac insufficiency (Fig. 6).

Heart Rate Behavior with Bradyarrhythmia

In our studies on the behavior of the spontaneous rate during exercise in different patient groups (Fig. 4a), we found that patients with bradyarrhythmia reached an average maximum rate of 116 bpm upon maximum individual exercise [11]. In half the cases the exercise was discontinued due to dyspnea. In the patient group with bradyarrhythmia the indication for rate-adaptive pacemaker therapy can be made contingent upon the course of the rate profile in the long-term ECG. Due to their restricted stroke volume reserve, these patients require adequate rate adaptation during exercise as an adaptive mechanism for increasing cardiac output. On the other hand, the overall situation of the patient must also be considered when deciding whether to use a rate-adaptive system. Due to an advanced myocardial insufficiency the range of physical performance is frequently not very pronounced. A study by

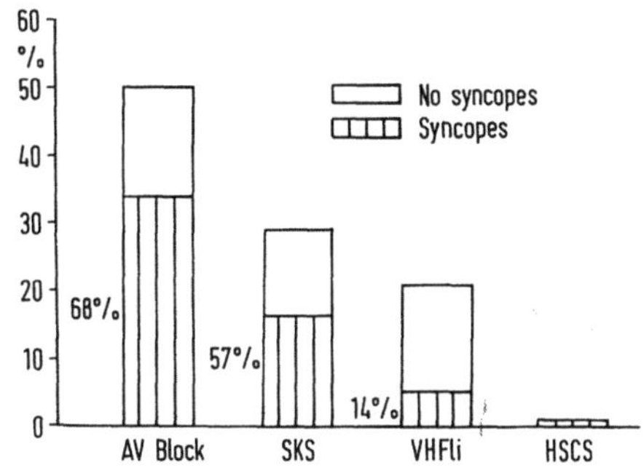

Fig. 6. Indication for implanting a pacemaker according to the underlying disease in patients receiving a pacemaker between 1970 and 1985 at the Rechts der Isar Medical Center, Technical University of Munich/ Germany.
The Percentage of patients in the various groups who had suffered a syncope before pacemaker implantation is shown by the lined bars. This percentage was highest (68%) in patients with an AV block, while it was only 14% in patients with atrial fibrillation (*VH Fli*). Altogether 2507 patients from our patient population were evaluated. *SKS*, sick sinus syndrome; *HSCS*, hypersensitive carotid sinus

Corbelli et al. [15] showed only a low increase in spontaneous rate during exercise in patients with atrial fibrillation, which was certainly also due to the high concomitant medication with pulse-influencing drugs (73% of the patients were given digoxin, 21% beta blockers, and 26% calcium antagonists). This study on pacemaker patients with bradyarrhythmia accordingly showed that three of the 19 patients examined would constantly have profited from a sensor, and that eight of the 19 would sometimes have profited, so that in a total of about 60% of the patients with atrial fibrillation a rate-adaptive pacemaker system would have been beneficial. [15] This agrees with our observations that in about 50% of patients with atrial fibrillation a rate-adaptive pacemaker system is the command variable for rate during exercise and that in these cases one can assume an indication for a rate-adaptive VVI-R system [11, 41].

The Status of DDD-R Pacing

Whereas the implantation of a dual-chamber pacemaker system (DDD) without additional sensor control is the method of choice for a total AV block with normal sinoatrial function, there have been problems in the past in terms of the optimal pacing mode for patients with disturbances not only in the AV node, but also in the sinoatrial node (binodal disease). An improved form of therapy for these patients was provided for the first time in 1986 by the clinical introduction of rate-adaptive dual-chamber pacemaker systems (DDD-R) [42].

Considerations in Favor of DDD-R Pacing

The following clinical aspects influence the decision in favor of a DDD-R system. *Improved Rate Response in Patients Requiring Additional Antiarrhythmic Therapy.* Along with the symptom of bradycardia, the so-called brady-tachy syndrome is a clinical feature of sick sinus syndrome. Suppression of the tachycardia by drugs is often the crucial factor for clinical manifestation of a bradycardia with a lack of rate increase during exercise. In patients with previously damaged AV conductivity, antiarrhythmic drugs can cause a further worsening in AV conduction. For these patients a DDD-R system offers the greatest flexibility even after implantation due to the possibility of selecting the individually most suitable pacing mode in the course of time (e.g., initially AAI-R, later DDD-R or DDI-R).

When Atrial Fibrillation Occurs and High-Grade AV Blockage Already Exists a DDD System Acts only as a VVI Pacemaker. Although improved pacemaker technology, programming possibilities, and atrial leads have certainly lowered the frequency of atrial fibrillation occurring in patients with an AV block today as compared with a few years ago [43], the possible occurrence of atrial fibrillation in patients with an AV block in the course of time is one of the strongest arguments for choosing a DDD-R system. This also holds for patients with primarily normal sinoatrial function, since one can then reprogram to the VVI-R mode if necessary. The same argument holds for "single lead" VDD systems, which are being increasingly used clinically and in which the backup of the VVI-R mode is an essential safety component.

Possible Dysfunctions in Atrial Leads over the Course of Time Can Be Solved in an Alternative Way. The number of sensing and pacing dysfunctions of atrial leads play a very minor part in experienced hands today. Nevertheless, disturbances in sensing and pacing functions cannot be entirely ruled out, sometimes due to previously existing damage in the atrial myocardium, sometimes to ischemic damage newly occurring in the atrial musculature over the course of time, and sometimes due to technical problems (lead break, defective insulation). In such cases one can select a VVI-R pacing mode or, in rare cases, also an DDI-R mode in order not to deprive the patient of rate modulation during exercise despite the disturbance in the atrium.

Detection of Inadequate Tachycardias Using a Sensor. Reentry tachycardias, atrial flutter, other pathological atrial tachycardias, and atrial fibrillation with resulting fast ventricular pacings have been a clinical problem of great importance since the introduction of DDD pacemakers. Numerous algorithms, programming proposals, and attempts to distinguish pathological from physiological rate increases have often failed to achieve the desired success in clinical practice, or have resulted in the compromise of a reduced maximum atrial tracking rate. These programmings have thus also restricted the maximum attainable upper limiting rate and the patient's exercise capacity.

In this area the use of a sensor will substantially contribute to simplifying and broadening the therapeutic possibilities in the future (Fig. 7). The purpose of the sensor is to ascertain whether the patient's state of activity justifies the corresponding

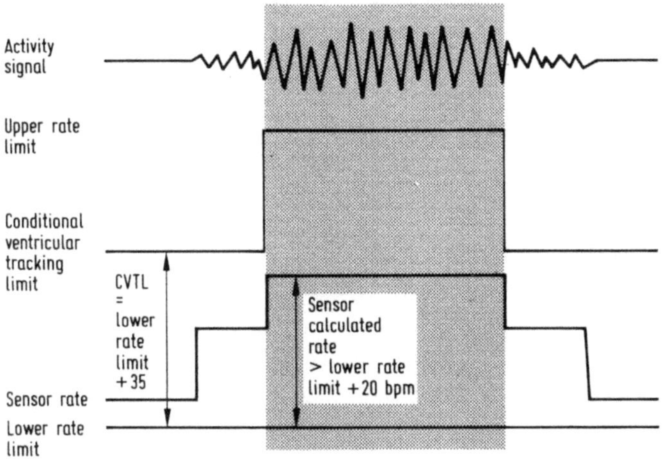

Fig. 7. The activity signal in the DDD-R pacemaker system Relay™ (Intermedics Inc. Angleton, TX, USA) serves two functions: (1) rate adaptation according to activity as already known from other activity-controlled pacemakers and (2) control of the maximum achievable rate in the DDD mode triggered by atrial signals. In this pacemaker the activity signal serves as a control means to select one of the two tracking limits. In case the sensor-indicated pacing rate is low and not higher than the lower rate + 20 bpm, atrial P waves can only be tracked up to the conditional ventricular tracking limit (*CVTL*) which is established at 35 bpm above the lower rate limit. The maximum CVTL is established by means of the Wenckebach phenomenon. This is in contrast to the mode switch in the Meta DDD-R pacemaker (from DDD to VVIR).

If the sensor-calculated rate indicates an instantaneous rate higher than 20 bpm above the lower rate limit, the CVTL ceases and the regular maximum upper rate limit in the DDD mode can be reached, triggered by atrial P waves. The novel feature of CVTL is important for maintaining *one* common upper rate limit for sensor indicated *and* for atrial triggered ventricular pacing rates since the use of separate upper rate limits (as applied in most other DDD-R systems) has the potential to create new pacing induced atrial rhythm disorders.

tachycardia. If not, a so-called conditional ventricular tracking limit is introduced, as in the case of a DDD-R activity pacemaker controlled by an accelerometer (Relay™ and Stride of Intermedics Inc., Angleton, TX, USA) [44]. The maximum attainable rate for the state in which the sensor indicates no physical activity is generally limited to values of 35 bpm above baseline pacing rate, i.e. 85–100 bpm. Physiological rate increases due to emotional or other metabolic changes are hereby permitted, even if the activity sensor does not detect them.

Other systems, such as the breathing-controlled Meta DDD-R, likewise are able to use the sensor as a criterion for distinguishing between physiological and pathological tachycardias. However, in the first generation of this pacemaker the automatic switchover from DDD to VVI-R was achieved in such a way that the occurrence of a few spontaneous atrial extrasystoles led to competitive pacing. This favored the occurrence of atrial flutter and fibrillation, as is known from experiences with DVI pacemakers in earlier years [45].

However, the use of a sensor for distinguishing between physiological and pathological tachycardias is one of the main reasons as to why a DDD-R system will presumably be implanted routinely in all patients in the future, instead of a DDD pacemaker as has happened up to now (Fig. 8).

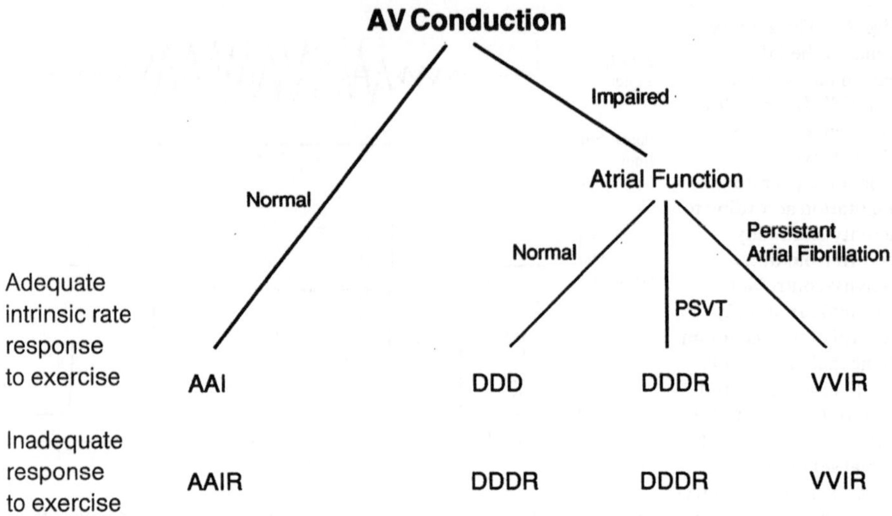

Fig. 8. An algorithm for determining the optimal pacemaker for the individual patient. Aside from the procedure of implanting a DDD system in patients with AV block, normal atrial functions, and chronotropic competence current developments show that a DDD-R system might presumably be implanted routinely in all of these patients in the near future. *PSVT*, paroxysmal supraventricular arrhythmias

This will only be possible, however, when the switchover modalities from atrially triggered pacing in the case of an inadequately high atrial rate to a mode with limited ventricular response will be applied in an automatic fashion in the majority of DDD-R pacemakers. Also the transition from the sensor-controlled function in the case of tachycardia back to a striktly DDD or VDD function requires further clinical validation [46].

Antiarrhythmic Effect of a Rate-Dependent Shortening of AV Delay and So-Called Rate Smoothing. Newer generations of DDD and particularly DDD-R pacemakers increasingly have the feature that the AV delay varies in a frequency-dependent fashion. This permits a frequency-related optimal upper rate limit to be reached in dual-chamber pacing as well, in analogy to the natural frequency dependence of the refractory period of myocardial cells. One can thus combine the advantages of a hemodynamically more favorable, longer AV time with a long postventricular atrial refractory period as protection against premature atrial extrasystoles, without limiting the maximum upper limiting rate unnecessarily.

Newer DDD-R systems, in which different maximum upper rate limits for DDD and the sensor can be adjusted independently of each other, additionally provide the possibility of so-called sensor-driven rate smoothing [47, 48]. However, considerable specialist knowledge is required for understanding the corresponding ECG findings.

Arguments Against Implanting DDD-R Pacemakers. Studies up to now have mainly shown no statistically significant improvement in the performance of DDD-R pacing over strictly DDD pacing [49, 50], although the selection of patients presumably plays the essential part here.

More complex programmings and higher demands on the physician's clinical knowledge do not exactly promote a wide acceptance of the systems. However, there are clear differences here between individual manufacturers.

The same argument holds for a higher current demand and therefore shorter life of the systems. Whereas the smallest DDD-R pacemakers currently weigh only 28 g, the majority of other DDD-R aggregates weigh between 30 and 50 g. This is mainly due to a relatively higher current demand which must be compensated for by a larger battery. The current demand for the various sensors also varies. In activity-controlled pacemakers with a piezoelectric sensor element (Elite, Medtronic, Minneapolis, MN, United States; Synchrony, Pacesetter, Sylmar, CA, United States; Relay, Intermedics, Freeport, TX, United States; Ergos 02, Biotronik, Berlin, Germany) the sensor itself requires no energy, but the circuit for evaluating the activity signals does. In the pacemakers Vigor DR (CPI, St. Paul, MN, United States) and Meta DDD-R (Telectronics, Lane Cove, Australia) the sensor itself consumes energy when detecting the measurement signals (5%–10% of the total current demand).

As far as the use of the sensor as a control instance for distinguishing between physiological and pathological tachycardias is concerned, this important path has been taken up to now by only two manufacturers (Intermedics Relay and Telectronics Meta DDD-R). Yet this discriminatory ability is one of the most valuable attributes of sensor control in dual-chamber pacemakers. The higher cost of a DDD-R system in comparison to a DDD system considerably influences the answer to the question of whether the potential clinical gain from the abovementioned points justifies the additional expense of a DDD-R system. However, in view of the current tendency of manufacturers to offer DDD and DDD-R pacemakers at the same price, there is less reason *not* to use DDD-R systems routinely in all cases in which a DDD systems appears sufficient at the time of implantation.

In our own hospital this year of 1992 we have begun using a pure DDD system only in exceptional cases and otherwise routinely use a DDD-R system. Some recent studies already have (51, 52) and future studies will show in how many cases the routine use of a DDD-R system has prevented complications in a noninvasive fashion, or has resulted in a long-term gain for the patients in comparison to the use of a DDD system.

References

1. Alt E, Stangl K, Blömer H (1986) Therapie mit frequenzadaptiven Herzschrittmachern. Herz Kreisl 18:556
2. Alt E (1988) Cardiac and pulmonary response during physical activity in normal patients. In: Santini M, Pistolese M, Alliegro A (eds) Progress in clinical pacing. Excerpta Medica, Amsterdam, pp 7-12
3. Nordlander R, Hedman A, Pehrsson SK (1989) Rate-responsive pacing and exercise capacity – a comment. PACE 12:749-751
4. Alt E, Völker R, Högl B, MacCarter D (1988) First clinical results with a new temperature controlled rate responsive pacemaker. Circulation 78; III:116-124
5. Alt E, Krieg HJ, Wirtzfeld A (1983) Verlauf bei 127 Patienten mit physiologischen Schrittmachersystemen. Z Kardiol 59:131
6. Alt. E, Zitzmann E, Heinz M, Gastmann U, Matula M, Lehmann M (1990) The effect of rate-responsive pacing on exercise capacity, serum catecholamines and other metabolic parameters. PACE 13:531
7. Pehrsson SK, Hjemdahl P, Nordlander R (1988) A comparison of sympathoadrenal activity and cardiac performance at rest and during exercise in patients with ventricular demand or atrial synchronous pacing. Br Heart J 60:212-220
8. Hatano K, Kato R, Hayashi H, Noda S, Sotobata I, Murase M (1989) Usefulness of rate-responsive atrial pacing in patients with sick sinus syndrome. PACE 12:16-24
9. Heinz M, Zitzmann E, Coenen M, Alt E (1990) Malfunctioning of DDD pacemakers despite correct functioning at routine pacemaker controls. PACE 13:560
10. Wilkoff BL, Corey J, Blackburn G (1989) A mathematical model of the cardiac chronotropic response to exercise J Electrophysiol(1989) 3/3:176
11. Heinz H, Wörl HH, Alt E, Theres H, Blömer H (1988) Which patient is most likely to benefit from a rate-responsive pacemaker? PACE 11:1834-1839
12. McBride JW, Reyes WJ, Medellin L, Lauer NY (1990) What is the need for rate-modulated pacemakers? PACE 13:504
13. Simonsen E (1987) Assessment of the need for a rate-responsive pacing in patients with sinus node dysfunction. A prospective study of heart-rate response during daily activities and exercise testing. PACE 10:418
14. Prior M, Masterson M, Morant VA, Castle LW, Maloney JD (1987) Do patients with sinus node dysfunction and permanent pacemakers require an additional chronotropic sensor? PACE 10:418
15. Corbelli R, Masterson M, Wilkoff BL (1990) Chronotropic response to exercise in patients with atrial fibrillation. PACE 13:179-187
16. Lau CHP, Wong CHH, Cheng CHH, Leung WH (1990) Importance of heart rate modulation on the cardiac hemodynamics during postexercise recovery. PACE 13:1277-1285
17. Sulke N, Pipilis A, Bucknall C, Sowton E (1990) Quantitative analysis of contribution of rate response in three different ventricular rate-responsive pacemakers during out of hospital activity. PACE 13:37-44
18. Seitz K, Stangl K, Wirtzfeld A, Delius W, Laule M (1990) Erlaubt die Sinusknotenerholungszeit Rückschlüsse auf die Belastungsadaptation im weiteren Verlauf? Herzschr Elektrophys 1:63, A37
19. Benchimol A, Ligett MS (1966) Cardiac hemodynamics during stimulation at the right atrium, right ventricle, and left ventricle in normal and abnormal hearts. Circulation 33:933
20. Cock CC, Fisser FC, Stockel L, Roos JP (1990) Rate-responsive pacing in patients after myocardial infarction and angina pectoris. PACE 13:1192
21. Kruse M (1988) Long-term improvements in functional capacity by AAI rate-responsive pacing. In: Santini M, Pistolese M, Alliegro A (eds) Progress in clinical pacing. Excerpta Medica, Amsterdam, pp 25-29
22. Griffin J (1991) The optimal pacing mode for the individual patient: the role of DDDR. In: Barold SS, Mugica J (eds) New perspectives in cardiac pacing, vol. 2. Futura, Mount Kisco, NY, pp 325-338
23. Rosenquist M, Brandt J, Schüller H (1988) Long-term pacing in sinus node disease. Effects of stimulation mode on cardiovascular morbidity and mortality. Am Heart J 116:16-22

24. Sutton R, Kenny RA (1986) The natural history of sick sinus syndrome. PACE 9:1110-1114
25. Kannel WB, Abbott RD, Savage DD (1978) Epidemiological features of chronic atrial fibrillation: the Framingham study. N Engl J Med 306:1018-1022
26. Wolf PA, Kannel WB, McGee DL (1983) Duration of atrial fibrillation and imminence of stroke: the Framingham study. Stroke 14:664-667
27. Perersen P, Madsen EB, Brun B (1987) Silent cerebral infarction in chronic atrial fibrillation. Stroke 18:1098-1100
28. Bathen JS, Rokseth R (1978) Embolism in sinoatrial disease. Acta Med Scand 203:7-11
29. Baller D, Wolpers H, Zipfel J (1988) Comparison of the effects of right atrial, right ventricular apex and atrioventricular sequential pacing on myocardial oxygen consumption and cardiac efficiency: a laboratory investigation. PACE 11:394-403
30. Edelstam C, Hjemdahl P, Pehrsson K, Aström H, Nordlander R (1990) Is DDD-pacing superior to VVI-R? Effects on myocardial sympathetic activity and oxygen consumption. PACE 13:1193
31. Kato R, Terasawa T, Gotoh T, Suzuki M (1988) Antiarrhythmic efficacy of atrial demand (AAI) and rate-responsive atrial pacing. In: Santini M, Pistolese M, Alliegro A (eds) Progress in clinical pacing. Excerpta Medica, Amsterdam, pp 15-24
32. Fairfax AJ, Lambert CD, Leatham A (1976) Systemic embolism in chronic sinoatrial disorder. N Engl J Med 295: 190-192
33. Ezekowitz M, Bridgers S, James K (1991) Interim analysis of the VA Co-operative study of stroke prevention in non rheumatic atrial fibrillation. Circulation 84/4 [Suppl II]:450
34. The Boston area anticoagulation trial for atrial fibrillation investigators: the effect of low-dose warfarin on the risk of stroke in patients with nonrheumatic atrial fibrillation. N Engl J Med 323:1505-1511
35. Rosenquist M, Obel IWP (1989) Atrial pacing and the risk vor AV block: is there a time for change in attitude? PACE 12:97-101
36. Camm AJ, Katritsis D (1990) Ventricular pacing for sick sinus syndrome – a risky business? PACE 13:695-699
37. Vardas P, Travill C, Williams M, Ingram A, Lightman S, Sutton R (1987) Atrial natriuretic peptide in complete atrioventricular block untreated and after VVI and DDD pacing. PACE 10:990
38. Hull RW, Snow F, Herre J, Ellenbogen KA (1990) The plasma catecholamine responses to ventricular pacing: implications for rate-responsive pacing. PACE 13:1408-1415
39. Edelstam C, Nordlander R, Wallgren E, Rosenquist M (1990) AAI-R pacing and exercise – what happens to AV conduction? PACE 13:1193
40. Alt E, Völker R, Wirtzfeld A, Ulm K (1985) Survival and follow-up after pacemaker implantation: a comparison of patients with sick sinus syndrome, complete heart block and atrial fibrillation. PACE 8:849-855
41. Stangl K, Wirtzfeld A, Alt E, Blömer H (1990) 30 Jahre Herzschrittmachertherapie: Eine Standortbestimmung. Z Kardiol 79:383-395
42. Kappenberger L, Hepes L (1986) Rate-responsive dual-chamber pacing. PACE 9:1110
43. Klementowicz P, Oseroff O, Anrews C, Furman S (1987) An analysis of DDD-pacing mode survival: the first 5 years. PACE 10:409
44. Relay technical manual (1991) Intermedics Inc Freeport TX, USA
45. Ilvento J, Fee J, Shewmaker S (1990) Automatic mode switching from DDDR to VVIR; a management algorithm for atrial arrhythmias in patients with dual-chamber pacemakers. Cardiostimulazione 8/4:256
46. Mugica J, Barold S, Ripart A (1991) The smart pacemaker. In: Barold SS, Mugica J (eds) New perspectives in cardiac pacing, vol 2. Futura, Mount Kisco, NY, p 545
47. Higano S, Hayes D, Eisinger G (1989) Sensor-driven rate smoothing in a DDD-R pacemaker. PACE 12:922-929
48. Hayes D, Higano S, Eisinger G (1989) Electrocardiographic manifestations of a dual-chamber, rate-modulated (DDDR) pacemaker. PACE 12:555-561
49. Vogt P, Goy J, Kuh M (1988) Single- versus double-chamber rate-responsive cardiac pacing: comparison by cardiopulmonary noninvasive exercise testing. PACE 11:1896-1901
50. Feuer J, Shandling A, Ellestad M (1990) Sensor-modulated dual-chamber pacing: too much of a good thing too fast? PACE 13:816-818

51. Lau CP, Tai YT, Fong PC, Li JPS, Leung SK, Chung FLW, Song S: Clinical experience with an activity sensing DDDR pacemaker using an accelerometer sensor. PACE 15: 334-343 (1992)
52. Lau CP, Tai YT, Fong PC, Li JPS, Chung FLW, Song S: The use of implantable sensors for the control of pacemaker mediated tachycardias: a comparative evaluation between minute ventilation sensing and acceleration sensing dual chamber rate adaptive pacemakers. PACE 15: 34-44 (1992)

II. Clinical and Functional Characteristics of Sensors Used for Rate-Adaptive Pacing

Activity-Sensing Rate-Adaptive Pacing

C. P. LAU[1]

Introduction

The idea of measuring body movement as a measure of activity level is not new, and has been used for quantifying and evaluating drug treatment in hyperactive children [1]. In the simplest form, the level of activity can be measured by an automatic mechanical "watch" (with the spring removed), and the "shaking" on the watch during body movement can be measured in terms of hours and minutes the watch goes through in a given time. The watch or mechanical accelerometer can be attached to either the waist or dominant hand of the child. Thus the detection of body movement can theoretically indicate exercise and Dahl [2] in 1979 published a patent on this principle. Because of the simplicity, this principle subsequently has been employed in rate-adaptive pacemakers and is one of the most important sensors available today.

Acceleration Forces on the Body During Different Types of Exercise

Since acceleration forces on the body during exercise are best detected by devices inside the pacemaker casing, Alt et al. [3, 4] and our group [5] have attempted to measure the body motion at the infraclavicular area using triaxially mounted accelerometers. We have mounted accelerometers on top of an externally attached pacemaker to define the acceleration signals at this level. The axes of the accelerometers used are referred to as "anteroposterior" (X), "lateral" (Y), and "vertical" (Z). Because of the sloping of the chest and the swaying of the body (and hence the pacemaker) during walking, these axes are not the same as horizontal (X or Y) or vertical (true Z) axes. The acceleration signals were transformed by fast Fourier method with respect to the frequency. The root mean square value of acceleration was used to quantify the acceleration force. The following findings have been made [5] that have been confirmed by others as well [3, 4, 8]:

[1] Division of Cardiology, Department of Medicine, Queen Mary Hospital, University of Hong Kong, Hong Kong

Axes Most Relevant to Detect Walking. A recording of acceleration signals in a typical subject during walking is shown in Fig. 1. It is apparent that either *Z* (vertical or upside-down axis) or *X* (horizontal or anterior-posterior axis) are useful to detect walking; on the other hand, the *Y* (lateral axis) axis is only useful to detect body swing. In the construction of a pacemaker, the *X* axis would be more practical than the *Z* axis because the "top" of the pacemaker can be variable, depending on how the pacemaker is implanted and is likely to be influenced by subsequent pacemaker rotation in the pocket, whereas the *X* axes will remain fixed over time.

Effects of Walking Speed and Gradient on the Acceleration Signals. Walking at an increased speed will induce a significant increase in amplitude and frequency of the acceleration signal (Fig. 2). Although walking upslope will also increase the acceleration forces, the increase is somewhat less than that induced by walking quickly.

Frequency Range of Acceleration Forces During Walking. During normal walking, the fast Fourier-transformed acceleration shows that the majority of the signal is

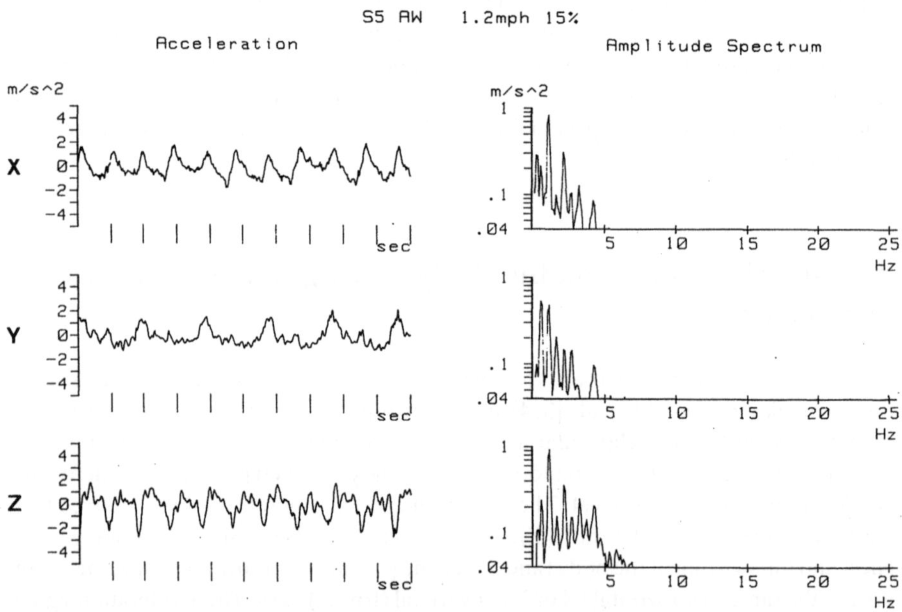

Fig. 1. Representative acceleration signals recorded in a typical subject during walking at 1.2 mph and 15% gradient on a treadmill. Each strip represents 10 s duration on the treadmill and each peak of the curves in the *X* and *Z* axes on the *left* represents one step on the treadmill. The number of peaks in the lateral (*Y*) axis is half of either that of the *X* or *Z* axis. This represents the swaying of the shoulder which occurred once per complete walking cycle. Fourier-transformed acceleration amplitude at different frequencies are shown on the *right*. Most of the acceleration froces are under 4 Hz. *X* = horizontal ~ anterior posterior axis, *Y* = lateral, *Z* = vertical axis. (From [5])

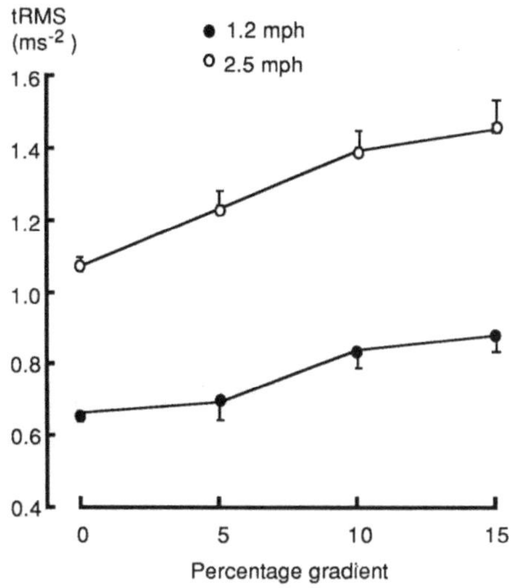

Fig. 2. Total root mean square acceleration (*tRMS*) in the *X* axis during walking at different speeds and gradients. tRMS describes the integral energy content of the acceleration signal. It increases as a function of both speed and gradient ($p < 0.001$). Each error bar represents 1 standard error of mean. (From [5])

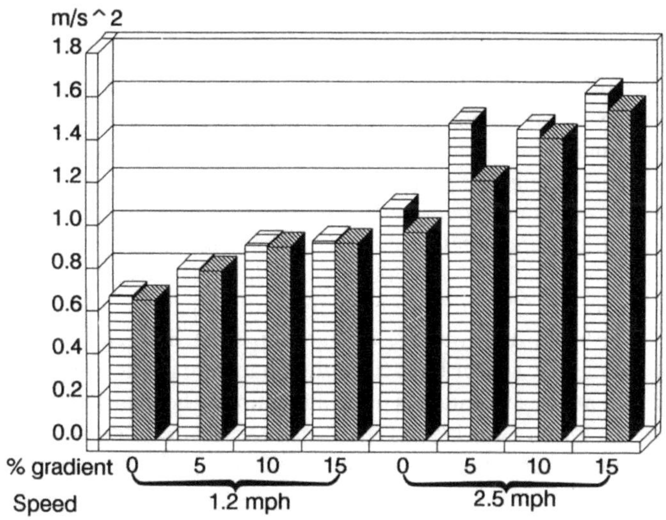

Fig. 3. Total root mean square acceleration (*tRMS*, ▤) and low pass root mean square acceleration (*RMS*, ▨ ; < 4 Hz) in a typical subject during treadmill exercises at different speeds and gradients (From [5])

under 4 Hz (Fig. 1). Relatively little signal will be lost by filtering, and filtering may also improve on the proportionality to the level of workload (Fig. 3).

Other Forms of Exercise. Appropriate increases in acceleration forces occur during running (Fig. 4). However, as the acceleration forces during arm exercise are small at the pectoral area, and particularly if the *X* axis is used, it follows that the forces measured during cycling and weight lifting would be lower than would be expected from the workload.

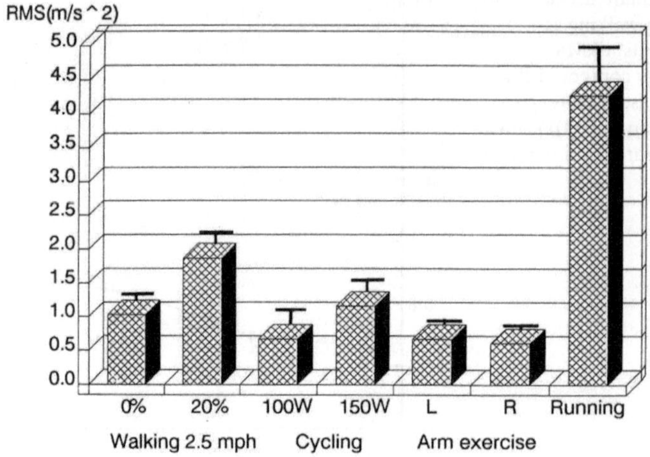

Fig. 4. Acceleration level (filtered root mean square, *RMS*) during different exercises. Arm exercise refers to the lifting of a 1 kg mass by 1 m up and down from the ground (From [5])

Advantages and Limitations of the Traditional Activity Sensing Principle

Activity-sensing pacemakers (Table 1) show the best approximation to sinus rhythm in the speed of onset of rate response [6]. Since it can be incorporated into the pacemaker casing, no special electrode is necessary and these pacemakers can be used during the upgrading of pacemakers without the need to change the electrode. There is no additional energy consumption to detect vibration (both using piezoelectric vibrational and accelerometer sensors). This principle is less liable to be affected by changes in patients' conditions than other methods of rate-adaptive sensing (e.g., the influence of QT sensing during myocardial ischemia).

The main disadvantage of traditional activity sensing by means of a vibrational piezoelectric sensor bonded to the inner side of the pacemaker can results from the fact that body vibration is more a function of how an activity is performed rather than of the level of workload [7]. At its best, the requirement of arm exercise and cycle ergometry are inadequately detected [4, 5]. Furthermore, ascending stairs gives a lower vibration signal than descending stairs. Thus the proportionality of this kind of activity sensing to different forms of exercise is only average. Furthermore, at the end of an exercise, vibration ceases immediately and an arbitrary rate decay curve has to be implemented which may not be adequate for the incurred metabolic debt. Nonexercise requirements such as anxiety reactions and Valsalva's maneuver cannot be detected using this principle. Environmental vibrations, such as those occurring during various forms of transport, may falsely trigger the pacemaker, especially if a wide frequency range is used for acceleration sensing. However, the new generation of accelerometer controlled devices applying a frequency filter for the detection of only low-frequency signals below 4 Hz seem to be more stable as far as their susceptibility to noise and nonphysiologic signals is concerned [3–5, 8–10].

Types of Activity-Sensing Pacemakers and Their Algorithms

Activitrax/Legend (Medtronic Inc. MN, United States)

This is the earliest activity-sensing pacemaker used clinically [11]. This pacemaker incorporates a piezoelectric crystal bonded to the inside of the pacemaker casing to detect body movement by means of detection of mechanical forces such as vibration and pressure on the pacemaker can originating mainly from the foot's impact on the ground when walking. Vibration levels above a programmable threshold are treated as counts, and the number of counts occurring within a given time can be interpolated as an increase in pacing rate by a series of programmable slopes of rate

Table 1. Comparison of the sensors and algorithms used in currently available activity-sensing rate-adaptive pacemakers

	Activitrax[a]	Legend[a]	Sensolog[b]	Ergos 01[d]	Relay/Dash[d]	Excel/ Vigor DR[e]
Sensor	Piezo-electric	Piezo-electric	Piezo-electric	Piezo-electric	Piezo-electric	Piezo-resistive Accelero-meter
Algorithm	Vibra-tional peak re-versal detection	Vibral-tional peak re-versal detection	Vibra-tional signal integra-tion	Vibra-tional signal integra-tion	Accelera-tion signal integra-tion	Accelera-tion signal integra-tion
Frequency band used	3-70 Hz	3-70 HZ	3-50 Hz	≤6 Hz	≤0.3-3 Hz	≦8 Hz
Onset and decay curves	–	+	+	+	+	
Rate monitor-ing	–	Histo-grams	Histo-grams, Instan-taneous rate	–	Histograms, Rate profile	Histograms Rate profile with the help of the port-able pro-grammer
Auto-program-mability	–	–	+	–	+	
Rate drop during sleep	–	–	–	–	+	–

[a] Activitrax and Legend: Medtronic Incorporation, MN, USA.
[b] Sensolog: Siemens Ltd, Sweden.
[c] Ergos 01: Biotronik, FRG.
[d] Relay: Intermedics Inc., TX, USA (refer to DDDR version).
[e] Excel: CPI Inc, St. Paul, MN, USA.

response. Thus the physician determine the rate response by selecting an appropriate combination of thresholds and slopes.

Clinical benefits of Activitrax have been extensively documented. Programming is simple and the commonest method is to adjust the threshold (commonly medium) and slope (refer to slope setting) to attain a pacing rate of 90–100 bpm during walking [11, 12, 13]. Compared with the VVI mode, activity-initiated rate-adaptive pacing enhances exercise capacity [13, 14], maximum oxygen consumption, and anaerobic threshold [14]. Symptoms such as problems with physical efforts [13] and breathlessness [15] are better in the rate-adaptive mode. This pacemaker has also been used successfully to achieve a rate increase in children [16–18].

Apart from the general limitations of vibrational activity sensing, the Activitrax algorithm, which counts the acceleration peaks to optimise rate adaptation, functions mainly via a "step counting" algorithm to determine the rate. Thus walking more quickly can increase the pacing rate, but walking upslope at the same speed will not (Fig. 5). Furthermore, since the algorithm utilises a curvilinear relationship between the acceleration pulses and the pacing rate, rates beyond 130 bpm are seldom achieved despite vigorous exercise [19]. Environmental vibrations can affect the pacing rate, but in general the effects are slight [20–22]. Direct pressure on the piezoelectric sensor can cause rate acceleration [23] and may become important if the patient lies on the pacemaker during sleep.

The Legend pacemaker is an improved model of Activitrax with wider programming facilities for rate adaptation. To overcome the excessively fast drop in rate in the Activitrax after exercise, several programmable rate-decay patterns are available. Furthermore, a more linear relationship between acceleration pulses and pacing rate is now used, so that the upper rate can be attained more easily, although the algorithm used for rate adaptation is otherwise similar [24].

Sensolog

Sensolog pacemakers (Siemens Pacesetter, Solna, Sweden) utilize a similar piezoelectric crystal for sensing activity. The incoming vibrational signals are integrated and preamplified, and the voltage generated is then converted into a rate response [25, 26]. The pacemaker can also automatically sample the pacing rates at different ranges into rate histograms, which are helpful for programming. Newer series also have an autoprogrammable option in which an automatic adjustment of the slope and threshold can be made once an arbitrary pacing rate is ascribed to an activity [27]. The Sensolog P49 is an investigational model which uses a nonpiezoelectric-sensing principle [28]. Early experience of this device is encouraging.

Comparison with the Activitrax

Both pacemakers detect mechanical forces by piezoelectric crystals and the frequency ranges used are similar (Activitrax, 3-70 Hz; Sensolog, 3-50 Hz) [26]. Bench testing shows that the Sensolog algorithm produces a proportional rate response to the level of external forces applied. On the other hand, the typical response of the Activitrax is

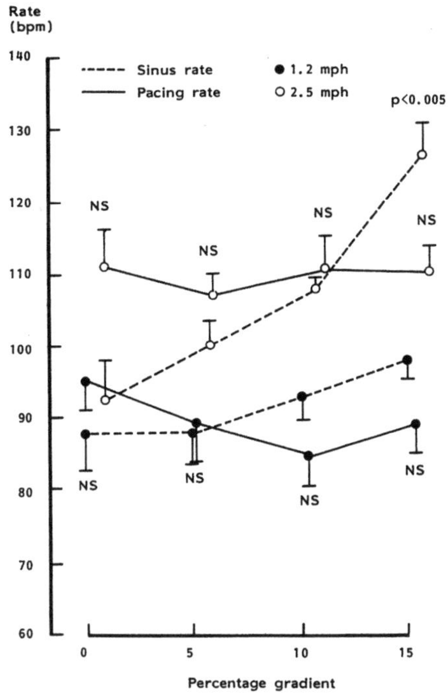

Fig. 5. Pacing rate of six subjects with externally attached Activitrax pacemakers during treadmill exercises at different speeds and gradients. Although there is an increase in pacing rate as the patients walk faster, there is no increase in rate as the subjects walk up steeper gradients. The sinus rate, on the other hand, shows an increase in rate to walking upslope and to walking faster (From [5])

Table 2. Effects of footwear in nine patients with implanted Sensolog pacemakers and externally attached Activitrax pacemakers during normal walking.

	No shoes	Hard Shoes	Soft Shoes
Activitrax	104 ± 4	102 ± 4	103 ± 4
Sensolog	104 ± 4	89 ± 3*	100 ± 4

The pacing rate of the Activitrax was reproducible whereas the rate achieved with the Sensolog was lower during walking with shoes, as mechanical signals are reduced.
* $p < 0.05$ compared with walking without shoes.

an "on-off" response, with the maximum rate achieved once the external force exceeds a certain level [26]. However, these in vitro testings were performed at a frequency of 10 Hz, which is significantly higher than the usual range of frequency during walking [4, 5].

In patients with implanted pacemakers, the rate responses of the two pacemakers behave very similarly. Both pacemakers do not significantly increase the pacing rate when a patient ascends an incline [25, 29], although there is a tendency for the Sensolog pacemaker to achieve a slightly higher rate during this exercise. External vibrations are likely to interfere with both pacemakers [25, 26, 29].

Since the Activitrax pacemaker mainly detects peak motion changes during walking, the response to arm exercise was less than that of the Sensolog [30]. On the other hand, signal integration is very susceptible to the nature of footwear the patient uses (Table 2), whereas the Activitrax algorithm is not. A less sensitive setting than they are determined by treadmill exercise is often required in patients with Sensolog pacemakers for ordinary activities.

Low-Frequency Acceleration Sensing

As the maximum frequency range of acceleration during daily activities is under 4 Hz [4, 5] it may be appropriate to put a low pass filter under this frequency. This has been achieved either with a piezoelectric crystal bonded to the innerside of the pacemaker case (Ergos, Biotronik, FRG) or with accelerometers (Dash or Relay, Intermedics, Angleton, TX, United States; Excel CPl, St Pauls, MN, United States – Table 1). In both cases, accelerations are integrated and the strength of the signal is used to effect a rate change.

Dash/Relay (Intermedics Inc)

Pacemaker description

These pacemakers detect activity using the accelerometric principle [8]. The accelerometer incorporates a piezoelectric crystal bonded to the circuit board of the pacemaker without attachment to the inside of the pacemaker casing (Fig. 6). This arrangement is in contrast to the attachment of the piezoelectric crystal in conventional types of activity-sensing rate adaptive pacemakers. The accelerometer is

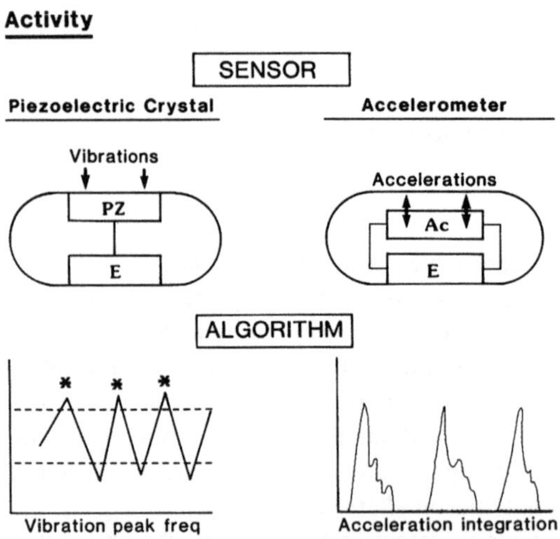

Fig. 6. Schematic representation of the types of activity sensing pacemakers. A piezoelectric crystal (PZ) is attached to the inside of one surface of the pacemaker case (which faces the muscle) to detect transmitted vibrations during exercise. In an accelerometer (Ac) based activity sensing device, the accelerometer is attached to the electronic circuit board (E) to detect accelerations. As a patient exercise, vibrations are generated, and the number of vibration peaks (*in lower left diagram) occurring above a programmable level is used to measure the level of activity in one version of the PZ system. A signal integration method on the strength of acceleration is used to relate the accelerations detected by the accelerometer into a rate change. As the accelerometer is not attached to the pacemaker case, it is therefore not susceptible to the influence of direct pressure. Reproduced with permission [8]

sensitive to accelerations of the low frequency range (0.5-3 Hz), and acceleration signals so derived during exercise are related to a rate change using a triphasic rate/acceleration relationship (Fig. 7). A relatively steep slope is used at low and high levels of exercise (phase I and III, respectively), with an intermediate gentle slope (phase II) to allow for relatively stable rate change during ordinary daily activities. The transition between phase II and III is known as the break point. Although increasing the overall slope of rate response affects the sensitivity to body movements during low and high levels of exercise, this intermediate rate response (as well as the break point) remains relatively unaffected.

Apart from the lower and upper rate, adaptation of the lower rate to nighttime pacing can be effected. Two separate lower rates can be programmed: one higher value during daytime and a lower value at sleep, using the built-in 24-hour clock to set the "sleeping" time. Rate response according to the sensor will be similar at the sleep rate except that the sensor driven rate begins from a lower resting value [8, 31].

Programming

The rate adaptive function can be optimized using a "tailor to patient" software. Programming of the sensor is effected by collecting acceleration signals during an ordinary daily activity such as walking for 3 minutes, and the physician can then ascribe a pacing rate to this activity level (commonly 95 beats/min). The current optimization algorithm only uses the maximum acceleration forces detected during these 3 minutes to represent the ordinary workload. This is liable to sampling error because the acceleration level tends to be high when the subject start walking on the

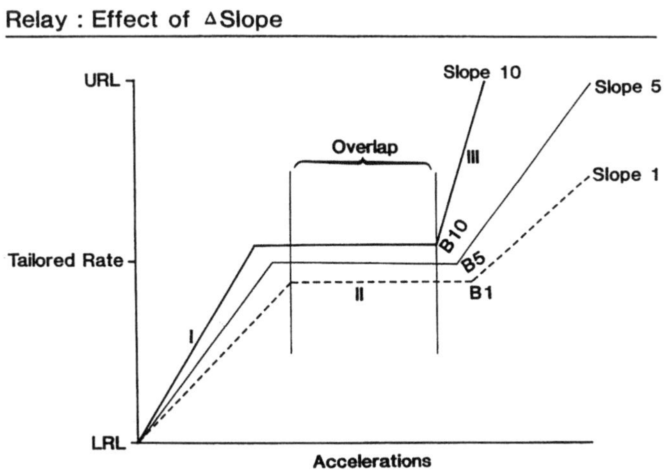

Fig. 7. Triphasic rate responsive curves of accelerometer based activity sensing pacemaker. Phase I and III represent low and high levels of accelerations respectively and are related to a steeper slope of rate change. Phase II represents ordinary activities at which the change in rate is small. The transition between Phase II and III is termed the breakpoint, which remained relatively constant at different slope values. Thus there is substantial overlap in rate changes during the ordinary level of acceleration despite the use of a different slope. B_1, B_5 and B_{10} = Breakpoints at slope 1,5 and 10 respectively, LRL = lover rate limit, URL = upper rate limit. Reproduced with permission [8].

treadmill. It is preferable to activate this optimization only when the subject has attained a stable stage of exercise. The acceleration signals collected correspond to phase II of the rate/acceleration curve. Depending on the patient and the anticipated daily activities, further optimization of the lower and higher workload ranges (Phases I and III) can be addressed separately using exercise at different workloads.

To assist rate adaptive programming, acceleration signals for an activity can be collected over a predetermined period of time (ranging from 15 minutes to 24 hours). The "calculated rate profile" software allows the rate response during this period to be calculated at different slope values, so that the desired slope response can be determined for a patient without the need to repeat the exercise. This feature significantly reduces the number of exercise testing required for rate optimization (Fig. 8).

Comparison with the piezoelectric sensing activity pacemaker

The rate adaptive characteristics of the accelerometer sensor in the Relay pacemaker has been compared with that of a piezoelectric sensor (Legend™) [8]. The acceleration sensor showed higher rate responses to jogging and standing from supine

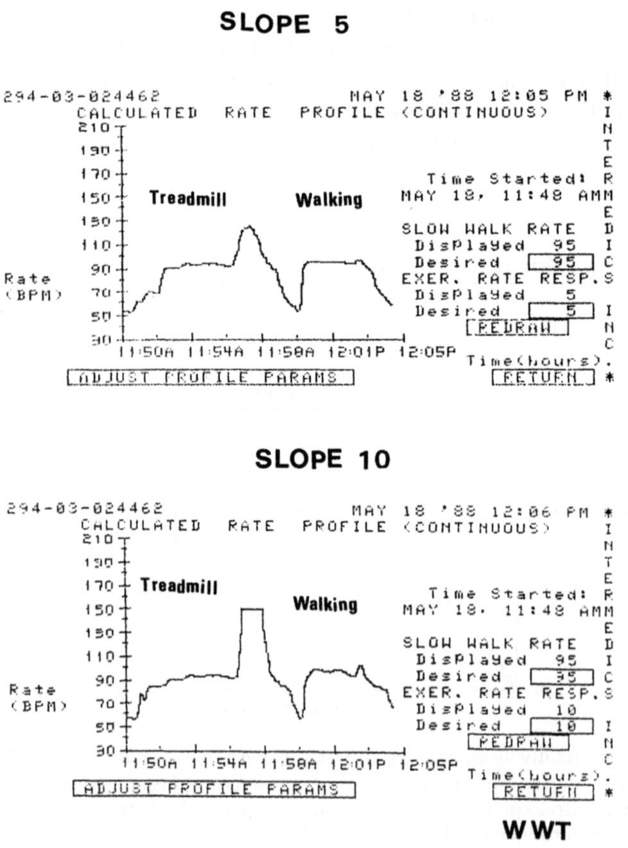

Fig. 8. Pacing rate profile in a patient with an activity sensing rate adaptive pacemaker using an accelerometer sensor during treadmill and walking exercise at a slope of "5". The projected pacing rate at slope "10" can be estimated graphically without requiring the patient to repeat the exercise. Note that by using a more sensitive slope, the maximum rate during treadmill can be reached without affecting the rate during walking

position, and less susceptibility to rate changes caused by direct pressure and tapping on the pacemaker. The use of a triphasic rate responsive curve with a relatively flat intermediate portion (Phase II) has increased rate stability during ordinary exercise (e.g. rate change was not affected by the nature of footwear). On the other hand, this has limited the rate response of the sensor to give an adequate rate response when the patient ascends a gradient. In addition, the upper rate during maximum exercise may not be reached in some patients whose acceleration level does not exceed the breakpoint on maximal exercise. As the breakpoint cannot be altered by a change in slope, maximum rate response can be limited in some patients during heavy exercise.

We have found that it is possible to make the breakpoint more sensitive by re-tailoring the tailored rate at a lower workload (Fig. 9). By collecting a lower level of acceleration forces to represent the ordinary workload, it is possible to enhance the rate response during lower levels of exercise. It is also possible to judiciously re-tailor the pacemaker to allow the upper rate to be reached during vigorous exercise without significantly increasing the rate attained during ordinary activities such as walking (Fig. 10). The availability of progammable breakpoint will enhance the usefulness of the complex rate adaptive curve used in this pacemaker.

Exel (Cardiac Pacemakers Inc)

Pacemaker description

The accelerometer in this device is an integrated silicon accelerometer suspended by four tiny bridges from the electronic circuit board. Low frequency body movements cause relative displacement of the silicon mass, which in turn affects the resistors located on the bridges. The elasticity of the accelerometer suspension will return the

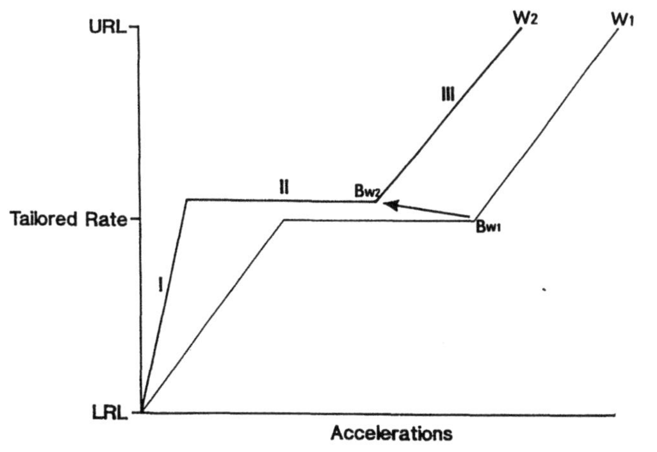

Fig. 9. Effect of re-tailoring on the breakpoint. W_1 is the workload used to represent ordinary daily activities. By tailoring at a lower workload (W_2), the breakpoint can be lowered resulting in an improved rate response. B_{w1} and B_{w2} are the breakpoints when the pacemaker is tailored at W_1 and W_2 respectively. Other abbreviations as in Figure 7. Reproduced with permission [8]

mass to the neutral position. Both the strength and amplitude of acceleration signals can be measured, and the accelerometer is most sensitive at the 1-8 Hz frequency band.

The rate responsive parameters include the activity threshold (1-8), the response factor (1-16), the reaction time (1-6), and the recovery time (1-8). Activity threshold is the minium level of activity which initiates a pacing rate response, and the magnitude of response can be adjusted by programming the response factor.

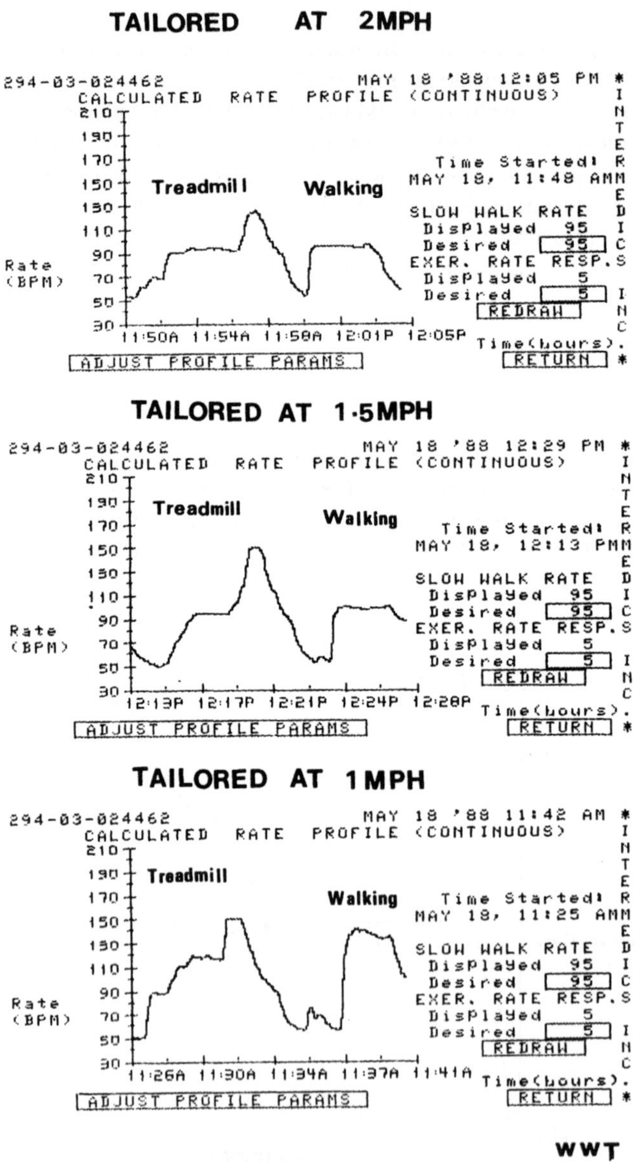

Fig. 10. Selected rate profiles obtained by telemetry of a patient with the accelerometer sensing DDDR pacemaker during graded treadmill exercise and walking. When the ordinary workload used for tailoring was walking at 2 mph (top panel), the maximum rate achieved with treadmill exercise was 128 bpm. When the pacemaker was re-tailored at a lower workload (1.5 mph, middle panel), the maximum programmed rate of 150 bpm was reached at maximum exercise without significantly affecting the rate attained during walking. When tailoring was performed at an even lower workload (1 mph, lowest panel), both the rate during treadmill and walking exercise would be affected. Reproduced with permission [8].

Clinical performance

Using an externally attached Excel pacemaker in 10 healthy volunteers (age 55-72 years), it was shown that there was a high correlation with the intrinsic heart rate of these volunteers with the pacemaker rates during treadmill exercise [32]. Compared with an externally attached piezoelectric crystal activity sensing pacemaker (Legend, Medtronic Inc), the accelerometer device showed better approximation to the sinus rate when both were programmed at nominal settings. However, both devices underestimated the normal sinus response during cycle ergometry and during staircase climbing. Whether individualized programming may enhance the rate response of both pacemakers remained to be examined. Early experience in implanted units showed appropriate rate response to a variety of daily activities.

Other Activity-Sensing Principles

Using a "tilt switch" principle, Alt et al. [33] reported the use of a mechanical sensor for detecting exercise. A mercury ball rolls over a disc with switches, and the rate of opening and closing of these switches by the mercury ball gives an index of body activity. Furthermore, the position of the mercury ball gives an indication of the posture of the body, and thus this sensor may be a good indicator of postural changes. Fortuitous sensing of arm movements are effected with both impedance-sensing respiratory-sensing pacemakers, the Biorate (RDP and MB pacemakers, Biorate, Bologna, Italy) and Meta (Telectronics Pacing Systems, Anglewood, CO, Unites States) [34, 35]. In both devices, arm movements will cause a relative displacement of the pacemaker and the impedance-sensing electrode, thereby causing an increase in impedance which would be interpreted by the pacemaker as an increase in breathing. This sensing of arm activity may improve the speed of rate response of these pacemakers.

Combination of Algorithms

As indicated in Table 2, one of the problems with acceleration integration is the susceptibility to small changes in acceleration due to, for example, the use of different footwear. On the other hand, the "step-counting" algorithm of the Activitrax is a robust means of activity sensing, although with less proportionality it is less liable to be triggered by environmental vibrations. A combination of these two algorithms may enhance the specificity and proportionality of this principle of rate-adaptive pacing [36].

Conclusion

Despite the relatively crude relationship to metabolic requirement, the excellent speed of onset of rate response and the simplicity of implementation have made activity sensing the most widely used form of rate-adaptive pacing. Activity sensing will almost certainly be one of the sensors to be included in combined sensor rate-adaptive pacemakers [37].

References

1. Schulman JL, Reisman JM (1959) An objective measure of hyperactivity. Am J Ment Defic 64:455-456
2. Dahl JD (1979) Variable rate timer for a cardiac pacemaker. US Patent 140 132
3. Alt E, Heinz M, Theres H, Matula M, Blömer H (1987) A new body motion activity-based rate-responsive pacing system. PACE 10:422, A65
4. Alt E, Matula M, Theres H, Heinz M, Baker R (1989) The basis for activity-controlled rate variable cardiac pacemakers: an analysis of mechanical forces on human body induced by exercise and environment. PACE 12:1667-1680
5. Lau CP, Stott JRR, Toff WD, Zetlein MB, Ward DE, Camm AJ (1988) Selective vibration sensing: a new concept for activity-sensing rate-responsive pacing. PACE 11:1299-1309
6. Lau CP, Butrous GS, Ward DE, Camm AJ (1989) Comparative assessment of exercise performance of six different rate-adaptive right ventricular cardiac pacemaker. Am J Cardiol 63:833-839
7. Lau CP, Mehta D, Toff W, Stott RJ, Ward DE, Camm AJ (1988) Limitations of rate response of activity-sensing rate-responsive pacing to different forms of activity. PACE 11:141-150
8. Lau CP, Tai YT, Fong PC, Li JPS, Leung SK, Chung FLW, Song S. Clinical experience with an accelerometer based activity sensing dual chamber rate adaptive pacemaker. PACE/PP2; 15:334-343
9. Zitzmann EM, Matula M, Alt E, Mentrup H, Heinz M (1990) A new dual-chamber rate-responsive pacing system sensitive to low-frequency acceleration. PACE 13:1217, A114
10. Silvermint EH, Salo RW, Meyerso SC, Burell JL, Freudenberg MW, Linder WJ, Maile KR, Nguyen HD, Zelkin B (1990) Distinctive characteristics of Excel VR rate-adaptive pacemaker with an innovative activity sensor. PACE 13:1210, A87
11. Humen DP, Kostuk WJ, Klein GJ (1985) Activity-sensing, rate-responsive pacing: improvement in myocardial performance with exercise. PACE 8:52-59
12. den Dulk K, Bouwells L, Lindemans FW, Rankin I, Brugada P, Wellens (1988) The Activitrax rate-responsive pacemaker system. Am J Cardiol 61:107-112
13. Lindemans FW, Rankin IR, Murtaugh R, Chevalier PA (1986) Clinical experience with an activity-sensing pacemaker. PACE 9:978-986
14. Benditt DG, Mianulli M, Fetter J, Benson DW, Dunnigan A, Molina E, Gornick CC, Almquist A (1987) Single-chamber cardiac pacing with activity-initiated chronotropic response; evaluation by cardiopulmonary testing. Circulation 75:184-191
15. Lipkin DP, Buller N, Frenneaux M, Ludgate L, Lowe T, Webb SC, Krikler DM (1987) Randomized crossover trial of rate-responsive Activitrax and conventional fixed-rate ventricular pacing. Br Heart J 58:613-616
16. Ladusans EJ, Tynan M, Jones O, Curry PVL (1986) Single-lead rate-responsive permanent cardiac pacing in very young children. Clin Prog Electrophysiol Pacing 4 [Suppl]:22 (abstr)
17. Kiel EA, Dungan NT, Westerman GR, Norton JB, Readinger RI, Van Devanter SH (1987) Ventricular rate-responsive activity pacing in children. Clin Res 35:51A (abstr)
18. Miller JD, Young ML, Atkins D, Wolff GS (1989) Rate-responsive ventricular pacing in pediatric patients. Am J Cardiol 64:1052-1053.

19. McAlister HF, Soberman J, Klementowicz P, Andrew SC, Furman S (1989) Treadmill assessment of an activity-modulated pacemaker: the importance of individual programming. PACE 12:486-501
20. Stangl K, Wirtzfeld A, Heinze H, Gobl G, Lochschmidt O (1986) Activitrax pacemaker: physiological rate response with a non-physiological sensor? In: Santini M, Pistolese M, Alliegro A (eds) Progress in clinical pacing. Centro Editoriale Publicitario Italiano, Rome, pp 124-132
21. Toff WD, Leeds C, Joy M, Bennet G, Camm AJ (1987) The effect of aircraft vibration on the function of an activity-sensing pacemaker. Br Heart J 57:573 (abstr)
22. Gordon RS, O'Dell KB, Low RB, Blumen IJ (1990) Activity-sensing permanent internal pacemaker dysfunctions during helicopter aeromedical transport. Ann Emerg Med 19:1260-1263
23. Wilkoff BL, Shimokochi DD, Schaal SF (1987) Pacing rate increase due to application of steady external pressure on an activity-sensing pacemaker. PACE 10:423 (abstr)
24. Mond H, Lire P, Hunt D (1990) A third generation activity pacemaker: is the rate-response algorithm superior? PACE 13:514 (abstr)
25. Lau CP, Tse WS, Camm AJ (1988) Clinical experience with Sensolog 703: a new activity-sensing rate-responsive pacemaker. PACE 11:1444-1455
26. Stangl K, Wirtzfeld A, Lochschmidt O, Basler B, Mittnachi A (1989) Physical movement sensitive pacing: comparison of two activity-triggered pacing systems. PACE 12:102-110
27. Mahaux V, Waleffe A, Kulbertus HE (1989) Clinical experience with a new activity-sensing rate-modulated pacemaker using autoprogrammability. PACE 12:1362-1368
28. Tse WS, Lau CP, Nadia S, Ward DE, Camm AJ (1988) Comparison of three activity-sensing rate-responsive pacemakers. PACE 11:799 (abstr)
29. Kubisch K, Peters W, Chiladakis L et al. (1989) Clinical experience with rate-responsive pacemaker Sensolog P703. PACE 11:1829-1833
30. Webb S, Lewis L, Morris-Thrugood J (1989) Activity-sensing pacemakers: clinical implications of different implant sites. In: Proceedings of the 4th Asian-Pacific symposium on cardiac pacing and electrophysiology, 20-23 August 1989, Singapore, 139
31. Lee MT, Baker R (1990). Circadian rate variation in rate-adaptive pacing systems. PACE 13:1797-1801.
32. Bacharech DW, Hilden JS, Millerhagen JO, Westrum BL, Kelly JM (1992). Activity-based pacing: comparison of a device using an accelerometer versus a piezoelectric crystal. PACE 15:188-196
33. Alt E, Matula M, Thilo R, Theres H, Heinz M, Blomer H (1988) A new mechanical sensor for detecting body activity and posture, suitable for rate-responsive pacing. PACE 11:1875-1881
34. Lau CP, Ritchie D, Butrous GC, Ward DE, Camm AJ (1988) Rate modulation by arm movements of the respiratory-dependent rate-responsive pacemaker. PACE 11:744-752
35. Lau CP, Ward DE, Camm AJ (1989) Single-chamber cardiac pacing with two forms of respiration-controlled rate-responsive pacemakers. Chest 95:352-359
36. Lau CP (1990) Activity-sensing rate-responsive pacing. PACE 13:819-820
37. Alt E, Theres H, Heinz M, Matula M, Thilo R, Blömer H (1988) A new rate-modulated pacemaker system optimized by combination of two sensors. PACE 11:1119-1129

Respiration

H. G. MOND[1]

Respiratory Rate

Respiration, and in particular respiratory rate is a simple biological parameter, first suggested as a sensor for rate-responsive pacing as early as 1966 [1]. Using normal subjects, as well as patients with a variety of respiratory diseases, Rossi et al. [2 ,3 ,4] demonstrated a good correlation between heart rate, respiratory rate, and oxygen uptake, irrespective of the underlying lung disease.

In order to demonstrate the effectiveness of using respiratory rate as a variable to control pacing rate, an external system was developed which was capable of altering the pacing rate of an implanted pulse generator in response to changes in respiratory rate [3]. Using exercise testing, patients pacing in the respiratory rate-responsive mode showed a significant improvement in exercise times compared to pacing in the VVI fixed-rate mode. The study demonstrated that in appropriate patients, a significant improvement in work capacity was possible with a respiratory rate sensor [3].

Following this work, a fully implantable system, the RDP1 (Biotec S.p.A., Bologna, Italy) was developed and first implanted in 1982 [5]. This pacing system measured respiratory rate using changes in electrical impedance between the pacemaker can and a separate auxiliary passive lead, implanted subcutaneously in the chest wall [2]. A constant current pulse train was sent from the tip of the auxiliary lead to the pulse-generator casing with chest wall movement altering the dipole length. The initial pacemaker model had a number of programmable features referable to the sensor only. There were three respiratory sensitivity threshold levels, with the most sensitive setting for patients with a low-resting tidal volume. There was a normal setting and a low sensitivity setting where deep breathing was required to activate the sensor. Although tidal volume was critical in determining the respiratory sensitivity threshold, it was not a component of the sensor algorithm and only respiratory rate was measured. As with other rate-responsive pacing systems, there were programmable slope settings which set the relationship between respiratory rate and heart rate.

Early clinical experience with the respiratory rate-responsive pacing system was encouraging [6–12]. Rossi et al. [6, 7] reported their experience with 143 patients including 23 patients with AAI rate-responsive pacing. Sensor malfunctions were

[1] The Royal Melbourne Hospital, Victoria, 3050, Australia

particularly common in the early generation models. Being a unipolar pacing system, myopotential inhibition was a common problem. Despite this, the authors reported a significant increase in exercise capacity with rate responsiveness in all patients in whom the system functioned. Because of the non-specificity of the sensor, this pacemaker system also demonstrated an increase in pacing rate with arm movements [13, 14].

The advantages of a respiratory rate-responsive pacing system are obvious. The sensor is simple and reasonably reliable. Any implanted lead, either in the atrium or ventricle can be used. The major disadvantage is the limitation of the sensor and algorithm to changes in respiratory rate and not to changes in tidal volume. Because of this, there is often a delay in rate responsiveness, particularly at low workloads [15]. A special sensor is necessary, but unlike other pacing systems with special sensors, this is not attached to the pacing lead. Implantation of the separate auxiliary lead is not particularly difficult, but does add to the operation time and patient discomfort both during and after the procedure. Complications with the auxiliary lead include nonsensing, skin erosion, and dislodgement due to sliding back into the pacemaker pocket [6, 7, 15, 16]. In order to overcome the disadvantage of a separate auxiliary lead, Rossi has recently reported the development of a unipolar pacing lead which also incorporates the sensor [5].

Apart from the initial enthusiasm, there has been little continuing work on the respiratory rate sensor for rate-responsive cardiac pacing. Problems with the auxiliary sensor and limitations of respiratory rate to accurately reflect physiologic changes in cardiac rate have impeded progress and widespread clinical use. The recently reported incorporation of the sensor onto the pacing lead is an advance, but has the disadvantage of requiring a special pacing lead.

Minute ventilation

Minute ventilation, the product of respiratory rate and tidal volume represents an excellent physiologic parameter for the demonstration of the metabolic demands of exercise. At rest, minute ventilation is in the order of 6 l/min increasing to 60 l/min with moderately severe exercise, and even up to 150 l/min in trained athletes at maximum exercise. Such changes in minute ventilation not only accurately reflect oxygen uptake but also changes in cardiac output and heart rate. Unlike a number of other sensors, minute ventilation also changes during stress and fever.

A number of workers have compared changes in heart rate with respiratory parameters and have found excellent correlation coefficients with minute ventilation, and less accurate ones with respiratory rate and tidal volume, particularly at low work levels [17–22]. It was not surprising therefore that minute ventilation was suggested as a physiologic and metabolic sensor for rate-responsive cardiac pacing.

Although respiratory rate and tidal volume can be measured accurately and easily by external means [22], the development of an implantable sensor has been more difficult. Nappholz et al. [23] investigated intravascular impedance techniques using an intravenous quadrapolar catheter positioned in the superior vena cava, and showed a high correlation coefficient between tidal volume and the measured electrical impedance. The impedance signal also showed inflections corresponding to breath direction, thereby allowing the measurement of respiratory rate.

This work was extended to using a pacing lead positioned at the apex of the right ventricle and another in the right atrium with a pectoral skin electrode serving as common ground [24]. Again, high correlation coefficients between intravascular impedance and minute ventilation were shown. Heinz et al. [25] investigated transthoracic impedance signals between the pacemaker pocket and pacing leads. Using a prepared algorithm to convert changes in impedance to changes in minute ventilation, a high correlation coefficient was shown between the measured changes in minute ventilation and directly measured values. This work confirmed the earlier extensive work of Nappholz et al. and justified further development of the minute ventilation rate-responsive pacing system.

Technical Means for Minute Ventilation Sensing

The minute ventilation rate-responsive pacing system (Telectronics META MV – metabolic minute ventilation – model 1202, Telectronics Pacing Systems, Englewood, Co, United States) utilises changes in minute ventilation as a sensed variable for adjusting pacing rate. The single-chamber bipolar pacemaker is multiprogrammable and suitable for both atrial and ventricular use.

To obviate the need for a special lead, a tripolar system was developed using a standard bipolar lead and the pulse-generator casing. The algorithm was obtained from animal and human studies and changes in pacing rate in comparison with sinus rhythm yielded a correlation coefficient of 0.85, and the time delay in rate response was 45 s [26]. A low-energy pulse (1 mA for 15 μs at 20 Hz) for the measurement of transthoracic impedance is generated between the ring electrode of the lead and the pulse-generator casing. The pulse is less than 10% of the threshold energy required for

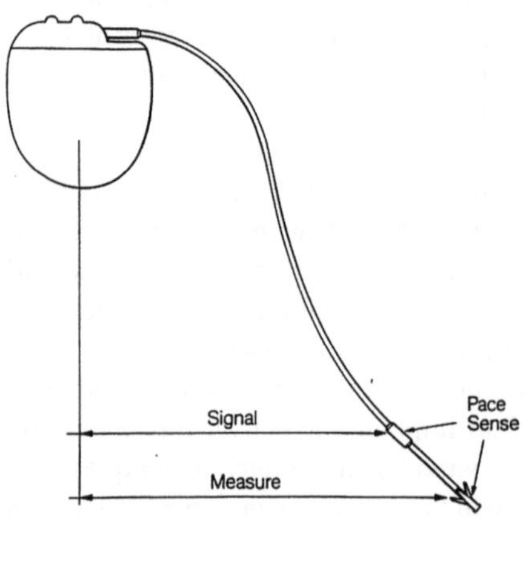

Fig. 1. The minute-ventilation, transthoracic impedance-sensing system. A standard bipolar lead lies at the apex of the right ventricle. Low-energy pulses are generated at the ring electrode and measurement of transthoracic impedance occurs between the tip electrode and the pulse generator casing

ventricular capture, is not generated from the lead tip, and is well below the levels which induce dangerous ventricular arrhythmias.

Measurement of transthoracic impedance is performed between the tip electrode and the pulse generator each 50 ms according to 20 measurement points per second (Fig. 1). Transthoracic impedance increases with inspiration, decreases with expiration, and its amplitude varies with tidal volume. The impedance signal thus comprises two components representing tidal volume and respiratory rate. The pulse-generator circuitry identifies the two signals and processes them to derive minute ventilation.

Two signal-averaging processes operate within the pulse generator; one with a short time constant of about 30 s, which allows for smooth rate changes, and the other with a long time constant of approximately 1 h. The difference between these two signal-averaging processes is used to monitor changes in minute ventilation which is continually updated. During prolonged exercise, the value of the long time constant will inappropriately reduce the pacing rate. To prevent this, the long-term data collection is frozen when the short-term value reaches 50% of the maximum impedance change. When the value falls below this threshold, both registers resume data processing. The relationship between the two time constants allows for the short time constant to maintain the upper rate limit during extended exercise, and also allows for rapid and maximal changes if exercise is recommenced after a short rest.

In addition to the rate-responsive and fixed-rate VVI modes, there is an adaptive mode used for determining the rate-responsive factor. The adaptive mode provides fixed-rate VVI or AAI pacing together with the minute-ventilation sensing function. Although analysis by the sensor of changes in minute ventilation takes place, there is no rate-responsive pacing in this mode.

Programming the minute-ventilation rate-responsive system ideally requires an exercise test. Apart from the upper and lower pacing rates, only one other function requires programming and this is calculated by the pulse generator. This is the rate-response factor (slope) which defines the changes in pacing rate in response to changes in transthoracic impedance. Fifty nine slope values are available. The higher slope

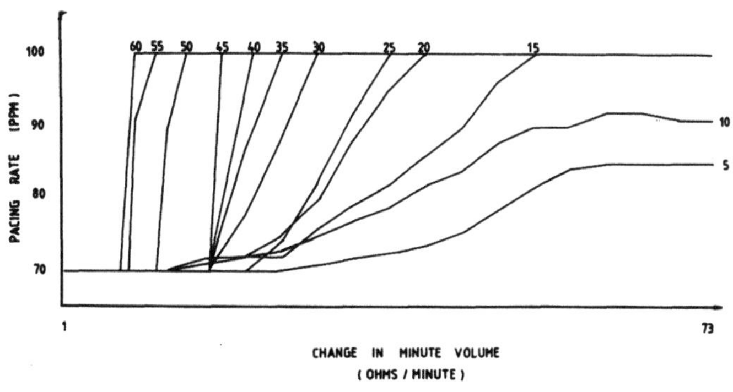

Fig. 2. Examples of slope values comparing pacing rate response (minimum rate 70 bpm, maximum rate 100 bpm) to changes in minute ventilation (volume). At a programmed slope, there is a specific change in pacing rate for a given change in minute ventilation as determined by changes in transthoracic impedance

values produce marked changes in pacing rate for only a small change in transthoracic impedance, whereas lower slope settings require large changes in transthoracic impedance to produce small changes in pacing rate (Fig. 2).

The optimal slope value can be determined for each patient and this is called the peak exercise function. Following pacemaker implantation, the pulse generator is programmed to the adaptive mode and the patient asked to rest for at least 1 h prior to exercise testing. In this mode, the rate-responsive sensing circuit adapts to the patient's individual respiratory characteristics. After an hour with the pulse generator still in the adaptive mode, a near maximal exercise test is performed. The suggested optimal slope value based on the patient's respiratory characteristics during exercise is calculated by the implanted pulse generator and programmer and displayed by the programmer. This is only the recommended slope value and the physician may choose any slope value either side of this, each level representing a change of about 10%.

Although helpful, it is not essential to perform an exercise test to program the slope value. A simpler method is to rest the patient for 1 h in the adaptive mode and then program on the rate-responsive function choosing a slope value usually between 15 and 25.

The minute-ventilation algorithm responds to respiratory rates between 3 and 60 breaths per minute and to changes of 50% in minute ventilation within 35 s. At the time of slope programming, the minimum or low rate (50–150 beats per minute) and maximum or upper rate (80–165 beats per minute) must be set. Once these three functions have been programmed, no further adjustments should be necessary.

In both the adaptive and the rate-responsive modes, the signals used to measure transthoracic impedance may be observed as interference on the ECG monitor or recording equipment. This can be inhibited with a magnet which temporarily disables the rate-responsive function (Fig. 3).

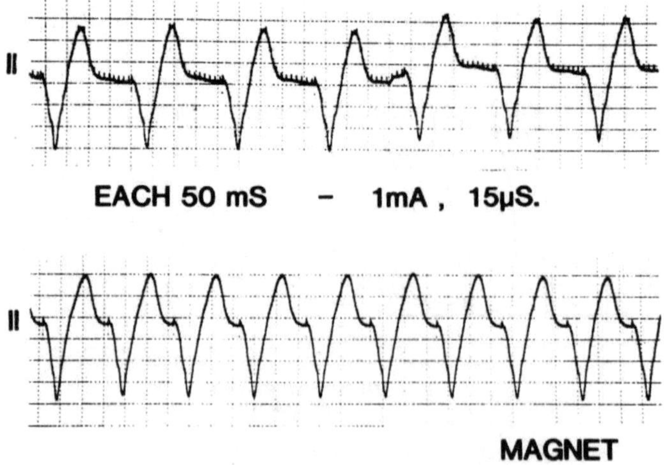

Fig. 3. ECG lead II from a patient with the minute-ventilation rate-responsive system. The signals used to measure transthoracic impedance can be seen each 50 ms. The signals disappear when a magnet is applied over the pulse generator

Clinical Experience with Minute Ventilation Controlled Rate Adaptive Pacing

Clinical experience with the minute-ventilation rate-responsive pacing system has demonstrated an excellent rate response to both exercise testing [27-35] and routine daily activities [32–35], although the rate response can be attenuated by talking continually throughout the exercise [31, 32]. Unlike the activity sensor, the

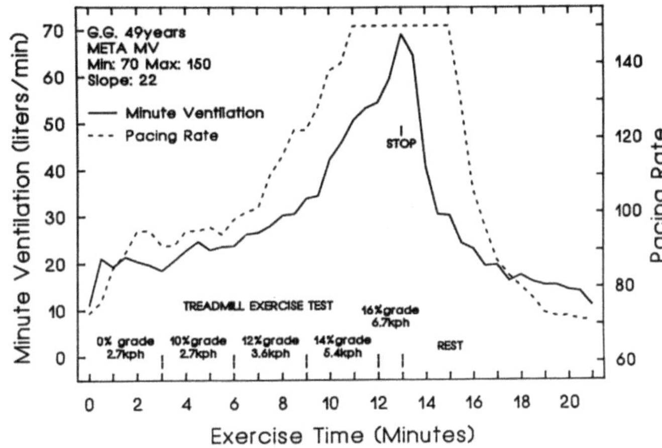

Fig. 4. Exercise test (modified Bruce protocol) to demonstrate the close relationship between measured minute ventilation and pacing rate with the minute-ventilation rate-responsive system. Minute ventilation was measured using a Fleisch head pneumotach with air flow converted to volume using a respiratory integrator

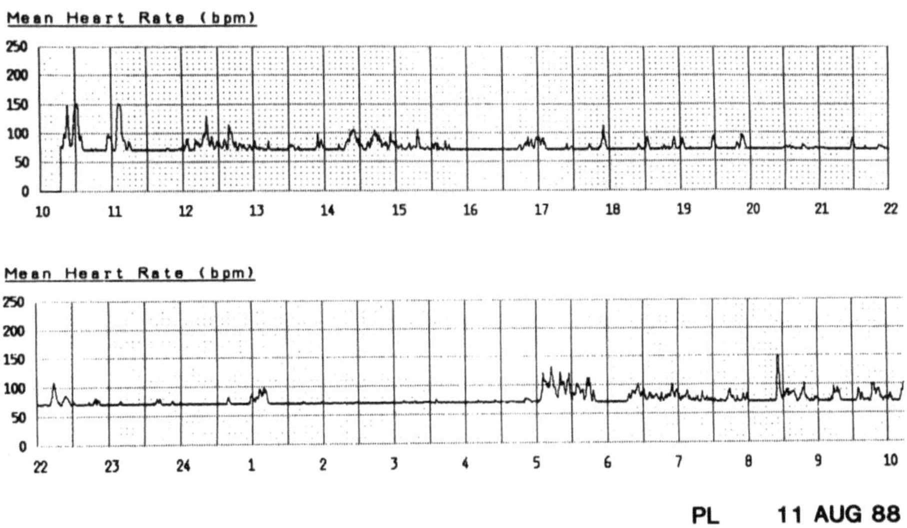

Fig. 5. Mean heart rate graph from a 24-h Holter monitor to demonstrate the pacing rate changes in a patient with the minute-ventilation rate-responsive system. With appropriate exertion the pacing rate rises to the upper rate limit of 150 bpm

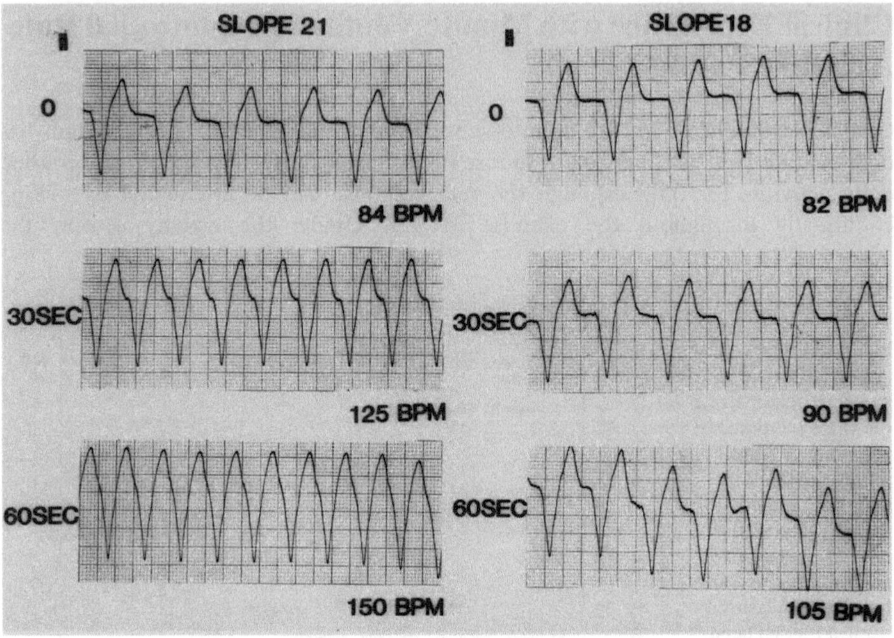

Fig. 6. Pacing rate tachycardia induced by arm movements in a patient with a minute-ventilation rate-responsive pacing system. With a slope of 21, the upper rate of 150 bpm was achieved in 60 s and the patient was symptomatic. By reducing the slope to 18, the same arm movements only achieved a pacing rate of 105 bpm at 60 s, and the patient had no further palpitations

programmed upper rate with the minute-ventilation rate-responsive pacing system can be readily achieved with a standard exercise protocol (Figs. 4 and 5) [29].

Minute-ventilation rate-responsive pacing has demonstrated superior exercise time compared to VVI pacing [29–32, 34, 35], and unlike activity rate-responsive pacing there is a more significant pacing rate increase during the ascending of stairs compared with descending [31, 32, 35]. The minute-ventilation rate-responsive pacing system has also been used successfully in the pediatric age group [36], during pregnancy, and delivery by cesarean section [37].

Because upper limb and in particular arm swinging will alter transthoracic impedance measurements, such movements will increase the minute-ventilation rate-responsive pacing rate (Fig. 6) [28, 32, 38, 39]. The increase in pacing rate, however, is not as significant as with the pure respiratory rate-responsive system [39]. Although of concern in some patients, the increase in pacing rate with upper limb movement is not necessarily a contraindication to the minute-ventilation rate-responsive system. With appropriate programming, such upper limb movements can be used to enhance the pacing rate response with specific activities such as walking.

Pacing complications related to the minute-ventilation sensor are rare and insignificant. Electrocautery will interfere with transthoracic impedance measurements, resulting in transient upper-rate pacing [40]. The manufacturer therefore recommends that the pacing system be programmed to the VVI mode prior to the use of electrocautery. Rare instances of sensing of the impedance-measuring pulses have been reported, resulting in asynchronous pacing due to interference reversion [41]. The problem, which was transient and occurred with particular lead models, was due to manufacturing residues on the anode having a capacitance effect with the impedance-measuring pulses. The build up of charge was sufficient to be sensed by the pacemaker.

An inappropriate rate response has been reported with the minute-ventilation rate-responsive pacing system in a patient with Cheyne-Stokes respiration [42]. The problem, however, was not the pacing system, but rather inappropriate programming of the slope value to 40 [43].

Ventilation Controlled DDD-R Pacing

The incorporation of the minute-ventilation sensor into a DDDR rate-responsive pacing system (Telectronics META DDDR Model 1250) has been very successful. An important change in the algorithm is an increase in the speed of response of either atrial or ventricular pacing at the commencement of exercise. This has now been reduced from 1 min to 0.5 min.

Unlike the activity sensor, the ability of the minute-ventilation sensor to reach high atrial pacing rates necessitates complex algorithms to control the atrioventricular delay and post-ventricular atrial refractory period. The maximum pacing (sensor-controlled) and tracking rates (VDD) are the same, which differs from at least one of the activity sensor systems where the atrial pacing rate may exceed the programmed atrial-sensing rate, creating a form of sensor-driven upper rate smoothing [44].

During rate-responsive dual-chamber pacing, the atrioventricular delay will continually adapt to changes in the metabolic-indicated rate during both atrial pacing

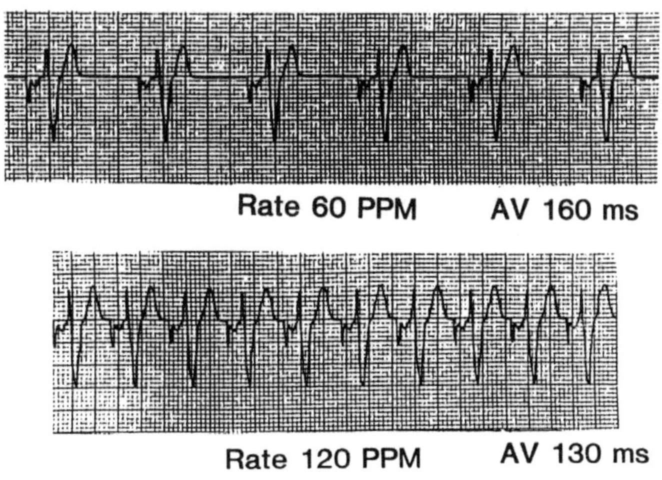

Fig. 7. ECG to demonstrate Auto A-V (adapt) with the dual-chamber minute-ventilation rate-responsive pacing system. At an atrial pacing rate of 60 bpm, the atrioventricular delay (*AV*) was 160 ms. Increasing the atrial pacing rate to 120 bpm shortened the AV to 130 ms

and sensing (Fig. 7). This is called the Auto A-V (adapt) and both normal and long atrioventricular delays are available. For example, with the normal program the atrioventricular delay will range from 103 to 155 ms with a metabolic-indicated rate range of 160–50 bpm. Autoadaptation of the postventricular atrial refrectory period (PVARP-adapt) to the metabolic-indicated rate, results in a decrease in this period with an increasing metabolic-indicated rate. The base or resting postventricular atrial refractory period is programmable.

Detection of P waves in the postventricular atrial refractory period by an atrial rate monitor, allows the pacing system to respond appropriately to supraventricular tachyarrhythmias and retrograde conduction. The complex algorithms required for this detection have yet to be fully clinically tested, although an appropriate response has been shown in patients with intermittent atrial fibrillation who automatically revert from DDDR to VVIR pacing.

Because of the large number of rate-responsive and nonrate-responsive modes available with this pacing system, a separate adaptive mode becomes cumbersome and therefore all nonrate-responsive modes are adaptive as well. Although a bipolar ventricular lead is necessary for the rate-responsive function, unipolar or bipolar pacing, and/or sensing in both chambers is programmable. To help extend the life of the pulse generator, atrial and ventricular voltage threshold measurements are available.

New developments in ventilation controlled pacing

In order to streamline and simplify the Telectronics Meta MV minute-ventilation rate-responsive pacing system, a number of new automatic or programmable functions are being incorporated into the second generation VVIR model. The smaller pulse generator will have programmable adapt times of 3 min or the current 1 h. Two programmable response times of 25 or 50 s will be available, together with a programmable rate acceleration factor and improved rate response curves that will overcome some of the limitations of the current Meta MV system. The system will also be combined with a second sensor, the ventricular depolarisation gradient, which will allow detection of the ventricular-paced evoked response. This will allow automatic ventricular threshold testing and setting of the ventricular output within a wide range of pacing amplitudes. Similary, ventricular sensitivity adjustments will also be automatic. The pacing system will automatically determine and adjust for lead polarity and the rate-responsive factor will be automatic or programmable. Telemetered histograms will hopefully obviate the need for exercise testing and Holter monitoring.

The minute-ventilation sensor has been incorporated into highly successful single- and dual-chamber rate-responsive pacing systems. Continuing developments will result in automatic features, which will simplify its use and help extend the life of the pulse generator.

Chorus RM

In addition to the ventilation contolled pacemakers from Biotec and Telectronics, Ela Medical (Montronge, France) has been starting clinicals with a new ventilation controlled DDD-R pacemaker (Chorus RM) by end of 1992. The new device (46 g, 55 x 52 x 8 mm) uses a 1.6 Ah battery and is multiprogammable in many ways. Ventilation is detected via the already known principle of impedance derived measurements of changes in transthoracic electrical resistance that varies with in- and expiration. Eight low-energy measuring pulses (0.15 ms duration, 400 μA amplitude) are applied each second between the pacemaker case and the distal electrode tip of a standard bipolar electrode. The impedance changes are measured between the proximal ring of the bipolar electrode and the pacemaker case. Ventilation rates between 6 and 45 respiratory cycles per minute can be detected and are turned together with the ventilation signal's amplitude into a pacing rate control signal.

The device has advanced automaticity function such as automatic calibration of the baseline ventilation (over a period of 6 min), automatic slope adjustment of the rate responsive factor depending on maximum exercise minute ventilation and average resting minute ventilation, and automatic mode switch from DDD to VVI-R if the maximum upper rate limit is exceeded for a pregiven time period.

Legend Plus

Another highly innovative device that uses two sensors – minute ventilation and body activity – for rate control has been introduced into clinical practice just recently (Legend Plus, Medtronic Inc., Minneapolis, MN, United States). The first of this new generation pacemaker had been implanted at the Rechts der Isar Medical Center in Munich/Germany in April 92 and by November 1992 more then 90 pacemaker have been implanted in clinical trials. The minute ventilation measurement is based on the measurement of transthoracic impedance variations between pacemaker case and a standard bipolar electrode. A 1.0 mA, 30 μs biphasic current pulse is applied 16 times per second between the ring electrode and the pacemaker case. The resultant voltage is sampled between tip and pacemaker case and processed by the pacemaker to determine thransthoracic impedance. The minute ventilation electrogram can be

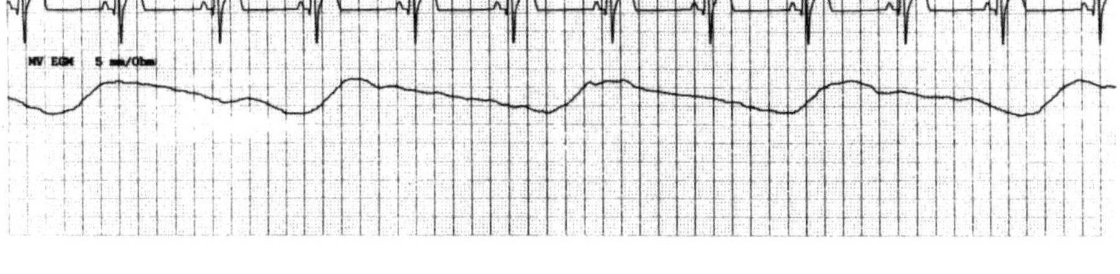

Fig. 8. MV Electrogram Transthoracic Impedance Waveform. The mm/Ohm scale of the transthoracic impedance refers to relative changes in impedance with ventilation over a baseline value.

displayed on-line from the pacemaker via telemetry on the 9760 programmer and recorded (Fig. 8).

The device programmer includes a simple initialization produce and a minute ventilation optimization protocol.

During a 100 sec initialization period with the patient of rest the pacemaker determines the baseline minute ventilation impedance signal. In order to determine an individualized rate responsive slope (from 1 to 16) a short individualized exercise protocol can be performed. The most appropriate minute ventilation rate response slope for the patient is recommended and displayed. The body activity sensor in this pacemaker functions similarly to the principle already known from traditional, activity controlled devices such as Activtrax and Legend: A piezoelectric sensor is bonded to the inside of the titanium shield and deflected by mechanical activity producing small electrical signals. A programmable Activity Threshold establishes the minimum magnitude above which these signals are detected and thereafter processed by Activity circuitry. The activity rate response setting can be selected from ten values that define incremental rate changes in response to detected body activity between a lower and upper rate limit.

The dual sensor rate responsive mode with both Activity and Minute Ventilation (MV) sensors active is shown in Fig. 9. The programmed lower rate is common for both the MV and Activity sensor. Each sensor has separate programmable upper rates: The Activity Rate for activity controlled rate adaption and the Upper MV Rate for the MV sensor.

Programming these upper rate limits to different values enhances the complementary function of the two sensors: Activity acts as the fast starter at onset of exercise, it's upper rate limit is preferably set to 100 to 110 bpm while MV takes the part of rate adaption with ongoing and more strenuons exercise. In this manner the pacemaker combines the quick response of activity to onset of exercise with the good workload proportionality of minute ventilation.

The MV upper rate limit is typically set to 135 bpm or above. Limited experience

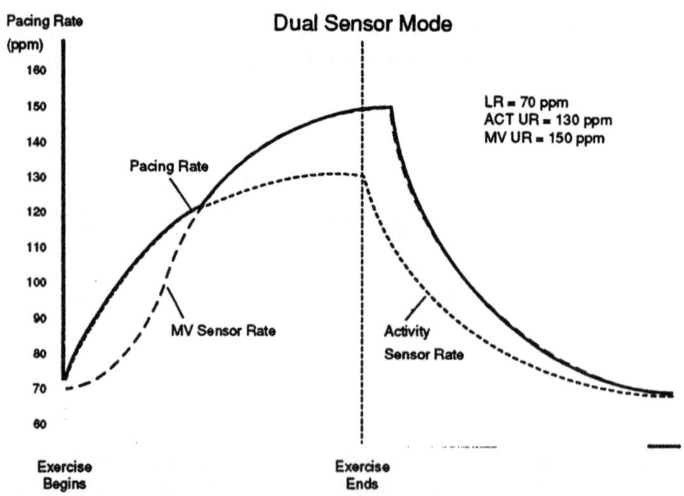

Fig. 9. Interaction of MV/ACT Sensors to Pacing Rate

from eight patients with the new legend plus at the Rechts der Isar Medical Center at Munich/Germany has shown so for a clear patient preferance for the dual sensor mode after being programmed in a single blind trial to eather of the sensors alone (MV or activity alone) or to the combined dual sensor mode. These data confirm the good results obtained with ten prototype impedance/ventilation minute ventilation and activity controlled pacemakers (45) that had been collected in the development phase of this new combination dual sensor device.

References

1. Krasner JL, Noukydis PV, Nardella PC (1966) A physiologically controlled cardiac pacemaker. J Assoc Adv Med Instrum 1:14
2. Rossi P, Plicchi G, Canducci G et al. (1983) Respiratory rate as a determinant of optimal pacing rate. PACE 6:502-507
3. Rossi P, Plicchi G, Canducci G et al. (1984) Respiration as a reliable physiological sensor for controlling pacing rate. Br Heart J 51:7-14
4. Rossi P, Aina F, Rognoni G et al. (1984) Increasing cardiac rate by tracking the respiratory rate. PACE 7:1246-1256
5. Rossi P (1990) The birth of the respiratory pacemaker. PACE 13:812-815
6. Rossi P, Prando MD, Magnani A et al. (1988) Physiological sensitivity of respiratory-dependent cardiac pacing: four-year follow-up. PACE 11:1267-1278
7. Rognoni G, Bolognese L, Aina F et al. (1988) Respiratory-dependent atrial pacing, management of sinus node disease. PACE 11:1853-1859
8. Rossi P, Rognoni G, Occhetta E et al. (1985) Respiration-dependent ventricular pacing compared with fixed ventricular and atrial-ventricular synchronous pacing: aerobic and hemodynamic variables. J Am Coll Cardiol 6:646-652
9. de Divitiis O, Santomauro M, Fazio S et al. (1985) Cardiac function in patients with breathing frequency controlled pacemaker. PACE 8:A-9
10. Tanaka S, Saigusa N, Osaka S et al. (1986) Evaluation of respiratory and cardiac function in patients with respiratory-dependent rate-responsive pacemaker. In: Belhassen B, Feldman S, Copperman Y (eds) Cardiac pacing and electrophysiology. Proceedings of the VIIIth world symposium on cardiac pacing and electrophysiology. Keterpress Enterprises, Israel, pp 75-80
11. Moracchini PV, Melandri F, Alfano G et al. (1986) Evaluation of the functional capacity in patients with a respiratory-dependent pacemaker: comparison with fixed-rate VVI pacing. Clin Prog Electrophysiol Pacing 4 [Suppl]:5
12. Henry L, Birkui P, Mugica J et al. (1986) Clinical experience of a pacer based on respiration. Clin Prog Electrophysiol Pacing 4 [Suppl]:5
13. Lau CP, Ritche D, Butrous GS et al. (1988) Rate modulation by arm movements of the respiratory-dependent rate-responsive pacemaker. PACE 11:744-752
14. Webb SC, Lewis LM, Morris-Thurgood JA et al. (1988) Respiratory-dependent pacing: a dual response from a single sensor. PACE 11:730-735
15. Melissano G, Preziuso M, Menegazzo G et al. (1987) Our experience with different rate-responsive systems. PACE 10:1221
16. Rossi P (1987) Rate-responsive pacing: biosensor reliability and physiological sensitivity. PACE 10:454-466
17. Alt E, Völker R, Wirtzfeld A (1985) Directly and indirectly measured respiratory parameters compared with oxygen uptake and heart rate. PACE 8:A-21
18. Heinz M, Alt E, Theres H, Oelker I, Zimmermann S (1990) Combination of multiple parameters for pacemaker rate control by intracardiac impedance measurement. PACE 13:1197
19. Pioger G, Vay F, Darwiche H et al. (1987) A comparative evaluation between minute ventilation and respiratory rate as indicators of activity for rate-responsive pacing. PACE 10:1224

20. Hettleman BD, Higginbotham MB, Cobb FR (1986) Minute ventilation, pulmonary artery oxygen saturation and temperature, and heart rate during exercise: profiles for physiological pacing. Clin Prog Electrophysiol Pacing 4 [Suppl]:7
21. Vai F, Bonnet JL, Ritter P et al. (1988) Relationship between heart rate and minute ventilation, tidal volume and respiratory rate during brief and low level exercise. PACE 11:1860
22. Alt E, Heinz M, Hirgstetter C et al. (1987) Control of pacemaker rate by impedance-based respiratory minute ventilation. Chest 92:247-252
23. Nappholz T, Lubin M, Maloney J et al. (1985) Measuring minute ventilation with a pacing catheter. PACE 8:785
24. Simmons T, Maloney J, Abi-Samra F et al. (1986) Exercise-responsive intravascular impedance changes as a rate controller for cardiac pacing. PACE 9:285
25. Heinz M, Alt E, Theres H et al. (1986) Impedance-based respiratory minute ventilation for control of pacemaker rate. Clin Prog Electrophysiol Pacing 4 [Suppl]:6
26. Nappholz TA, Maloney JD, Simmons T et al. (1987) A two-year research study of minute ventilation as an indicator for rate-responsive pacing. PACE 10:1222
27. Fee JA, Schultz K, Fischer S et al. (1988) Preliminary clinical results of the Meta MV rate-responsive pacemaker. PACE 11:810
28. Beckers J, Waleffe A, Kulbertus H et al. (1988) Preliminary experience with a new impedance-derived respiratory parameter pacemaker as an indicator for rate-responsive pacing. PACE 11:797
29. Mond H, Strathmore N, Kertes P et al. (1988) Rate-responsive pacing using a minute-ventilation sensor. PACE 11:1866-1874
30. Lau CP, Antoniou A, Ward DE et al. (1988) Initial clinical experience with a minute-ventilation sensing rate-modulated pacemaker: improvements in exercise capacity and symptomatology. PACE 11:1815-1822
31. Lau CP, Drysdale M, Ward D et al. (1988) Clinical experience of Meta: a minute ventilation-sensing rate-responsive pacemaker. PACE 11:507
32. Lau CP, Antoniou A, Ward DE et al. (1989) Reliability of minute ventilation as a parameter for rate-responsive pacing. PACE 12:321-330
33. Jordaens L, Berghmans L, van Wassenhove E et al. (1989) Behavior of a respiratory-driven pacemaker and direct respiratory measurements. PACE 12:1600-1606
34. Kay GN, Bubien RS, Epstein AE et al. (1989) Rate-modulated cardiac pacing based on transthoracic impedance measurements of minute ventilation: Correlation with exercise gas exchange. J Am Coll Cardiol 14:1283-1289
35. Lau CP, Wong K, Leung WH et al. (1989) A comparative evaluation of a minute ventilation-sensing and activity-sensing adaptive-rate pacemakers during daily activities. PACE 12:1514-1521
36. Yabek SM, Wernly J, Chick TW et al. (1989) Use of a minute ventilation-sensing, rate-adaptive pacemaker in children. Circulation 80:II-390
37. Lau CP, Lee CP, Wong CK et al. (1990) Rate-responsive pacing with a minute ventilation-sensing pacemaker during pregnancy and delivery. PACE 13:158-163
38. Seeger W, Kleinert M (1989) An unexpected rate response of a minute ventilation-dependent pacemaker. PACE 12:1707
39. Lau CP, Leigh-Jones M, Kingwell S et al. (1988) Comparative evaluation of two respiratory-sensing rate-responsive pacemakers. PACE 11:487
40. van Hemel NM, Hamerlijnck RPHM, Pronk KJ et al. (1989) Upper limit ventricular stimulation in respiratory rate-responsive pacing due to electrocautery. PACE 12:1720-1723
41. Wilson JH, Lattner S (1988) Apparent undersensing due to oversensing of low-amplitude pulses in a thoracic impedance-sensing, rate-responsive pacemaker. PACE 11:1479-1481
42. Scanu P, Guilleman D, Groiller G et al. (1989) Letter to the editor. PACE 12:1963
43. Kertes P, Mond H (1990) Letter to the editor. PACE 13:948
44. Higano ST, Hayes DL, Eisinger G (1989) Sensor-driven rate smoothing in a DDDR pacemaker. PACE 12:92-929
45. Theres H, Alt E, Zimmermann S, Heinz M, Oelker I, Huntley S (1991) Intracardiac impedance: an advanced concept for combination of multiple parameters for pacemaker rate control. PACE 14:692 (abstr)

Intracardiac Pressure for Rate-Adaptive Pacing

C.P. Lau[1]

Introduction

Arterial pressure increases during exercise and emotionally related stresses, and thus can theoretically be used as a sensor in a rate-adaptive system for determining the physiological need for an increase in rate. However, for long-term use in implantable devices, sensors have to be implanted on the right side of the heart. Thus the detection of the right atrial and ventricular pressure, and pulmonary arterial pressure are alternative approaches to detecting the consequences of exercise. Besides the use in rate-adaptive pacemakers, implantable sensors for the measurement of intracardiac hemodynamics may also be useful for improving the detection of ventricular tachycardias. The use of pacing therapy for hemodynamically stable ventricular tachycardia and defibrillation in the event of pacing induced acceleration into unstable ventricular tachycardia / fibrillation constitute recent tiered therapy for implantable antitachycardia pacers with cardioverter-defibrillator backup. Successful tiered therapy requires accurate hemodynamic detection capability and an intracardiac pressure sensor is a potentially very useful parameter.

Right Atrial Pressure

Cohen [1] suggested the theoretical use of right atrial pressure as a parameter for rate-adaptive pacing in 1984. In the normal individual, right atrial pressure increases slightly during the onset of moderate exercise due to increased mean circulatory filling pressure. The increase in autonomically mediated inotropic effect and in heart rate thereafter, tend to reduce the right atrial pressure. This is compensated for by an increase in venous return consequent upon the increase in muscular blood flow and muscular contraction during exercise, which leads to an increase in the mean atrial pressure within the first minute of exercise. It is postulated that the increase in right atrial pressure would be more in the absence of a rate increase in patients with

[1] Division of Cardiology, Department of Medicine, University of Hong Kong, Queen Mary Hospital, Hong Kong

bradycardias. As an increase in rate leads to an increase in cardiac output with a consequent reduction in right atrial pressure, a potential negative feedback control is theoretically possible.

This sensor has not been evaluated clinically. The right atrial pressure will change as a result of the central venous loading condition. Heart failure will increase the atrial pressures, which may lead to an adverse increase in rate (positive feedback) if the right atrial pressure is used for rate adaptation.

Right Ventricular Pressure

The rate of rise of ventricular pressure has been of interest to investigators for many years [2, 3]. This first derivative of the ventricular pressure (dp/dt) is influenced by the ventricular filling pressure, the contractile state of the heart, and the heart rate. Wiggers [4] demonstrated that when venous return caused an increase in left ventricular end-diastolic pressure, dp/dt also increased. When inotropic agents like epinephrine, digoxin, and isoproterenol were administered, dp/dt increased despite a fall in ventricular end-diastolic pressure [5]. Conversely, when myocardial ischemia occurred, the slope of the ventricular pressure rise decreased in the face of a rising end-diastolic pressure. Dp/dt was also increased by an increase in heart rate, the "treppe" effect which was originally described by Bowditch [6].

The sensing of right ventricular dp/dt as an indicator of exercise has been studied [7, 8]. A unipolar pacing electrode (Model 6220, Medtronic), which contained a piezoelectric sensor behind the tip, was used. The sensor was attached to a deflectable diaphragm and the unit was hermetically sealed. Changes in the right ventricular pressure caused a deflection of the diaphragm and a piezoelectric effect, the derived pressure was then differentiated to yield the dp/dt. The maximum dp/dt was found to correlate ($r = 0.81$) with the atrial rate in four dogs with induced complete heart block, paced at a constant ventricular rate. An investigational unit based on this principle has been constructed.

Pacemaker Description and Implantation

The Deltatrax maker (Model 2503, Medtronic) is a ventricular-demand pacemaker modified from a dual-chamber unit. The maximum dp/dt is determined on a beat-to-beat basis during a 200 ms interval after a sensed or paced event, and the value of the dp/dt max computed from a moving average of 10 beats is used for rate adaptive pacing. The atrial channel has been adapted to receive right ventricular pressure signals from the special lead which was described above. Thus the ventricular rate is determined by the signal input from the right ventricular pressure.

The pressure waveform can be assessed by telemetry using the electrogram channel. For investigational purposes, this can be externally differentiated by a custom-built device to yield a dp/dt signal for analysis.

Implantation followed the routine procedure. In order to ensure that the electrode

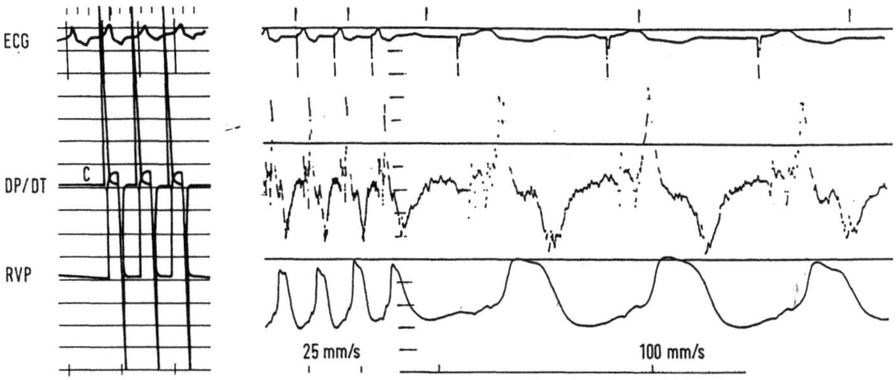

Fig. 1. Electrocardiogram (*ECG*) and right ventricular pressure (*RVP*) in a patient with a right ventricular dp/dt-sensing pacemaker. The right ventricular pressure was assessed by telemetry and externally differentiated into its first derivative (DP/DT)

functioned normally, the right ventricular pressure waveform was measured, either directly from the lead or indirectly from the pacemaker after connection (Fig. 1).

The use of medical adhesive at the connection between the pacemaker and the electrode is advisable as the failure of insulation might lead to electrode malfunction.

Clinical Performance

Exercise response

A limited number of implants were produced for investigational purposes [9–11, 11a–c]. A substantial increase in right ventricular pressure and dp/dt occurred during exercise (Fig. 2). The right ventricular pulse pressure and dp/dt values increased significantly from rest to exercise (Table 1). Using either a fully implanted Deltatrax pacemaker or an externally triggered dp/dt sensing device in 17 patients, pacing rate increased from 71 ± 6 to 115 ± 24 bpm ($P < 0.05$) (Fig. 3). For those with implanted pacemakers, the pacing rate was highly correlated with estimated oxygen consumption during exercise ($r = 0.93 \pm 0.04$). Exercise in the VVI mode tends to have a larger increase in dp/dt max and higher atrial rate than in the VVIR mode, suggesting recruitment of contractility reserve during VVI pacing (Fig. 3). Exercise time was prolonged from 6 to 13 min during paired exercise tests in the VVI and VVIR mode. The speed of rate response of the pacemaker was rapid [11a], although slightly slower than rate adaptive pacemakers using the activity sensing principle. The recovery rate decay after exercise was physiological, and usually took 5-6 minutes for the rate to return to the resting level [11b]. Holter monitoring showed pacing rate changes for the resting state to nearly twice that level during daily activities [11c].

Table 1. Right ventricular pressures and heart rate at rest and during exercise in the VVI and VVIR modes. Reproduced with permission [11c]

Mode	Rate (bpm)	$+dP/dt_{max}$* ($mmHg.sec^{-1}$)	$-dP/dt_{max}$** ($mmHg.sec^{-1}$)	Pulse † (mmHg)	Peak ‡ (mmHg)	T+dP/ dt_{max}§ (msec)	T-dP/ dt_{max}§§ (msec)
VVI PACING							
Rest	74 ± 9	194 ± 68	176 ±26	12.9 ± 5.8	18.1 ± 8.0	112 ± 23	334 ± 74
Exercise	88 ± 18	413 ± 275	346 ± 257	17.2 ± 8.7	33.9 ± 18.2	81 ± 53	318 ±107
VVIR PACING							
Rest	82 ± 13	223 ± 55	222 ± 66	13.6 ± 4.8	22.6 ± 10.8	106 ±30	324 ± 70
Exercise	119 ± 13	405 ± 181	335 ± 180	17.6 ± 6.5	32.1 ± 12.4	119 ± 12	299 ± 52

* Maximum positive right ventricular dP/dt

** Maximum negative right ventricular dP/dt

† Systolic right ventricular pressure minus end-diastolic pressure

‡ Maximum right ventricular pressure minus minimum pressure in cardiac cycle

§ Time from QRS detect to $+dP/dt_{max}$ in msec

§§ Time from QRS detect to $-dP/dt_{max}$ in msec

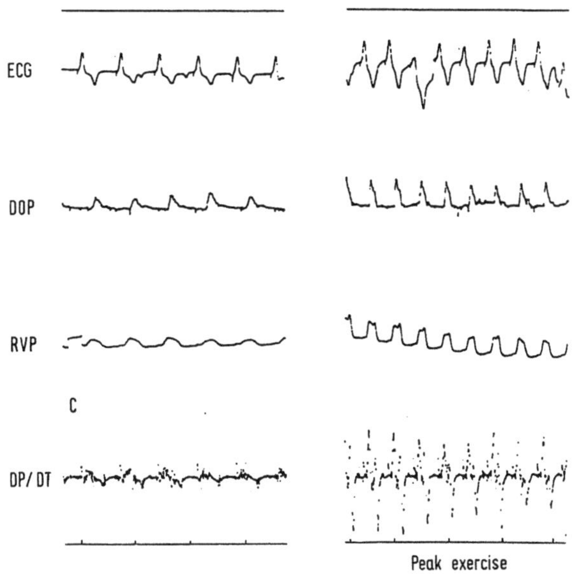

Fig. 2. Selected recordings of a patient with a dp/dt-sensing pacemaker during exercise. The right ventricular pressure (*RVP*), as assessed by telemetry, increased and showed a more rapid upstroke during exercise. The peak dp/dt also increased. The increased dp/dt was used to increase the pacing rate. Doppler recording of the aortic blood flow (*DOP*) was also included. *ECG*, electrocardiogram; *DP/DT*, First derivative of right ventricular pressure (externally differentiated from RVP)

Non exercise related influences on dp/dt max

These include the effects of changes in automatic tone and preload on maximum dp/dt:

1. Upright tilt: While right ventricular preload tends to decrease when a subject adopts upright posture, the expected reduction in maximum dp/dt is counteracted by the increase in sympathetic activities and an appropriate rate increase in a dp/dt sensing pacemaker usually occurred [11b-11c]. An average of 6 bpm increase was reported. On the other hand, a rate reduction of 12 bpm was reported in another patient [11c], although in the clinical setting this decrease could be prevented by increasing the backup rate using the 'rate-offset'.
2. Responses to respiratory maneuvers and amylnitrate: These tests examined the relative effects of mechanical (preload) versus autonomic reflex activities. Both hyperventilation and the Valsalva maneuver resulted only in minor changes in pacing rate (maximum change in maximum dp/dt about 15%) [11c]. This lack of response to changes in intrathoracic pressure may be partially explained on the basis that the pressure changes might have occurred outside the right ventricular pressure sensing window. An appropriate tachycardia occurred in response to amylnitrate, as a combination of autonomic response and a reduction in afterload.
3. 'Treppe' effect: A mild increase of maximum dp/dt when the pacing rate was increased at rest was noted (e.g. maximum dp/dt increased from 262 ± 96 mmHg/s at 40 bpm to 337 ± 81 mmHg/s at 70 bpm), although the changes were not statistically significant [11b]. No cases of positive feedback pacemaker tachycardia had been observed.

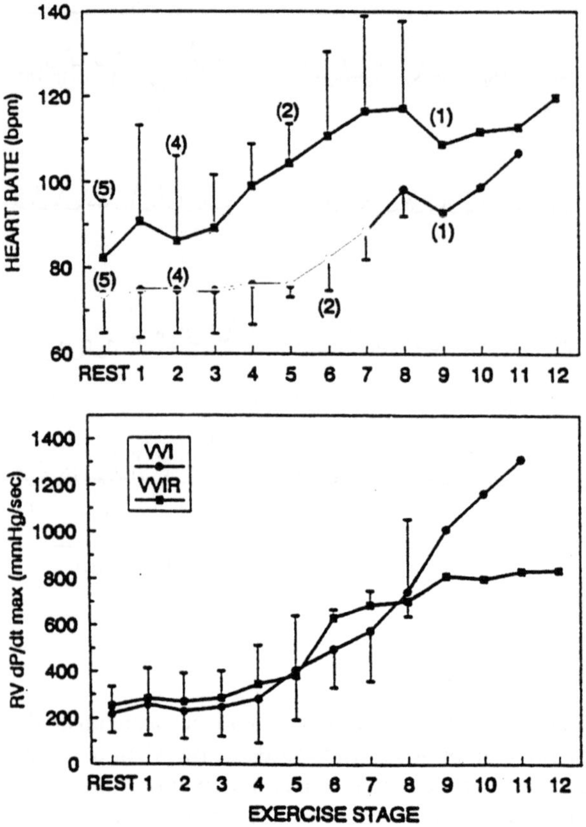

Fig. 3. Summary of the exercise heart rate and right ventricular maximum dp/dt during exercise in the VVI and VVIR modes. Pacing rate achieved was significantly higher during treadmill exercise in the VVIR mode using the modified Naughton protocol. Note the higher maximum dp/dt during peak exercise in the VVI mode suggesting a higher sympathetic state when a similar exercise was performed at a fixed rate. Reproduced with permission [11c]

Follow-up results

In one study [11b], a positive correlation between the right ventricular systolic pressure and dp/dt max was found ($r = 0.93$), and the right ventricular systolic pressure was suggested to be useful to predict the rate response setting. In an unrandomized observation, patients programmed to VVIR mode had an improvement in New York Heart Classification Status on dyspnea. This study suggested that additional rate adaptive settings may be required for fine tuning of the rate adaptive response.

A number of technical problems have been encountered in the early dp/dt system. These include the electrostatic damage (generated from opening of the packaging of the lead) of the pressure sensor and insulation problems between the electrode-pacemaker connection. The presence of the piezosensor on the electrode limits the extent at which the guide wire can be inserted although in general the positioning of the electrode is easily achieved. Burying of the sensor into the myocardium may erroneously increase the dp/dt value. A decrease in telemetered pressure amplitude was observed in 2 devices due to insufficient current to operate the sensor [11c]. This technical problem is now corrected. Circuitry crosstalk resulted in limitation of upper rate response in some units. Electrical interference from the operation of a two-way radio resulted in a transient rate increase in one patient, due to the generation of erroneously high dp/dt signal. This phenomenon required no change in the pacemaker setting in this patient. Long-term stability of the sensor is a potential problem, but recent experiments in canine implants over one year showed reproducible pressure waveforms in 4/6 implants, and satisfactory rate adaptation during exercise and isoproterenol infusion was achieved [12]. Satisfactory function in man has been observed in some patients for up to 5 years [11c]. Further studies in a broad rage of patients with pulmonary disease, right ventricular failure and autonomic dysfunction will be needed.

Advantages and limitations

The advantages of the dp/dt sensing principle are its high proportionality to workload, sensitivity to non exercise requirement and the ability to noninvasively obtain intracardiac hemodynamics. The limitations are mainly the requirement of a special pacing lead. Early dp/dt sensing devices have a number of technical problems and the long term stability of the sensor remains to be assessed.

Future applications

Besides useful in achieving rate adaptation, intracardiac pressure sensing can be used as an indicator of right ventricular capture [13]. For example, a reduction in the maximum dp/dt of right ventricular pressure (to 35% in one study) is an indicator of failure of ventricular capture. This may allow an automatic reduction in the pacing output so that pacing with the minimum energy expenditure can be effected. Right ventricular pressure may also be useful in giving diagnostic data with respect to pulmonary disease and heart failure, with signals being acquired by telemetric transmission to allow long term adjustment of therapy. As mentioned before, right ventricular pressure can be used to reflect changes of arterial pressure during ventricular tachycardia, with one study quoting a correlation of right ventricular pulse pressure with mean arterial pressure of 0.68 [14]. This concept has been postulated to be useful for the detection of hemodynamically unstable ventricular tachycardias [15, 16].

Other Methods of Sensing Intracardiac Pressures

Intravascular Doppler ultrasound has recently been used to measure intracardiac blood flow. Using a 3-F catheter with microsized Doppler crystals in the right ventricle of open-chest dogs [17], it was shown that ventricular blood flow speed was closely related to the dp/dt, and that relative changes in cardiac output can be reliably determined. Proper alignment of the ultrasound probe to the blood flow is essential in this approach and it may be technically difficult to achieve this in an implantable system. Ascending aortic flow was measured by other Investigators [18] with an ultrasound probe in the superior vena cava and right atrial junction. The crystals operated from 5 to 8 MHz with a peak power of 20 mW and are suitable for chronic implantation. A baseband signal processor optimized the signal to noise ratio during each cardiac systole. Ascending aorta Doppler can thus be used as a measure of stroke volume and contractility (by assessing flow acceleration).

Intracardiac impedance has been used to measure respiration [19] and stroke volume [20]. These parameters can be simultaneously derived using a standard bipolar-pacing electrode, with impedance current being sensed between the proximal electrode and an epicutaneous patch [21]. A low-pass filtered component reflects minute ventilation and a high-pass component yields signals pertaining to stroke volume (from which the preejection period can be derived). It is also postulated that the right ventricular volume parameter bears a positive correlation to the ventricular pressure, and thus this measurement may also indirectly give an indication of the right ventricular/pulmonary pressure [22]. The high-pass signal changed rapidly at the onset of exercise, although the signal was not proportional to the workload. This can be advantageously combined with the low-pass signal which although slow in reacting to exercise is proportional to workload. Thus the use of impedance measurement will allow the derivation of many cardiorespiratory data using a single sensor and standard pacing electrode. If this theoretical system proves effective in practice, it may open up the possibilities of using multiple cardiorespiratory parameters for rate-adaptive pacing, as well as using them for fine-tuning therapy for patients with cardiac or respiratory disease.

Conclusion

Intracardiac pressure measurement is a feasible method of rate-adaptive pacing, although still technically challenging. Intracardiac pressure sensing might be useful not only for rate-adaptive pacing, but also in the field of tachycardia detection and for monitoring patients with cardiac and respiratory diseases.

References

1. Cohen TJ (1984) A theoretical right atrial pressure feedback heart rate control system to restore physiologic control to the rate-limited heart. PACE 7:671-677
2. Patterson SW, Piper H, Starling EH (1914) The regulation of the heart beat. J Physiol (Lond) 48:465-513
3. Frank O (1959) On the dynamics of cardiac muscle. Am Heart J 58:282-317
4. Wiggers CJ (1927) Studies on the cardiodynamic action of drugs: I. The Application of the optical methods of pressure registration in the study of cardiac stimulants and depressants; II. The mechanism of cardiac stimulation by epinephrine. J Pharmacol Exp Ther 30:217

5. Wiggers CJ, Stimson B (1927) Studies on the cardiodynamic actions of drugs: III. The mechanism of cardiac stimulation by digitalis and g-strophanthin. J Pharmacol Exp Ther 30:251
6. Bowditch HP (1871) Uber die Eigenthumlichkeiten der Reizarbeit, welche die Muskelfasern des Herzens zeigen. Ber Verh Koniglich Sachsischen Ges Wissenschaften Leipzig 23:852
7. Bennett TD (1985) Dynamic characteristic of alternative physiological pacing. PACE 8:294 (abstr)
8. Anderson KM, Moore AA, Bennett TD (1986) Sensors in pacing. PACE 9:954-959
9. Sutton R, Sharma A, Ingram A, Camm J, Lindemans F, Bennett T (1987) First derivative of right ventricular pressure as a sensor of an implantable rate-responsive VVI pacemaker. PACE 10:1210 (abstr)
10. Sharma AD, Yee R, Bennett T, Erickson M, Beck R, Sutton R, Klein G (1987) The effects of ventricular pacing on right ventricular maximum positive dp/dt: implications for a rate-responsive pacing system based on this parameter. PACE 10:1228 (abstr)
11. Sharma A, Bennett T, Sutton R, Ericson M, Yee R, Klein G (1988) Randomized single-blind assessment of rate-responsive pacing based upon maximum positive right ventricular dp/dt during treadmill exercise. PACE 11:487 (abstr)
11a. Lau CP, Butrous GS, Ward DE, Camm AJ (1989) Comparative assessment of exercise performance of six different rate adaptive right ventricular pacemakers. Am J Cardiol 63:833-839
11b. Ovsychcher I, Guetta V, Bondy C, Porath AVI (1992) First derivative of right ventricular pressure, dp/dt, as a sensor for a rate adaptive VVI pacemaker: initial experience. PACE 15:211-218
11c. Bennett T, Sharma A, Sutton R, Camm AJ, Erickson M, Beck R (1992). Development of a rate adaptive pacemaker based on the maximum rate-of-use of right vertricular pressure (RV dp/dt max). PACE 15:219-234
12. Erickson MK, Bennett TD (1990) Right ventricular pressure for rate control: one year experience with dp/dt pacemaker in heart-blocked dogs. Rev Eur Technol Biomed 12:33
13. Bennett TD, Sharma A (1990) Right ventricular pressure parameters for pacemaker automatic capture detection. Rev Eur Technol Biomed 12:17
14. Lu B, Wood M, Ellenbogen KA, Valenta HL Jr (1990) Correlation of an invasive measure of right ventricular pressure and mean arterial pressure. Biomed Sci Instrum 26:137-140
15. Cohen TJ, Lien LB (1990) A hemodynamically responsive antitachycardia system. Development and basis for design humans. Circulation 82:394-406
16. Ellenbogen K, Lu B, Kapadis K, Wood M, Valenta H (1990) Usefulness of right ventricular pulse pressure as a potential sensor for hemodynamically unstable ventricular tachycardia. Am J Cardiol 65:1105-1111
17. Laule M, Stangle K, Wirtzfeld A, Heinze R, Erhardt W, Schmalfeld B (1990) Intracardiac echo-Doppler-measurement: a new parameter for rate-responsive pacing? Rev Eur Technol Biomed 12:33 (abstr)
18. Valenta HL, Wrigley RH, Ellenbogen KA, Lu B (1991) A new hemodynamic sensor for pacemakers and defibrillators. PACE 14:659 (abstr)
19. Valenta H Jr, Nappholtz T, Maloney J, Simmons T, McElroy P (1986) Correlation of heart rate with an intravenous impedance, respiratory sensor. Biomed Sci Instrum 22:7-12
20. McGoon MD, Shapland E, Salo R, Pederson B, Olive A (1989) The feasibility of utilizing the systolic pre-ejection interval as a determinant of pacing rate. J Am Coll Cardiol 14:1753-1758
21. Theres H, Alt E, Zimmermann S, Heinz M, Oelker J, Huntley S (1991) Intracardiac impedance: an advanced concept for combination of multiple parameters for pacemaker rate control. PACE 14:692 (abstr)
22. Alt E. (1991) Cardiac and pulmonary physiological analysis via intracardiac measurements with a single sensor. US Patent No. 5,003,976, 2. April 1991

Mixed-Venous Oxygen Saturation

K. STANGL[1] and E. ALT[2]

Introduction

Mixed-venous oxygen saturation (SO_2) refers to the percentage of hemoglobin with oxygen in the binding sites in the right ventricle and the pulmonary artery. The utilization of this physiological parameter as a regulating variable in a rate-adaptive pacemaker system was first proposed by Wirtzfeld [32–34]. SO_2 pacemakers were first implanted in humans in 1988 (P55, Siemens Company, Solna, Sweden) [28]. Somewhat later the Faerestrand group [8–10] began a series of implantations (Oxylog, Medtronic Inc., Minneapolis, United States) as well.

Physiological Considerations

Under physiological conditions, adult hemoglobin (HbA) is the specific transport protein of the blood for oxygen. Hemoglobin is a tetramer consisting of four polypeptide subunits with molecular weights of approximately 17 000. These four polypeptide chains are each divided into two a and b chains. The O_2 binding takes place through the reversible addition (oxygenation) of the O_2 molecule to the bivalent iron of the prosthetic heme groups of the hemoglobin $(HbO_2)^4$. Based on weight, 1g hemoglobin binds 1.34 ml oxygen (Hüfner number).

The relation between the O_2 partial pressure and the degree of hemoglobin occupation at the O_2-binging sites is described by the oxygen-binding curve (Fig. 1).

The curve, expressing the affinity between O_2 and hemoglobin, is modulated by so-called "allosteric effects". This term embraces changes in the quaternary structure of the hemoglobin that result from changes in affinity modulators such as proton concentration (Bohr effect [4, 5]), carbon dioxide partial pressure (pCO_2), 2,3-diphosphoglycerate concentration (2,3-DPG) in the erythrocyte [3, 14], and temperature [2].

An expression of the reduced hemoglobin affinity to oxygen is the rightward shift of the oxygen-binding curve. As apparent from Fig. 1, the rightward shift makes higher

[1] First Medical Clinic, Charité, Humboldt University, 1040 Berlin
[2] First Medical Clinic, Technical University of Munich, 8000 Munich 80

Fig. 1. Rightward shift of the oxygen-binding curve. A drop in the pH value, an increase in temperature (*T*) and carbon dioxide partial pressure (pCO_2), and the increase in 2,3-diphosphoglycerate (2,3-DPG) lead to a rightward shift in the oxygen-binding curve with decreased affinity of the hemoglobin to oxygen. P_{50} = O_2 pressure at which 50% of hemoglobin binding sites are occupied; PO_2 = Oxygen pressure

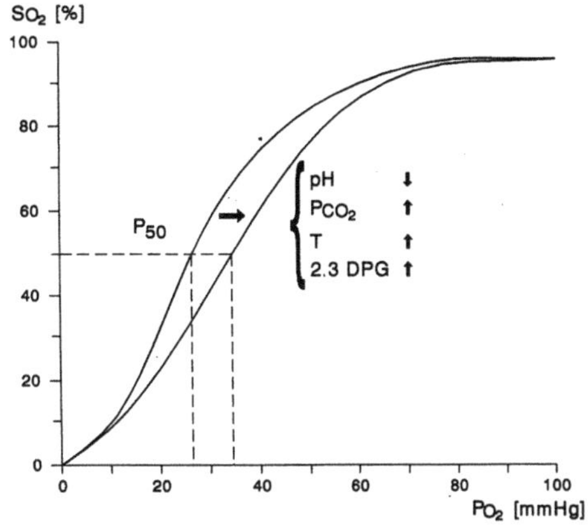

oxygen partial pressures necessary to reach oxygenation of the hemoglobin. Conversely, oxygen is released at higher partial pressures in the tissue. The quaternary structure of the hemoglobin changes in accordance with oxygenation, the quaternary structure of the oxygenated hemoglobin being referred to as the relaxed (R)-form and that of the deoxygenated hemoglobin as the tensed (T)-form. The R-form and the T-form differ in that the affinity to oxygen is about 300 times greater in the R-form.

Summing up, the decrease in the oxygen affinity of hemoglobin is – from a teleological point of view – an useful mechanism of the body for adapting to changing exercise. The exercise-induced decrease in affinity leads to easier oxygen release and thus to an improved oxygen supply in metabolically active tissues, such as the striped musculature.

Technical Considerations of SO_2 Measurement

SO_2 of the blood is determined by the principle of reflection oximetry. By this method two light pulses with wavelengths of 660 nm and 850 nm are released into the blood and the reflected light's intensity measured. As apparent from Fig. 2, at the 660 nm wavelength the reflection factor of oxygenated hemoglobin (Hb-O_2) is twice as great as that of deoxygenated hemoglobin (Hb). By contrast, the reflection factors of Hb-O_2 and Hb are the same at 850 nm (isobestic point).

At present, semiconductor probes are used in the two oxygen pacemakers currently under clinical investigation. The optical sensor is positioned directly at the place of measurement and connected to the pacemaker via an electric lead. Both systems work in pulse interval modes, i.e.; they are always switched on for a short time (0.1-1 ms) in synchronism with the ECG or pacing pulse. The relation between the on and off states results in the low power consumption in the range that is necessary for these systems.

The first sensor system (P55, Siemens Company) with an analog-measuring signal is shown in Fig. 3. It contains only light-emitting and -receiving elements. The

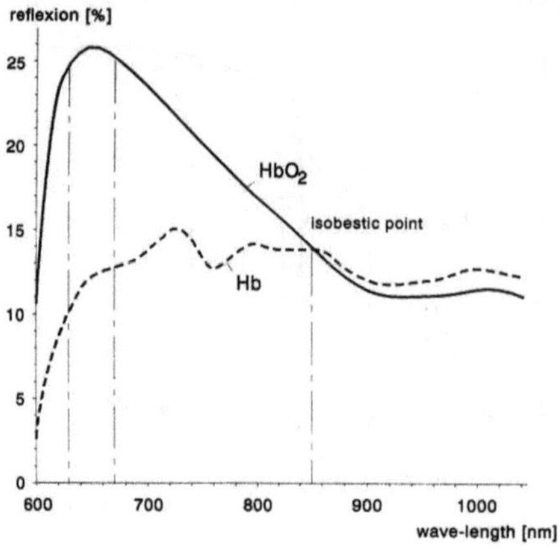

Fig. 2. Absorption spectra of oxygenated (*Hb-O*$_2$) and deoxygenated hemoglobin (*Hb*). The isobestic point refers to the wavelength of equal absorption

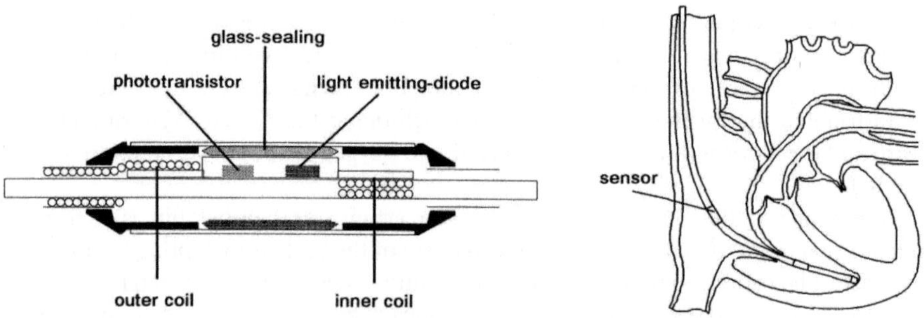

Fig. 3. Cross section through the sensor with the light-emitting diode and phototransistor. The measuring amplifier is integrated in the pacemaker can

advantage of this sensor structure is its low power consumption (< 3 μA). Also, it can compensate for a data drift due to deposits within a wide range.

The second system (Oxylog, Medtronic Inc.) for determining the absolute oxygen value contains a measuring amplifier integrated into the sensor. This sensor converts the measuring signal directly into a binary-coded signal. The advantage of this circuit is its high signal to noise ratio, its disadvantage is its relatively high power consumption. Also, the sensor's ability to compensate for a measured range drift due to coating of the surface might be limited.

Dynamic Behavior

Delay Times. The delay time of a parameter is defined as the time span between the beginning of the change in exercise level and the moment when 10% of the parameters total change in signal associated with the maximum exercise level is reached. It is thus the measurement of how fast a parameter reacts to changes in exercise. The mean delay times of SO_2 under physiological conditions in volunteers (n = 15) and pacemaker patients (n = 18) has been found to range from 8 to 12 s [29].

Time Constants. The time constant of a parameter is defined as the period of time between the beginning of the exercise and the moment when 67% of the parameters total change in signal is reached. It is the unit for calculating the time until a new balance forms. In volunteers and patients as discribed above [29], we found time constants between 15 s in the low-load range and 45 s in the high-load range. The SO_2 curve with exercise was found to have an exponential relationship to workload in each individual case with a rapid drop in SO_2 at start of exercise and a more flat decline in SO_2 with ongoing exercise.

Static Behavior

Functional Relationship: SO_2 and Workload. The relationship between SO_2 and workload in 18 patients with DDD pacemakers with reference to the pacing mode is shown in Fig. 4a.

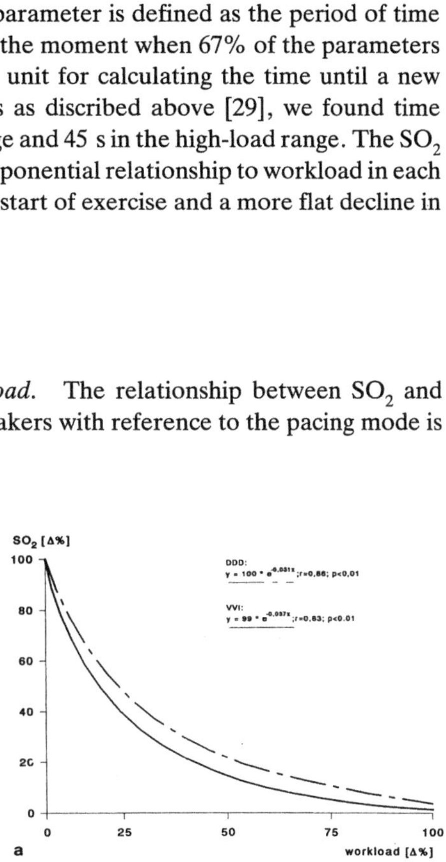

Fig. 4a. Functional relation between the percentage change in performance and oxygen saturation (SO_2) in patients with DDD systems with an AV block III (n = 18) standardized to the individual range of performance (100%)

In the VVI mode the average saturation values were always significantly below those in DDD pacing. For both pacing modes an exponential relationship exists between SO_2 (y) and workload (x):

VVI: $y = 29 \times e^{-0.068} \times x + 41;$ $r = 0.68; p < 0.001$

DDD: $y = 24 \times e^{-0.049} \times x + 49;$ $r = 0.53; p < 0.001$

Sensitivity. Sensitivity is the first derivative after workload and refers to the ability to discriminate between changes in exercise. The sensitivity curve of SO_2 to changes in load (Fig. 4b) follows an exponential function in each case:

VVI: $y = 2.0 \times e^{-0.068} \times x$

VDD/DDD: $y = 1.2 \times e^{-0.049} \times x$

The highest sensitivity is accordingly reached in the low- and medium-load ranges

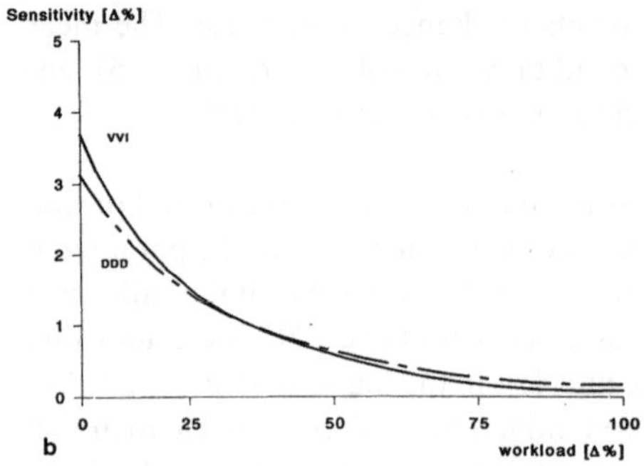

Fig. 4b. Corresponding sensitivity curves in those patients tested in Fig. 4a

and dies out in the high-load range in accordance with the exponential function. About 80% of the total change in SO_2 are seen with the initial 50% of a given workload, while the reminder 50% of ongoing workload effect only about 20% of the total change in SO_2 seen with exercise (Figs. 4a and 4b). Therefore, SO_2 is a very sensitive parameter for low and medium load workloads, but less sensitive with more strenious work.

Rate Optimization

Rate optimization is possible with SO_2 due to the feedback according to Fick's principle. In 1988 Heinze et al. [15] developed a method permitting automatic selection of the hemodynamically optimal pacing rate (Fig. 5). In this case the lowest rate at rest at which an "adequate" cardiac output is reached is set to 60/min. The plateau formation of cardiac output shows that this rate is adequate and that a further increase in the rate will not lead to any further increase in cardiac output. During submaximal exercise by a patient with severe coronary heart disease, the rate/cardiac output relation shows the rate of 110/min to be the critical rate above which no further increase, but decrease, in cardiac output occurs. Accordingly, the maximum pacing rate of the pacemaker is set to this limiting rate.

Final Assessment

Physiology. SO_2 is a complex physiological variable that is determined using Fick principle by oxygen consumption, cardiac output, and the hemoglobin content of the blood. It is thus a predominantly exercise-dependent control parameter. Furthermore, it contains information about the hemodynamic effects of rate changes so as to permit an optimizing rate adaptation (Fig. 5). Its additional dependence of affinity-modulating factors, such as proton concentration (pH value), temperature, and 2,3-DPG does not involve any negative influence on the load-specific form of reaction described above, since the decrease in hemoglobin affinity is a process by which the body adapts to exercise.

A first nonspecific influence is an exercise-independent temperature increase due to fever or an isolated metabolic acidosis (e.g., diabetic coma). A second exercise-independent factor is the hemoglobin content of the blood. A crucial influence from changes in concentration must be expected, particularly in the case of loss of blood and/or a decrease in the O_2-binding sites of the hemoglobin, as occurs in smokers due to the occupation of the Hb by carbon monoxide. The resulting rate increase in an SO_2-regulated pacemaker system should not be considered a false adjustment; it corresponds instead to the reaction of a person with a sound heart in this situation.

Dynamics. With its delay times of about 10 s, SO_2 is a fast-reacting parameter. Since SO_2 additionally has a fast time constant, it quickly reaches the steady state. Due to these characteristics SO_2 has a dynamic behavior similar to sinus rhythm. [29]

Diagnostic Value. According to Fick's principle, mixed-venous SO_2 is, as a determinant, a specific indicator of the hemodynamic and respiratory situation of the body. It therefore has an independent diagnostic and prognostic value beyond its suitability as a pacemaker-regulating variable.

SO_2 is thus a component of intensive care monitoring. Its high-informative power for assessing the hemodynamics of intensive care patients [6, 12], for arrhythmias [23], and for therapeutic drug monitoring [13, 17, 20] and nursing measures [1, 25] has often been described. Also, SO_2 can be used profitably in intra- and postoperative monitoring [19, 24, 31]. SO_2 is useful not only as a hemodynamic-measuring variable, but also for controlling and finely tuning ventilation (e.g., best PEEP) [7, 11, 21, 22, 27, 30]. Furthermore, the association of SO_2 with hemodynamic parameters and with

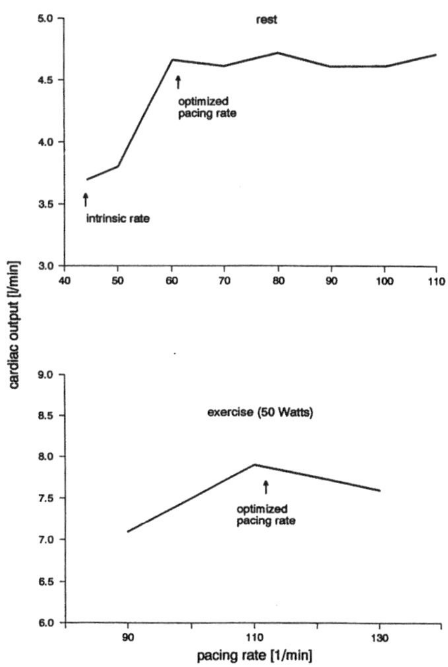

Fig. 5. Hemodynamic self-optimization in a patient with an implanted P55

the patient's overall clinical situation, permits valuable prognostic statements to be made [12, 16, 18, 20, 26].

Problems. The essential problem of the system must be seen in the long-term stability of the optical measurement. This is determined by the mechanical stability of the optical sensor catheter and the lasting transparency of the sensor window. The development of sensors sealed hermetically in glass has crucially contributed to guaranteeing mechanical stability. Although the question of the optical window being coated with fibrin cannot be answered definitevely today, experiences with human implantations over 3 years seem to be encouraging in this respect.

The limitation of somewhat lower sensitivity to medium to high-load exercise might be overcome by combination with a complementary second parameter in the future [29, 35].

References

1. Baele PL, McMichan JC, Marsh HM et al. (1982) Continuous monitoring of mixed venous oxygen saturation in critically ill patients. Anesth Analg 61:513
2. Barcroft J, King WOR (1909) The effect of temperature on the dissociation curve of blood. J Physiol (Lond) 39:374
3. Benesch R, Benesch RE (1967) The effect of organic phosphates from the human erythrocyte on the allosteric properties of hemoglobin. Biochem Biophys Res Commun 26:162
4. Bohr CH (1904) Theoretische Behandlung der quantitativen Verhältnisse bei der Sauerstoffaufnahme des Hämoglobins. Zbl Physiol 23:682
5. Bohr CH (1904) Die Sauerstoffaufnahme des genuinen Blutfarbstoffes und des aus dem Blute dargestellten Hämoglobins. Zbl Physiol 23:688
6. De La Rocha AG, Edmonds JF, Williams WG et al. (1978) Importance of mixed-venous oxygen saturation in the care of ciritically ill patients. Can J Surg 21:227
7. Divertie MB, McMichan MB (1984) Continuous monitoring of mixed venous saturation. Chest 85:423
8. Faerestrand S, Skadberg BT, Anderson K et al. (1988) Rate-responsive guide by central venous oxygen saturation. Cardiostimulatione 4:2218
9. Faerestrand S, Ohm O (1990) Central venous oxygen saturation at rest and exercise during bradycardia and rate-responsive pacing. PACE 13:529
10. Faerestrand S, Ohm O (1990) The implanted central venous oxygen saturation sensor can modulate the pacing rate on long-term basis. PACE 13:1195
11. Fahey PJ, Harris K, Vanderwarf C (1984) Clinical experience with continuous monitoring of mixed-venous saturation in respiratory failure. Chest 86:748
12. Goldman RH, Klughaupt M, Metcalf T et al. (1968) Measurement of central venous saturation in patients with myocardial infarction. Circulation 38:941
13. Hansen JF, Hessle B, Christensen NJ (1978) Enhanced sympathetic nervous activity after intravenous propranolol in ischemic heart disease: plasma noradrenaline splanchnic blood flow and mixed-venous oxygen saturation at rest and during exercise. Eur J Clin Invest 8:31
14. Hasart E, Roth W, Jagemann K et al. (1973) 2,3 Diphosphoglyceratkonzentration in Erythrozyten und körperliche Belastung. Med Sport (Basel) 13:112
15. Heinze R, Hoekstein KN, Liess HD et al. (1988) Automatische Anpassung frequenzgeregelter Herzschrittmacher an die cardiale Förderleistung der Patienten. Biomed Tech (Berlin) 39 [Suppl]:19
16. Jameson WRE, Turnbull KW, Larieu AJ et al. (1982) Continuous monitoring of mixed-venous oxygen saturation in cardiac surgery. Can J Surg 25:538

17. Kandel G, Aberman A (1983) Mixed venous saturation: its role in the assessment of the critically ill patient. Arch Intern Med 143:1400
18. Kawakami Y, Kishi F, Yamamoto H et al. (1983) Relation of oxygen delivery, mixed venous oxygenation, and pulmonary hemodynamics to prognosis in chronic obstructive pulmonary disease. N Engl J Med 308:1045
19. Kazarian KK, Del Guercio LRM (1980) The use of mixed venous blood gas determinations in traumatic shock. Ann Emerg Med 9:179
20. Krauss XH, Verdoux PD, Hugenholtz PG et al. (1975) On-line monitoring of mixed venous saturation after cardiothoracic surgery. Thorax 30:636
21. LaFarge CG, Miettinen OS (1970) The estimation of oxygen consumption. Cardiovasc Res 4:23
22. Lutch JS, Muray JF (1972) Continuous positive-pressure ventilation: effects on systemic oxygen transport and tissue oxygenation. Ann Intern Med 76:193
23. Lee J, Wright F, Barber R et al. (1972) Central-venous oxygen saturation in shock: a study in man. Anesthesiology 36:472
24. Prakash O, Meij SH, Clementi G et al. (1978) Cardiovascular monitoring with special emphasis on mixed-venous oxygen measurements. Act Anaesth Belg 3:253
25. Rah KH, Dunwiddle WC, Lower R (1984) A method for continuous postoperative measurement of mixed-venous oxygen saturation in infants and children after open heart procedures. Anesth Analg 63:873
26. Scheinman MM, Brown MA, Rapafort E (1969) Critical assessment of use of central venous oxygen saturation as a mirror of mixed venous oxygen in severely ill cardiac patients. Circulation 40:165
27. Springer RR, Stevens PM (1979) The influence of PEEP on survival of patients in respiratory failure. Am J Med 66:196
28. Stangl K, Wirtzfeld A, Heinze R et al. (1988) First experience with an oxygen-controlled pacemaker in man. PACE 11/II:1882
29. Stangl K, Wirtzfeld A (1990) Gemischtvenöse Sauerstoffsättigung. In: Stangl K, Heuer H, Wirtzfeld A (eds) Frequenzadaptive Herschrittmacher. Physiologie, Technologie, Klinische Ergebnisse. Steinkopff, Darmstadt, p 187
30. Suter PM, Fairley HB, Isenburg MD (1975) Optimum end-expiratory airway pressure with acute pulmonary failure. N Engl J Med 292:284
31. Theye RA, Tuohy GF (1964) The value of venous oxygen levels during general anesthesia. Anesthesiology 26:49
32. Wirtzfeld A, Goedel-Meinen L, Bock T et al. (1981) Central venous oxygen saturation for the control of automatic rate-responsive pacing. Circulation 64 [Suppl. IV]:299
33. Wirtzfeld A, Heinze R, Liess HD et al. (1983) An active optical sensor for monitoring mixed-venous oxygen saturation for an implantable rate-regulating pacing system. PACE 6/II:494
34. Wirtzfeld A, Heinze R, Stangl K et al. (1984) Regulation of pacing rate by variations of mixed-venous oxygen saturation. PACE 7/II:1257
35. Alt E, Theres H, Heinz M, Matula M, Thilo R, Blömer H (1988) A new rate-modulated pacemaker system optimized by combination of two sensors. PACE 11:1119

Central Venous Blood Temperature

E. ALT[2], K. STANGL[1], and H. THERES[1]

Introduction

The suitability of central venous blood temperature for rate control of cardiac pacemakers is based on the fact that under physical exercise the overall metabolic rate of the organism increases. An increased metabolic rate also effects an increase in heat production.

A liter of oxygen burned produces about 5 kcal total metabolic energy. In hormonally healthy persons this energy is converted into 22±4% mechanical energy and into 78±4% thermal energy, with a constant relationship under working conditions. The heat produced thus correlates directly with the total metabolic rate. The increased amount of heat during exercise is conducted by the blood which serves as a transporting and conducting medium. Within a broad range of environmental temperatures, the temperature regulation of the body is most accurately controlled by hypothalamic regulatory mechanisms that control heat production and heat dissipation.

By means of a small thermistor (resolution 0.01 °C) that can be totally incorporated into the stimulation electrode, central venous blood temperature can be measured with high accuracy.

In healthy persons, the central venous blood temperature exhibits an exercise behavior as shown in Fig. 1. This exercise-induced increase in body temperature has been known for more than 30 years [1]. With strong and prolonged physical stress, like in marathon runners, rectal temperatures of up to 41 °C are known [2].

Temperature Physiology

With everyday routine physical exercise, there is a small decrease in blood temperature at the onset of exercise. As the majority of the heat produced at the commencement of exercise is used to warm up the working muscles, only a small amount of heat is conducted by the blood at the beginning of muscular work. Additionally, the concomitantly increased perfusion of the limbs transports an increased amount of cold blood from the body surface to the heart, resulting in an

[2] First Medical Clinic, Technical University of Munich, 8000 Munich 80, FRG
[1] First Medical Clinic, Charité, Humboldt University, 1040 Berlin

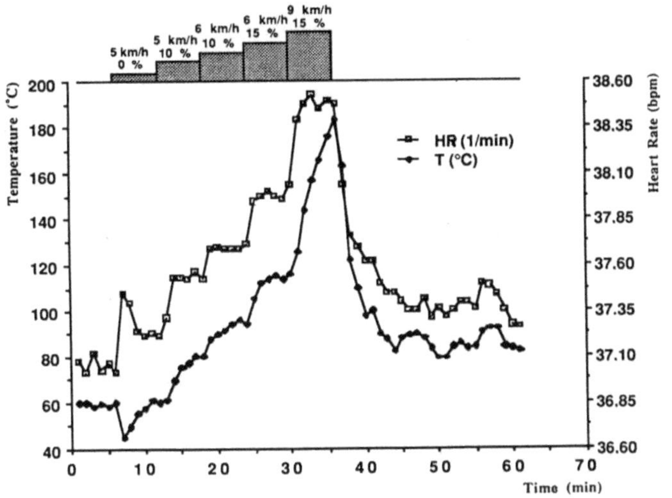

Fig. 1. Temperature (*T*) and heart-rate (*HR*) patterns in a healthy volunteer during increasing workload on the treadmill. The heart rate (bpm, upper line) and right ventricular blood temperature (°C) (lower line) measured by means of a thermistor electrode are shown. At the onset of exercise, there is a initial and prompt decrease in temperature, but at higher workloads, the temperature shows a curve parallel to the heart rate. After cessation of exercise, there is a fast decrease in heart rate and blood temperature. In the recovery phase, the blood temperature level being higher than the initial value due to the increased metabolic turnover after maximum work loads. The heart rate shows a behavior comparable to an elevated recovery pulse after exercise as well.

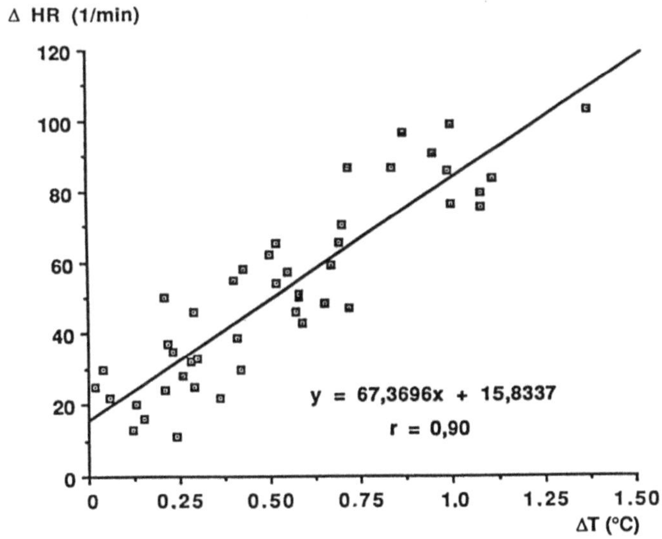

Fig. 2. Correlation between the change in heart rate relative to an initial value (Δ HR) and the change in blood temperature relative to a basal value (ΔT). There is a good correlation ($r = 0.9$) of heart rate and temperature for treadmill exercise with increasing work loads. Pooled data from 11 healthy volunteers and from 12 pacemaker patients with AV block, DDD pacemakers and correct functioning sinus node.

initial drop in blood temperature. With repetitive exercise, this initial "dip" is no longer present [3–6].

With longer lasting exercise of a least 3 min duration, a good correlation between the relative increase in heart rate and the relative increase in central blood temperature has been found (Fig. 2) [7–11].

While there is a linear and straight correlation between temperature changes and heart rate changes with ongoing and increasing workloads, there is a different behavior

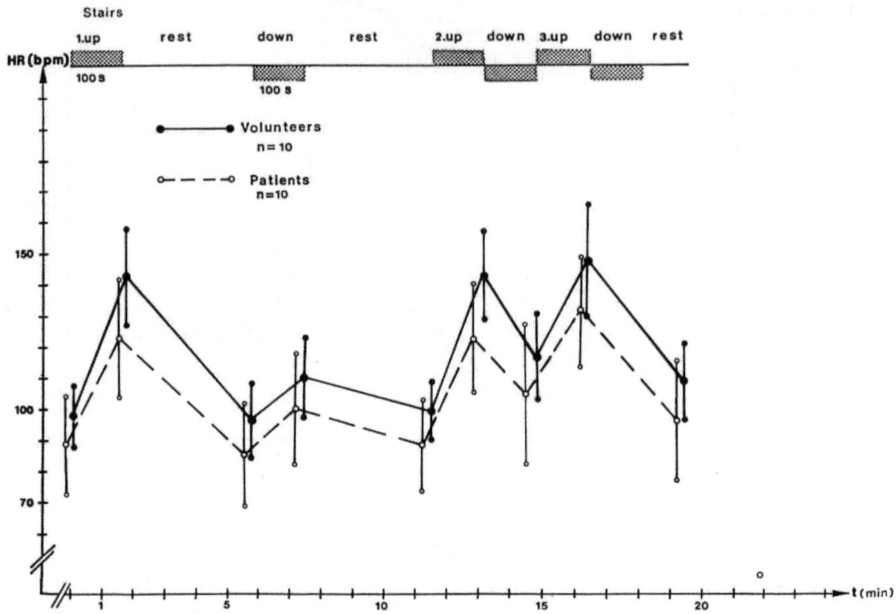

Fig. 3a Course of 3a heart rate (*HR*) and 3b central venous blood temperature (T) in ten healthy young volunteers and in ten pacemaker patients. In all patients DDD pacemakers were implanted except in one, where a VVI pacemaker was placed. This patient exhibited an adequate intrinsic rate increase with exercise and in the other nine pacemaker patients a normal rate behavior was present due to atrial synchronous pacing at complete AV block.

The volunteers and patients were made to walk up- and downstairs three times (five flights of stairs within 100 s). With the second, and in particular the third walk the central venous temperature rose to higher values compared to the first walk upstairs. Pacemaker patients exhibited a more pronounced increase in blood temperature with exercise compared to the volunteers, despite virtually the same physical work (nearly same body weight) performed by both groups.

The cumulative behavior of temperature increase with repetitive exercise has to be considered by a temperature-controlled pacemaker through the application of an "intelligent", nonlinear algorithm

Table 1. Summarized results of relative increase in heart rate and central venous blood temperature in 11 volunteers and 12 pacemaker patients (DDD) compared to the data at rest.

	Volunteers			Patients	
Workload (W)	ΔHR (l/min)	ΔT (°C)	Workload (W)	ΔHR (l/min)	ΔT (°C)
50	26	0.21	25	30	0.27
100	52	0.57	50	38	0.44
150	74	0.84	75	42	0.58
200	86	1.02	100	67	0.78

ΔHR, change in heart rate compared to the resting heart rate
ΔT, change in temperature compared to the resting temperature

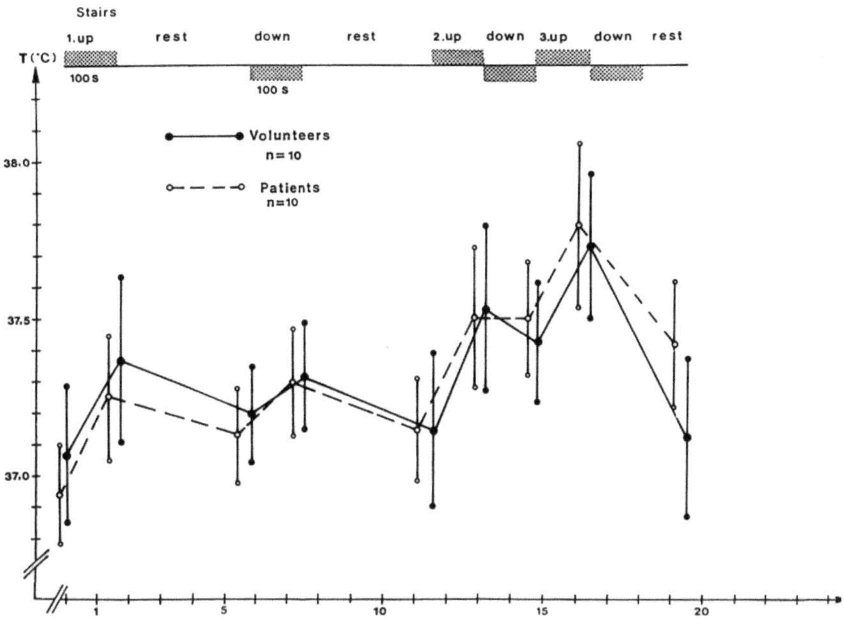

Fig. 3b Course of central venous blood temperature

Table 2. The slope (change per min.) of heart rate and temperature with different workloads

Workload (W)	No.	Average slope of heart rate (bmp/min)	Average slope of temperature (°C/min)
50	14	15.63±8.37	0.0573±0.0232
100	14	9.54±4.54	0.0784±0.0227
150	12	8.47±2.57	0.0829±0.0250
Decrease after exercise	14	–24.08±4.31	–0.2416±0.0655 –0.2416

The opposite behavior of a relatively fast increase in the heart rate with 50 W compared to the slower increase in temperature should be noted. With higher workloads this relationship changes. For effective rate control therefore the algorithm has to compensate for this opposite behavior by a substantially nonlinear slope featuring high gain at start of exercise and considerably lower gain with ongoing and higher workloads.

with repetitive exercises (Figs. 3a, b) [12]. The variations in heart rate with each single climbing of the stairs are about the same in healthy persons as in cardiac patients. Also, the central venous blood temperature shows a similar relative increase with each exercise, but each consecutive increase tops the previous increase resulting in the highest temperature after the third stress period. This is due to the fact that temperature does not return to the basic value with shortterm breaks between repetitive exercise. Additionally, the increase in temperature with a given exercise is not only a function of the external workload, but it is also influenced by the maximum achievable exercise capacity of the individual (Table 1) [3]. Also the speed of increase in temperature (slope of temperature over time, $\Delta T/dt$) varies with the workload (Table 2) [12].

Temperature Behavior in Pacemaker Patients and Control Algorithms

While the above-mentioned correlations between temperature changes and heart rate changes with constantly increasing workloads hold true for healthy persons, there is a different temperature response in patients with heart failure. Fig. 4 shows the temperature response in a female patient with heart failure performing exercises (climbing stairs). This example depicts that typically the overall temperature behavior and the heat dissipation mechanisms after the end of exercise are impaired in patients with heart failure. Their body temperature often reacts to the onset of exercise with an exaggerated and prolonged initial dip and remains relatively elevated for a substantial period after the end of exercise. Therefore, a sophisticated algorithm is needed to effect the correct control of the pacing rate by the measurement of central venous blood, despite individual variations such as different temperature slopes, different extent of temperature variations, different response time, and different temperature patterns in patients with heart failure [13].

A temperature-controlled pacemaker system (Nova MR VVI-R, Circadia DDD-R, Intermedics Inc., Angleton, TX, United States) developed in cooperation with our group, makes use of the observation that changes in central venous blood temperature under resting conditions have a different correlation to heart rate variations when

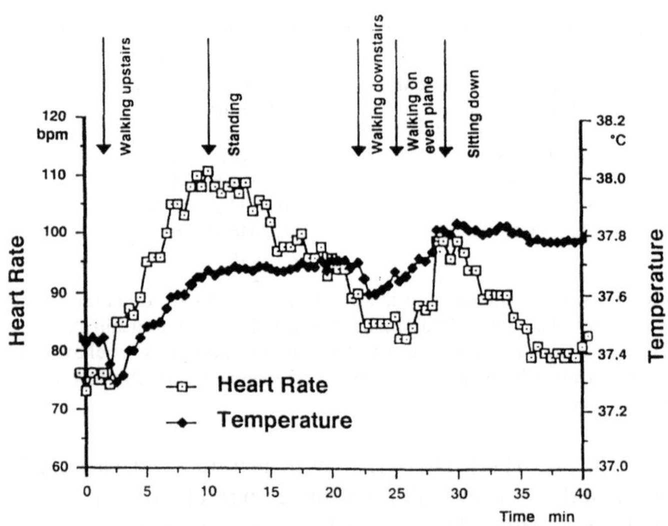

Fig. 4. Response to exercise of temperature and heart-rate patterns in an 80-year-old woman with a temperature-controlled rate-adaptive pacemaker (Nova MR, Intermedics Inc.). There is an initial temperature dip at the onset of climbing stairs; at the end of the staircase the temperature levels out. On the way downstairs there is again a slight initial temperature dip followed by a further increase. After the end of exercise the temperature remains elevated and shows only a slow decrease. This temperature pattern is typical of patients with impaired cardiac function. The temperature values and pacing-rate values were telemetered from the implanted pacemaker. The pacing-rate response shows that the initial temperature dip was detected correctly by the pacemaker, whereupon it induced an increase in heart rate to 85 beats/minute (according to the control algorithm), and this was followed by a further increase in the pacing rate on the way upstairs. The decrease in the pacing rate after the end of exercise despite a constant temperature is correct, as is the rate decrease after climbing stairs

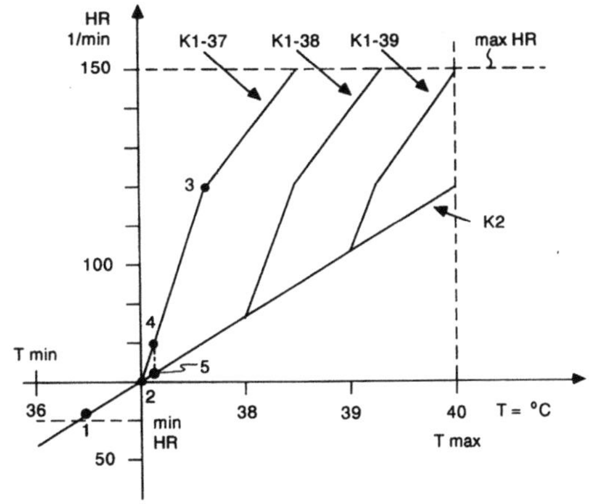

Fig. 5. Typical relationship between temperature (*T*) changes and heart rate (*HR*). The *line K2* depicts the relationship between absolute blood temperature and heart rate and corresponds to slow temperature changes, such as diurnal variations or fever. The *steep lines* (K1-37, K1-38 and K1-39) show the correlation between blood temperature changes and relative changes in heart rate under exercise conditions, taking into account the rate of change in temperature. The decision as to which of the two lines should be used for the pacemaker for rate control is made by constantly checking the rate of temperature change. Empirical observations have shown that the rate of temperature change with physical exercise significantly exceeds the rate of temperature changes in the case of diurnal variations or fever. *1*, shows a low temperature and heart rate at night; *2*, temperature and heart rate awakening in the morning; *3*, temperature and heart rate walking outside with physical exercise; *4*, exercise ceases and temperature has almost returned to the starting point; *5*, heart-rate response when the slightly elevated temperature remains constant when the rate drops back after exercise. Note the nonlinear response of heart rate to temperature with different levels of exercise

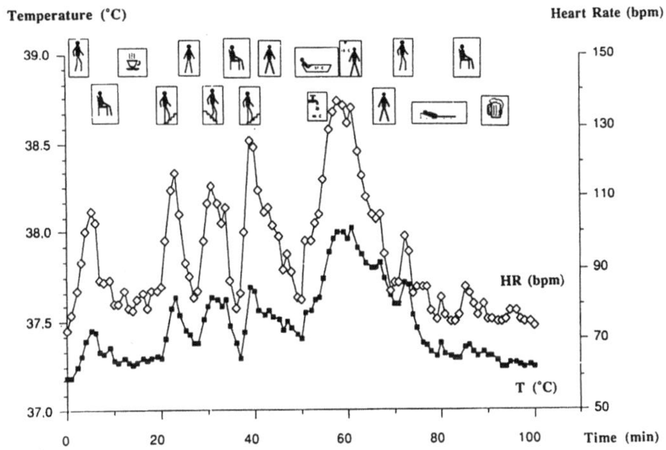

Fig. 6. Pacing rate (*HR*) and blood temperature (*T*) in a 63-year-old male patient with an implanted Nova MR temperature-controlled rate-adaptive pacemaker in an atrial position (AAI-R). The symbols show different kinds of activities within the follow-up of 100 min. A warm (37 °C) tub causes no considerable rate change while a hot (40 °C) tub effects a rate increase to more than 130 bpm. But this rate increase was not even noticed by the patient as the heart rate normally reacts to this thermal load to the body in a similiar way. The pacing rate and the intracardiac temperature were telemetrically obtained from the implanted pacemaker and continously recorded by an external recording (Teac R 71) device

compared to temperature changes under physical exercise. A control algorithm (Fig. 5) takes these varying correlations of temperature to heart rate into account and uses both. The absolute blood temperature and the relative change in blood temperature over a baseline value are both employed for rate control[14]. The change over time ($\Delta T/dt$) is used as a switch from the rest to the exercise correlation.

By means of the combination of relative temperature changes and absolute temperature values, the complex pattern of central venous blood temperature under different conditions can be covered effectively and turned into a beneficial rate response (Fig. 6) [14, 15].

There are two other pacemaker systems currently available that use the central venous blood temperature for rate control (Thermos; Biotronik, Berlin, Germany, and Kelvin 500, Cook, Leechburg, PA, USA). Initial experiences with the Kelvin system have been published recently following the first multicenter study [16]. While the first algorithm of the Biotronik Thermos could not cover the varying temperature profile resulting in only limited clinical value, the second generation algorithm is very similar to the Intermedics' algorithm.

Advantages and Disadvantages of Temperature-Controlled Pacing

The major advantage of rate control by central blood temperature is based on the fact that this parameter permits an insight into metabolic processes of the organism. Thus, rate control is feasible not only under conditions of physical exercise, but also during fever or metabolic variations due to, for example, changes in posture or to emotional stress.

The major disadvantage of the central blood temperature concept is that it requires a special pacing lead containing a thermistor. Initial experience with non standard electrodes of this type have shown that all three companies (Intermedics, Biotronik, and Cook) had problems with long-term stable detection of the temperature signal [17–18]. This was due primarily to the fact that high-quality insulation of the thermistor and stable electrical connection to the pacemaker is required in order to provide reliable long-term measurement with low current consumption (in the range of microamperes). Problems also originated from the tripolar lead and connector system which is still required to perform temperature measurements within the right ventricle at the moment. Since the bifurcated lead connector is still an "exotic" lead concept, it has not yet been widely accepted by the medical community.

Another disadvantage of temperature is its potentially slow reaction at the start of exercise. As temperature often decreases at the start of exercise, only pacemakers that can detect this initial dip and increase the rate by means of a so-called dip-response algorithm are capable of reacting within 15–30 s after commencement of exercise. Experience in the past has shown that the dip response is a beneficial way of shortening the reaction time of temperature-controlled pacemakers. A further advantage of the dip response is the ability of those pacemakers to react to changes in body posture, from supine to upright with a physiologically correct increase in pacing rate. Nevertheless, our data indicate that about only 50% of all initial temperature dips are correctly detected and turned into an increase in pacing rate by pacemakers currently in use [19, 20]. This holds especially true for patients with congestive heart failure, if they exercise with low workloads. For the future the combination of activity – as a fast-reacting parameter – with the slower reacting, but more physiologically adequate parameter temperature seems to be capable to enhance the concept of temperature controlled rate adaptive pacing considerably (Fig. 7) [21].

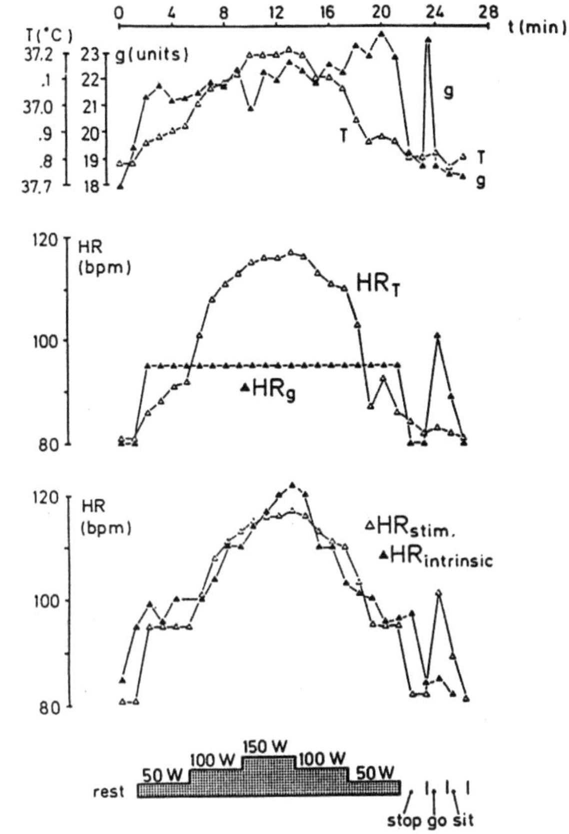

Fig. 7. Results with bicycle ergometry of increasing and decreasing workloads of 50, 100, 150, 100, and 50 W over 4 min each. In the volunteer RK the values of the acceleration sensor (*g*) in the *upper tracing* show an increasing course despite a reduction in workload. Since the volunteer was tired towards the end of the study, the acceleration values increased, following more intensive motion of the volunteer's body. Temperature in contrast features a more load dependent course (T) with an increase and a decrease depending on the workload. Neither of the pacing rates calculated according to only one of the parameters (HR_T, HR_g, middle tracing) is quiet correct. But the combination of both parameters (HR_{stim}) yields a rate response very similar to the course of the intrinsic sinus rate (lower tracing) ($HR_{intrinsic}$) *HR*, heart rate; *T*, temperature; *t*, time

The Future

In the future a flexible and small-diameter temperature lead (5-F) containing only one standard-sized tripolar connector could be a way of overcoming some of the currently existing objections in the medical community to use "exotic, non standard" leads [22]. New developments and concepts of this kind are currently being investigated.

References

1. Nielsen M (1938) Die Regulation der Körpertemperatur bei Muskelarbeit. Skand Arch 79/13:230-254
2. Maron MB, Wagner JA, Horvath SM (1977) Thermoregulatory responses during competitive marathon running. J Appl Physiol 42/6:909-914
3. Alt E, Hirgstetter C, Heinz M, Blömer H (1986) Rate control of physiological pacemakers by central venous blood temperature. Circulation 73/6:1206-1212

4. Alt E, Hirgstetter C, Heinz M, Theres H (1986) Measurement of right ventricular blood temperature during exercise as means of a rate control in physiological pacemakers. PACE 9/II:970-977
5. Brundin T (1975) Temperature of mixed venous blood during exercise. Scand J Clin Lab Invest 35:539-546
6. Brundin T (1978) Effects of betaadrenergic-receptor blockade on metabolic rate and mixed-venous blood temperature during dynamic exercise. Scand J Clin Lab Invest 38:229-232
7. Saltin B, Hermansen L (1966) Esophageal, rectal and muscle temperature during exercise. J Appl Physiol 21/6:1757
8. Nielsen B (1966) Regulation of body temperature and heat dissipation at different levels of energy and heat production in man. Acta Physiol Scand 68:215-227
9. Griffin JC, Jutzy KR, Claude JP et al. (1983) Central body temperature as a guide to optimal heart rate. PACE 6:498-506
10. Laskovics A (1984) The central venous blood temperature as a guide for rate control in pacemaker therapy. PACE 7:822-831
11. Hirgstetter C, Alt E, Theres H, Heinz M, Blömer H (1987) The exercise-induced increase in central venous blood temperature is a function of both work load and individual's maximum exercise capacity. PACE 10:1213
12. Alt E, Hirgstetter C, Heinz M, Theres H, Blömer H (1988) Central venous blood temperature for rate control of physiological pacemakers. J Cardiovasc Surg 29:80-88
13. Alt E, Theres H, Voelker R, Hirgstetter C, Heinz M (1987) Temperature-controlled rate-responsive pacing with the aid of an optimized algorithm. J Electrophysiol 6:481-489
14. Alt E, Völker R, Högl B, Blömer H (1987) Function of the temperature-controlled Nova MR pacemaker in patient's everyday live: preliminary clinical results. PACE 10:1206
15. Winter UJ, Holz B, Berge PG, Alt E, Treese N, Zegelman M, Klein H, Henry L (1990) Bicycle ergometry in the temperature-guided pacemaker Nova MR: comparison of the SSI- and SSI-R-mode. PACE 13:1215
16. Faernot NE, Smith HJ, Sellers D, Boal B (1989) Evaluation of the temperature response to exercise testing in patients with single-chamber, rate-adaptive pacemakers: a multicenter study. PACE 12:1806-1815
17. Volosin KJ, O'Connor WH, Fabiszewski R, Waxman HL (1989) Pacemaker-mediated tachycardia from a single-chamber temperature-sensitive pacemaker. PACE 12:1596-1599
18. Arakawa M, Kambara K, Ito H, Hirakawa S, Umaeda S, Hirose H (1989) Intermittent oversensing due to internal insulation damage of temperature-sensing rate-responsive pacemaker lead in subclavian veinpuncture method. PACE 12:1312-1316
19. Heinz M, Alt E, Hirgstetter C, Theres H (1987) The special behavior of central venous blood temperature at the onset of exercise -- disturbance or beneficial supplement for temperature-controlled rate-responsive pacemakers? PACE 10:1213
20. Heinz M, Alt E, Hirgstetter C, Theres H, Högl B (1988) Das Verhalten der zentralvenösen Bluttemperatur bei Belastungsbeginn -- Störfaktor oder sinnvolle Ergänzung temperaturabhängiger frequenzadaptiver Schrittmachersysteme? Herzschrittmacher 8:19-29
21. Alt E, Theres H, Heinz M, Matula M, Thilo R, Blömer H (1988) A new rate-modulated pacemaker system optimized by combination of two sensors. PACE 11:1119
22. Alt E, Höcherl H, Theres H, Heinz M (1990) A new multipolar pacemaker electrode connector based on bipolar IS 1 standard. PACE 13:1189

The QT Interval

A. F. Rickards[1], W. Boute[2], and M. J. S. Begemann[2]

Introduction

The QT interval as a sensor for rate-adaptive pacemakers was first mentioned in 1981. Initial testing showed that the QT interval shortened during exercise in patients with complete heart block and constant-rate ventricular pacemakers. A pacemaker capable of measuring and timing the evoked endocardial T wave was designed. Basically this pacemaker measures the stimulus to T wave interval.

The first generation of QT interval-sensing pacemakers showed encouraging results, but were hampered by two factors. The evoked T wave was sometimes difficult to detect because it was masked by polarization potentials which are generated at the electrode-tissue interface when a pacing pulse is delivered. It required the design of a special, dual-stimulus fast-recharge to eliminate these polarization potentials.

Secondly, the first algorithm was based on a linear relationship between the pacing interval and the QT interval. A relatively slow start in the rate increase at the beginning of exercise and non-exercise-related rate variations were sometimes reported and these phenomena could mainly be addressed to the linear type of algorithm.

Latest Generation QT Interval-Sensing Pacemakers

Later investigations showed that the relationship between the pacing interval and the QT interval is non-linear and this had significant consequences for the type of algorithm used in these pacemakers. The parameter that converts changes in the QT interval into changes in heart rate is known as the slope. A high slope causes the change in pacing rate to be fast and pronounced when the QT interval changes. Conversely a low slope causes a slower and smaller change in the pacing rate. The slope was constant in the first generation while it is rate-dependent in the latest generation of QT interval-sensing pacemakers (Fig. 1).

Comparing the two different slopes, constant and rate-dependent, can help to

[1] Royal Brompton and National Heart Hospital, Sydney Street, London SW3 6NP, UK
[2] Vitatron Medical B.V., Technical Division, 6950 AB Dierens, Netherlands

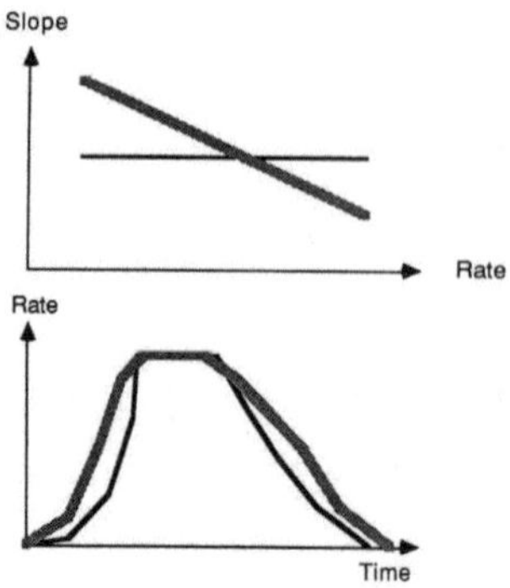

Fig. 1. The inverse relationship of slope and heart rate (high slope with lower heart rates, decreasing slope with higher heart rates) provide a more adequate rate profile (*top* figure, *bold* line) compared to the linear slope used with older generations of QT interval pacemakers

explain the difficulties mentioned earlier. At low-pacing rates the constant slope was lower than the rate-dependent slope, causing the slow response at the onset of exercise. However, at higher-pacing rates the situation was inverse, causing the pacing rate to increase rapidly to the upper rate limit.

The rate-dependent slope is relatively high at low-pacing rates, causing a faster response when exercise starts. The slope decreases as the pacing rate increases causing a more gradual approach towards the upper rate limit.

The QT interval is influenced by both metabolic demand (independent of heart rate) and heart rate itself. If the heart rate increases, the QT interval will decrease and vice versa (positive feedback). Any increase in metabolic demand will shorten the QT interval; the pacemaker will react by increasing the pacing rate. However, this increase in pacing rate will again cause the QT interval to shorten further. Will this loop not result in an endless increase in the pacing rate until the programmed upper rate limit is reached? The answer is no, providing that the slope is programmed correctly.

The fact that the QT interval is also heart rate dependent can provide the pacemaker with valuable information concerning the maximal allowable slope that causes a stable rate response. The next example will illustrate this.

Setting of the Slope (Change in Pacing Rate Following Changes in QT Interval)

The QT interval in a given patient was measured at rest and at different pacing rates. The rate dependency of the QT interval was found to be 1 ms pulses per minute (ppm), in other words, every ppm heart rate increase will cause the QT interval to shorten by 1 ms (heart rate influence). We assume a low and constant level of exercise that causes a constant exercise related, QT interval-shortening of 1 ms. At two different slope settings we will obtain different types of rate response (Fig. 2 and Table 1).

From this example it can be seen that the slope of 0.8 ppm/ms results in a stable and limited rate response to this low-level constant exercise, while the slope of 1.2 ppm/ms tends to accelerate the pacing rate faster and faster until the programmed upper rate limit is reached. In general the maximum slope that still produces a stable rate response is set by the inverse of the QT interval rate-dependency.

Table 1. Rate dependency of the QT interval

Slope ppm/ms	QT interval (ms) Rest	Exercise	Rate (ppm) Rest	Exercise	Difference
0.8	400.0	399.0	70.0	70.8	+0.8
	399.0	398.2	70.8	71.4	+0.6
	398.2	397.6	71.4	71.9	+0.5
	397.6	397.1	71.9	72.3	+0.4
1.2	400.0	399.0	70.0	71.2	+1.2
	399.0	397.8	71.2	72.4	+1.4
	397.8	396.4	72.4	74.1	+1.7
	396.4	394.7	74.1	76.1	+2.0

The QT interval rate-dependency can be easily measured by simply pacing at two different rates and measuring the subsequent QT intervals. From this information the pacemaker can calculate and automatically set its slope parameter value close to the maximal value to obtain the fastest possible rate response.

Effects Other than Metabolic Needs and Heart Rate

It is also known that the QT interval is influenced by many factors other than metabolic demand and heart rate. Various types of antiarrhythmic drugs have the ability to change the QT interval. However, most of these influences only affect the absolute length of the QT interval. The pacemaker is designed to react only on relative changes in the QT interval, no matter what the absolute value is.

Secondly, when taken orally, all antiarrhythmic drugs have a very slow effect on the changes of the QT interval. A numerical filter as part of the rate-adaptive algorithm eliminates these extremely slow changes and only passes relatively fast changes – as a result of exercise and/or emotional stress – to the algorithm to cause a rate response.

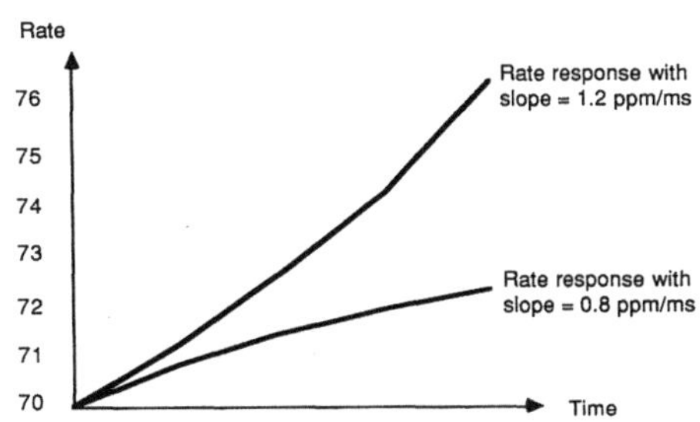

Fig. 2. A slope of 1.2 ppm/ms shortening of the QT interval conditions a too fast and too extensive rate increase resulting in rate oscillations between the lower and upper pacing rate limits. Since the pure rate associated with the shortening of the QT interval is 1 ms/ppm, a slope of 0.8 ppm/ms provides a stable and workload-related increase in pacing rate

Using the QT Interval for Automatic Adjustment of the Refractory Period

The T wave is the electrocardiographic marker for the myocardial repolarization phase. Therefore, the end of the T wave also marks the end of the myocardial refractoriness and from this time on one can expect early depolarizations (PVCs). QT interval-sensing pacemakers detect the downslope of the evoked T wave. The pacemaker's pace-refractory period automatically ends 25 ms after the detection of the T wave on a beat-to-beat basis. Such algorithm implies that the pace-refractory period is relatively long when the patient is at rest and shortens automatically during exercise. This then guarantees the detection of early PVCs indipendent of the current pacing rate by means of this automatic adjustment of the refractory period.

Combining QT Interval Sensing with Activity Sensing

After more than 8 years of experience with different types of sensors it has become clear that none of the sensors presently available has ideal characteristics. Advanced sensors, such as oxygen saturation might approach the requirements of an ideal sensor, but a highly specialized lead, the deminished sensitivity to more rigorous exercise, the lack of long-term stability and reliable data slow the introduction of such systems. Combining sensors are the logical next step.

The best combinations would be a physiological sensor and an activity sensor. All of the presently available physiological sensors (QT interval, temperature and minute ventilation) show a somewhat delayed response when exercise starts. However, when exercise continues these sensors provide excellent information which is highly proportional with the workload level. In addition, these sensors provide the pacemaker with information after the cessation of exercise, enabling the pacemaker to decrease the pacing rate according to the metabolic needs of the patient. Adding an activity-type sensor offers the possibility of improving the onset of rate response if the algorithm is designed to use the activity information, especially at low-pacing rates. As the pacing rate increases the information from the physiological sensor should become more and more important (Sensor Blending).

Sensor cross-checking is another important aspect of multisensor systems. Important conclusions can be drawn if only one of the sensor indicates activity while the others do not. For example, if the activity sensor indicates body activity and the physiological sensor does not confirm this we most probably are dealing with external vibration type artefacts. The pacemaker then could respond (after the initial rate increase caused by the activity sensor) by slowly decreasing the rate towards the rate that is indicated by the physiological sensor.

In September 1990 the first dual-sensor investigational pacemaker was implanted in a patient, combining QT interval sensing and activity sensing in a single pacemaker system. Topaz^{TM}, the first dual sensor pacemaker combining QT and activity has now been released for routine application in Europe. Several hundred of this innovative devices have been implanted by end of 1992 with excellent clinical results.

Closed-Loop Rate-Adaptive Pacemaker Based on the Ventricular Evoked Response

I. SINGER[1], B. M. STEINHAUS[2], and J. KUPERSMITH[3]

Ventricular Depolarization Gradient

The concept of the ventricular gradient was first proposed by Wilson et al. in the early 1930s [1]. Briefly, Wilson's gradient hypothesis states that by integrating surface electrocardiographic tracings, indirect measures of activation and recovery dispersion can be derived. Based on the analyses of the surface ECG tracings, it has been demonstrated that the area under the QRS complex reflects the spatial distribution of ventricular activation times, and that the QRST integral reflects the spatial distribution of action potential durations. Both measures represent true physical gradients which can be represented by a vector which has a magnitude and a direction. The QRS integral magnitude reflects the activation time difference from sites of early to sites of late activation. The QRS integral vector direction is from sites of early to sites of late activation. Similarly, the QRST integral vector direction is from sites of short to sites of long action potential duration. The magnitude of the QRST vector reflects action potential dispersion within the myocardium.

The gradient concept has been applied to develop a fully automatic pacing system. The rate-adaptive pacing scheme is based on a gradient analysis of the paced ventricular evoked response obtained from a permanent transvenous pacemaker lead. The ventricular depolarization gradient (Gd) is the peak negative amplitude of the time integral of the evoked potential and represents the area under the evoked (pacemaker-induced) R wave (Fig. 1). Pacing rate and either physiological or exercise stress produce opposing effects on Gd [2]. In addition, recent studies suggest that an intrinsic mechanism may exist that maintains Gd constant during homeostatic disturbances [2]. This finding has been employed in a closed-loop rate-adaptive pacing system. A decrease in Gd results in an increase in paced heart rate, while an increase in Gd results in a decrease in paced heart rate. True closed-loop control is thus possible due to the negative feedback effect of heart rate.

[1] Cardiovascular Division; University of Louisville School of Medicine, Louisville, Ky, USA
[2] Telectronics Pacing Systems, Englewood, Co, USA
[3] Department of Medicine, Michigan State University, East Lansing, MI

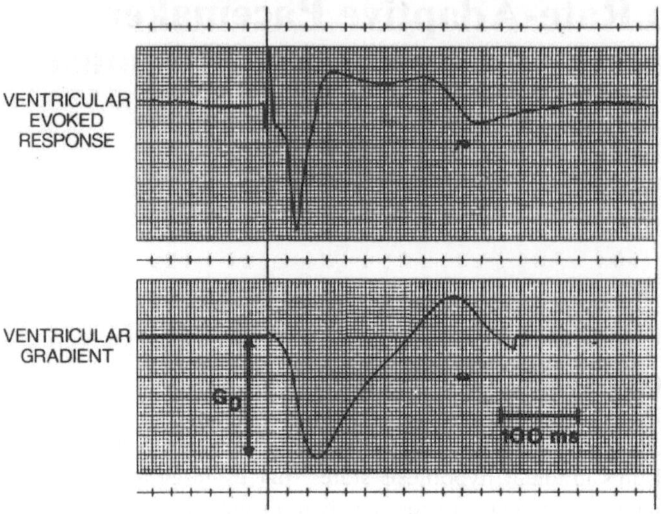

Fig. 1. The ventricular-evoked response and its gradient. The ventricular depolarization gradient (*Gd*) is the peak negative amplitude of the evoked response integral and represents the area under the evoked R wave. (From [2])

Effects of Exercise Stress, Pacing Rate and Other Interventions on Ventricular Depolarization Gradient

Callaghan et al. studied the effect of exercise stress and pacing rate on Gd [2]. In heart-blocked dogs paced at a fixed rate, exercise stress caused a decrease in Gd. The mean percent change was –10.8 ± 4.0% (range –4.5% to –16.7%). The response time from exercise onset to the time of maximum change in Gd ranged from 19.0 to 40.0 s (mean 27.9 ± 6.6 s). Postexercise recovery was uniformly longer in duration than the exercise-onset response time and ranged from 33.3 to 84.0 s (mean 54.1 ± 16.4 s). On the other hand, an elevation in pacing rates in dogs at rest produced a significant increase in Gd.

Epinephrine infusion in pentobarbital-anesthetized dogs produced a decrease in Gd which was dose-dependent [2]. Doubling the epinephrine concentration from 2.5 to 5.0 μg/kg increased the Gd change by 22% at the paced heart rate of 150 beats per minute (bpm). At a higher pacing rate of 190 bpm, the doubling of epinephrine concentration increased Gd change by 71%. Thus, epinephrine decreases the depolarization gradient in a dose-dependent fashion.

Callaghan et al. studied the effects of pentobarbital anesthesia on the change in Gd in response to increased pacing rate [2]. Pentobarbital was found to attenuate sensitivity of Gd to paced heart rates by an average of 38%.

In the same study [2], the effect of exercise on Gd was studied in healthy dogs with intact conduction. The mean percent change in the Gd was –0.24% (range –2.7% to 1.85%) and was not significantly different from the resting state. Thus, Gd remains largely unchanged during exercise in healthy dogs with normal conduction.

Mechanisms Underlying Changes in the Ventricular Depolarization Gradient

Recent studies have shown that Gd, in addition to being inversely related to conduction velocity [1], is also directly related to the ventricular mass [3, 4]. Exercise at a fixed heart rate causes an increase in sympathetic tone and circulating catecholamines. Catecholamines increase myocardial contractility [5,6] and thus, exercise leads to an increase in venous blood return and an increase in end-diastolic dimensions [7]. The resulting decrease in ventricular wall thickness, in addition to the reported direct effect of catecholamines to increase conduction velocity [8–11], would account for the decreased Gd measured during exercise and during epinephrine infusion. In contrast, increased pacing rate at rest would decrease the diastolic filling time, stroke volume [12, 13], and end-diastolic dimensions. Thus, the expected increase in ventricular wall thickness, as well as the effect of high-rate pacing to reduce conduction velocity [14], would account for the increased Gd measured during increased pacing rate. The factors which attenuate this effect by pentobarbital anesthesia have not been fully identified, but may be related to the influence of the anesthesia on changes in ventricular volume with changes in pacing rate. A similar blunting of the hemodynamic responses to isoproternol by pentobarbital anesthesia has been reported [15].

Prism-CL Model 450A Rate-Responsive Pacemaker

The Gd concept was incorporated in the design of the Prism-CL model 450A ventricular rate-responsive pacemaker. High-fidelity recordings of the ventricular-evoked response are acquired from a three electrode system comprised of the pacemaker case and the two electrodes of a bipolar endocardial lead. Alert period sensing is bipolar (tip^+, $ring^-$). Stimulation is unipolar (tip to case), followed by a brief electronic short-circuit of the output amplifier of 10 ms (charge dump). This permits a passive discharge of the output-coupling capacitor and reduces poststimulus polarization. An evoked response window occurs following the charge dump during which the evoked response may be amplified and integrated. Evoked-response sensing is unipolar from the ring electrode (referenced to the case), Fig. 2. Since the ring electrode is not used for stimulation, its tissue interface is not polarized by the stimulus.

Two unique features of Prism-CL pacemaker are: (1) rate-responsive pacing based on a closed-loop system using the concept of depolarization gradient of the endocardial-evoked response, and (2) automatic output regulation.

The rate response is controlled by Gd. The effect of exercise and emotional stress on Gd are opposite to the effect of an increase in heart rate on Gd and they establish a physiological negative feedback mechanism. The paced rate is adjusted to maintain a constant Gd. The Gd is also called the rate control parameter (RCP) and the constant "target" RCP is analogous to a set point in any control system. The RCP is measured every fourth cycle and compared to the target RCP.

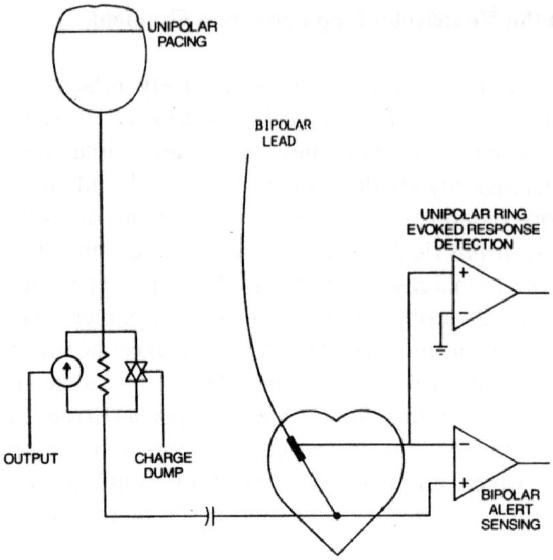

Fig. 2. The evoked-response detection method: pacing is unipolar with charge dump, and alert-period sensing is bipolar. Following charge dump, the unipolar ventricular-evoked response is amplified and electronically integrated from the ring electrode. (From [2])

If the measured RCP is less than the target RCP, the pacing rate is increased. If the measured RCP is greater than the target RCP, the pacing rate is decreased.

The target RCP is automatically determined by an initialization process of approximately 20 paced beats when rate response is first programmed on automatic. An automatic calibration procedure adjusts the target RCP to compensate for shifts in baseline conditions due to lead maturation or to the possible effects of drug therapy.

Automatic capture verification and threshold search provide output regulation of the pacemaker. Capture verification automatically checks for successful ventricular capture following pacing. If loss of capture is detected, the pacemaker output is incrementally increased on a beat-by-beat basis until capture is regained and a pacing safety margin added. A 10 mA/1ms backup pulse is issued at every cycle where loss of capture is detected. The threshold search occurs approximately every 12 h and determines the pacing threshold where capture is consistently obtained (Fig. 3). If the

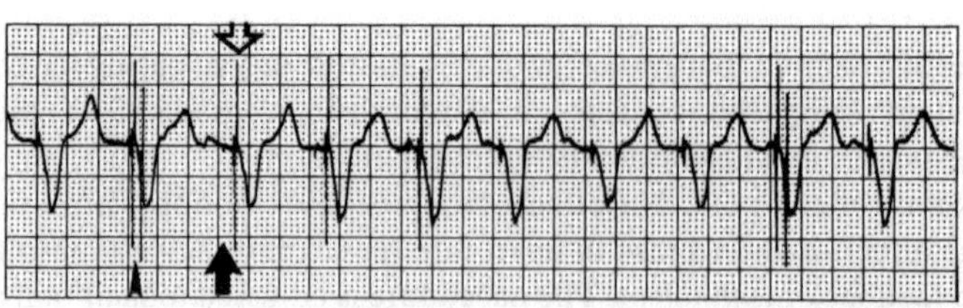

Fig. 3. An example of a threshold test. Each noncaptured beat (*thick black arrow*) is followed by a back-up pulse (*thick white arrow*) until the output is augmented sufficiently to regain capture. Double lines (*small dark arrowhead*) represent a "signature" to indicate the beginning and the end of the test

capture threshold plus the pacing output safety margin exceed the maximum output values for evoked response detection (5 mA/1ms), "STAT SET" safety pacing is initiated (10 mA/1ms).

Clinical Results with Prism-CL 450A Pacemaker

Phase 1 clinical trials of the Prism-CL model 450A pacemaker began in September 1988 in Europe and have subsequently been expanded to the United States and Canada. The device is in phase 2 of the clinical study at the beginning of 1991. The initial experience with the pacemaker has already been reported [16-18]. As of March 1990, 123 patients have received a Prism-CL pacemaker. The average age of the patients was 71±11 years (43-83 years) with the male to female ratio being 2:1. The left ventricular ejection fraction was 54±17% (12%-80%) and according to the New York Heart Association functional classification 25% of the patients belonged to class 1, 52% to class 2, 19% to class 3, and 4% to class 4. The average number of days postimplant was 303 (5-592). The diagnosis was sick sinus syndrome in the majority of patients (44%). Other diagnoses included second or third degree heart block (23%), symptomatic sinus arrest (17%), chronotropic incompetence (14%), and carotid hypersensitivity (2%). The majority of patients are alive (95%). The causes of death in the six patients were congestive heart failure (3), pulmonary emboli unrelated to the pacemaker lead (1), noncardiac cause (1), and an unexplained cause in one patient, who died during sleep.

Response to Exercise. Phase 1 patients underwent rigorous treadmill testing within 1 month of the implant date. In all patients, the paced heart rate increased appropriately from the mean baseline rate of 75 ± 9 bpm to a maximum paced heart rate of 127 ± 14 bpm ($p < 0.0001$). The upper rate was limited by the programmed limit which was left to the investigator's discretion. A representative example of an exercise response is illustrated in Fig. 4.

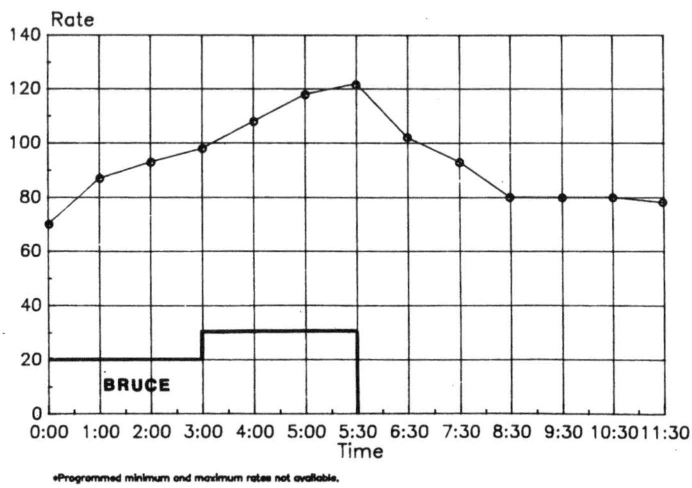

Fig. 4. An example of a typical exercise response in a patient with the Prism-CL 450A pacemaker 29 days after implant. Note a prompt and brisk response to exercise and appropriate rate deceleration with exercise termination. *Ordinate* represents paced heart rate (BPM) and *abscissa* time

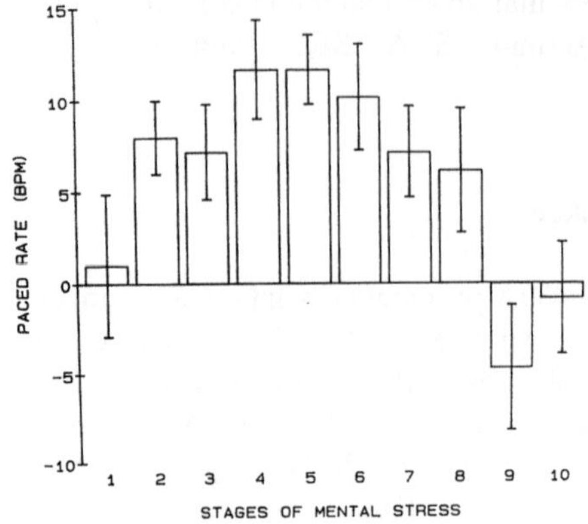

Fig. 5. Heart-rate response to mental stress. Stages of mental stress protocol are plotted on the *abscissa* and paced heart rates (adjusted to the baseline pacing rate) on the *ordinate*. Changes in peaked heart rates are significant ($p < 0.05$, analysis of variance)

Response to Mental Activity/Stress. The heart-rate response to mental stress has been studied in patients implanted with Prism-CL pacemakers [16–18]. In one study [18, 19], eight patients were tested using a mental stress protocol while resting supine in a quiet environment with dimmed lighting to minimize the external sensory input. The protocol consisted of ten stages: baseline recording (stage 1), performing difficult arithmetic tasks (stages 2-6), talking about a stressful event (stage 7), talking about a positive event (stage 8), thinking positive thoughts with no talking (stage 9), and reassurance of the patients test performance by the test coordinator (stage 10). Results are summarized in Fig. 5. In response to mental stress, whether due to performing difficult arithmetic tasks or talking about either stressful or positive events, the paced heart rate increased, although the magnitude of the rate increase differed from patient to patient. Similar responses to mental stress were also reported by Paul et al. [17]. In response to positive thinking the paced rate decreased, while in response to reassurance the rate returned to near baseline values.

These findings suggest that the Gd can be modulated by sympathetic autonomic response. The specific mechanism of the pacing rate changes due to mental stress has not been identified, but is most likely related to changes in Gd secondary to changes in either circulatory or locally released catecholamines [2].

Response to Postural Changes. The heart-rate response to postural changes was assessed using a tilt table by Paul et al. [17]. When patients were tilted from a standing to a supine position a prompt increase in paced rate was observed. When the baseline rate was elevated, there was a prompt decrease in paced rate when patients were tilted from supine to standing. The mechanism of these paradoxical effects have not been studied, but may be due to alterations in right ventricular preload causing changes in end-diastolic ventricular dimensions.

Response to a Beta$_1$-Selective Antagonist (Esmolol). The heart-rate response to the beta$_1$-selective blocker esmolol was studied in six Prism-CL patients who were in a supine resting state (Fig. 6) [18]. Bolus infusion of esmolol (500 μ/kg) over 1 min increased the mean paced heart rate from 70 ± 7 to 85 ± 6 bpm ($p < 0.05$). Peak

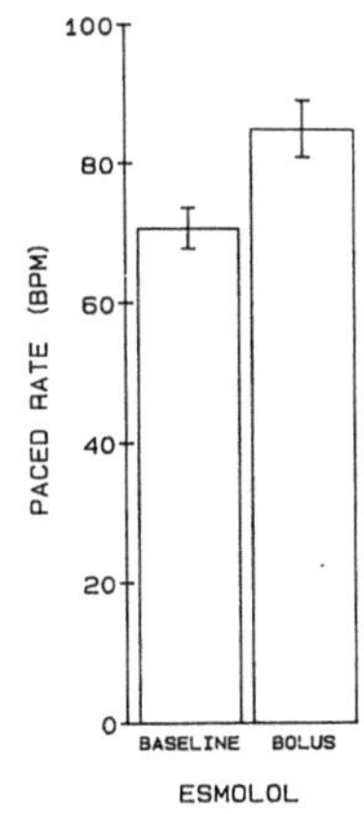

Fig. 6. Response to bolus infusion of esmolol. Paced heart rate is shown on the ordinate and increased significantly in response to esmolol (mean ± SE), $p < 0.05$

paced heart rates similarly increased during esmolol infusion of 75–125 μg/kg per minute (69 ± 5 vs 84 ± 11 bpm, $p < 0.05$). Continuous blood pressure monitoring showed no significant changes in systolic or diastolic blood pressures during either the bolus or continuous esmolol infusions.

Esmolol is an ultrashort time-constant beta_1-selective antagonist (t 1/2 of 9 min) [20]. In a normal heart, esmolol would decrease both the sinus and atrioventricular nodal intrinsic rates. In the patients with implanted Prism-CL pacemakers, a paradoxical effect occurred where esmolol infusion increased the pacing rate. The increased pacing rate suggests that esmolol may have a direct effect in decreasing Gd. This hypothesis was tested in dogs by recording evoked potential waveforms at a fixed pacing rate during control saline infusion and bolus infusion of esmolol. Shown in Fig. 7 are example unipolar waveforms from the tip electrode (panel A) and from the ring electrode (panel B) of a bipolar pacing catheter in the right ventricular apex. Comparing the waveforms during control (solid lines) with the waveforms post esmolol infusion (broken lines) demonstrates that esmolol infusion reduces the Gd recorded from both the tip and ring electrode. This finding was supported in the three other dogs studied. The results provide a mechanism for the increased pacing rate in the patients with Prism-CL pacemakers following infusion of esmolol. It is interesting to note that propranolol, another beta antagonist, does not effect the Gd in this manner. The underlying effect of esmolol on the factors which alter Gd and the reason for the difference between esmolol and propranolol are unknown, although alteration in myocardial contractility or alteration in right ventricular preload can be suspected.

Response to Antiarrhythmic Drugs. Although the effects of antiarrhythmic drugs on Gd are unpublished, theoretical considerations suggest that agents which alter myocardial conduction velocity would influence rate response based on the Gd measurement. For example, the rapid infusion of an antiarrhythmic drug which decreases conduction velocity, e.g., amiodarone or any class 1 antiarrhythmic drug, would tend to increase Gd and thus decrease the pacing rate. Since the RCP automatic calibration adjusts the target RCP in the direction of the drifts in RCP, it is unlikely that orally administered antiarrhythmic drugs would result in any significant and/or substained alteration in pacing rate.

Limitations of the Prism-CL Pacemaker

During the clinical trial with the Prism-CL pacemaker, several limitations became apparent. The most troubling feature was that the pacemaker automatically switched to fixed rate (STAT-SET) pacing at the maximal output (10 mA/1ms). The STAT-SET mode was appropriate in some patients due to lead dislodgement (3%), but in some patients it was inappropriate (13%) [18]. Although this did not result in any adverse patient reaction, in those patients in whom STAT-SET occurred, the pacemaker did not have the intended rate-responsive function until after reprogramming the pacemaker. The major cause of STAT-SET was the inaccurate classification of captured ventricular beats as noncaptured beats. An example of this false-negative capture classification is shown in Fig. 8. In some patients, the resulting output augmentation inappropriately resulted in triggering the STAT-SET pacing mode when the output exceeded the 5 mA/1ms threshold. This limitation was due to the 60 ms time window for capture recognition in the pacemaker (software version 20.5). When this problem was recognized, the time window for capture recognition was extended to 75 ms (software version 20.6).

Although this helped to decrease the number of patients with false-negative capture classifications, a further extension of the time window was necessary for the correct capture detection in some patients. The most recent pacemaker software allows the

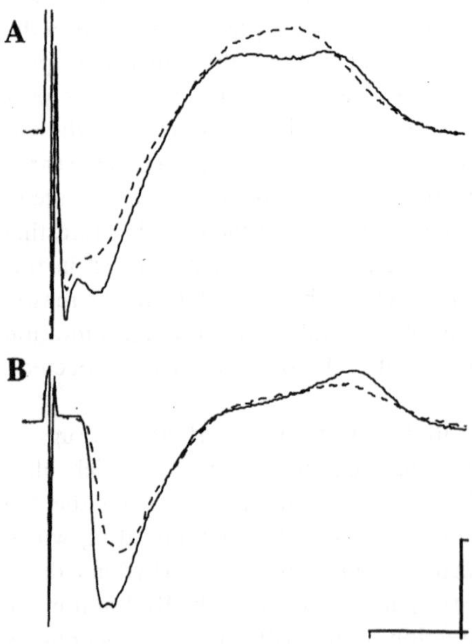

Fig. 7. Evoked potential recordings during control (*solid lines*) and during infusion of esmolol (*broken lines*) from the catheter tip (*panel A*) and catheter ring (*panel B*) Pacing Stimulus can be seen as the first fast deflections from the baseline. Calibration bars are 50 ms and 15 mV

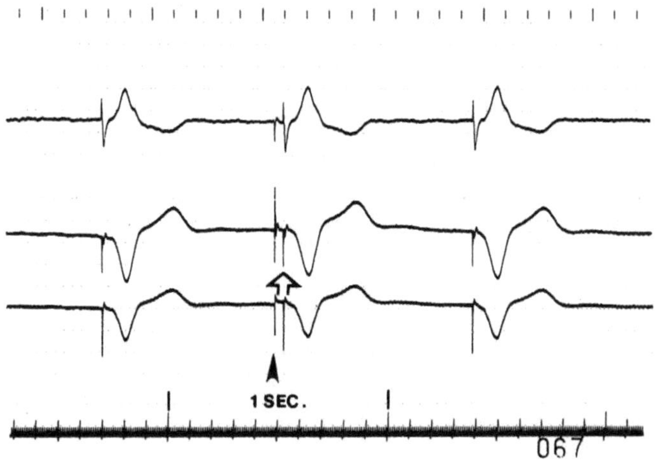

Fig. 8. An example of a false-negative classification of a captured beat. Note that despite an appropriate ventricular capture (*black arrow*) the beat was classified as non-capture and a backup pulse was issued (*open arrow*). Survace leads I, II and aVf are shown

physician to program the interval up to 125 ms. Another cause of STAT-SET was low RCP values. Because of design limitations in the pacemaker, RCP values below 160 μV/s could not be reliably measured and automatically triggered the STAT-SET pacing mode.

Nevertheless, in the majority of patients, the algorithms performed reliably and appropriately. Based on a recent review of the data [18], the majority of patients have both the rate response and autothreshold functions turned on and both algorithms functioned appropriately (Table 1).

Future Developments

Future developments of rate-adaptive pacing based on the ventricular-evoked response will allow rate response using a unipolar pacing lead. In this application, polarization artifact due to the pacing stimulus must be minimized to the level that accurate evoked potential recordings during depolarization can be obtained from the same electrode site as that used for stimulation. In this regard, promising results have been reported which utilize a triphasic stimulus pulse and an automatic algorithm that issues a test stimulus in the refractory period to balance out the polarization artifact [21, 22]. The evoked potentials shown in Fig. 7 were obtained using a computer-based

Table 1. Percentage of Prism-CL patients with algorithm enabled depending on the type of software implemented

Software version	No. of patients	RR (%)	AT (%)	RR+AT (%)	STAT-SET (%)
20.5	22	82	77	55	32.1
20.6	101	86	93	70	11.2

RR, rate-responsive function; *AT*, automatic threshold adjustment.

pacing system emulator which executed such an algorithm. The polarization artefact was successfully balanced out and resulted in an accurate recording of the evoked potential from the ring electrode, as well as from the tip electrode. This type of system will also provide a robust automatic threshold verification algorithm. Note that the morphology of the evoked potential from the tip-pacing site does not show the characteristic poststimulus isoelectric time seen in the evoked potential from a nearby ring electrode (refer to Fig. 7). Thus, for automatic output regulation, the patient-to-patient variability in the capture time window setting for the Prism-CL pacemaker will not be an issue when using the evoked potential from the tip. This development, as well as new hardware designs which allow a much greater range in RCP values, will allow the utility of the pacing system to be applied to a wider range of patients.

Future development will also extend evoked potential recordings and rate response to dual-chamber pacing systems. In one application, evoked potentials recorded from atrial-pacing catheters will be able to provide automatic output regulation for pacing the atrial chamber. Preliminary research results have been reported [23]. In other applications, dual-chamber pacing with a decreased atrioventricular delay could be utilized to remove the ambiguity in the ventricular-evoked potential due to fusion beats.

Future research studies will need to fully explore and identify the independent factors which are responsible for the modulation of the ventricular-evoked response Gd parameter. Factors such as lead maturation, cardioactive drugs, hemodynamic changes, and other influences separate from sympathetic tone need to be studied in humans.

Undoubtedly, these studies will lead to future developments utilizing the evoked potential waveform which go beyond the applications in rate-responsive pacing. For example, the evoked potential could be used for "noninvasive" drug monitoring and control of cardiac antiarrhythmic drugs which influence myocardial conduction velocity. Obviously, it is an exciting time for research into the relatively new and unexplored evoked potential parameter of cardiac electrophysiology.

References

1. Wilson F, Macleod AG, Barker P et al. (1934) The determination and the significance of the areas of the ventricular deflections of the electrocardiogram. Am Heart J 10:46-61
2. Callaghan F, Vollmann W, Livingston A et al. (1989) The ventricular depolarization gradient: effects of exercise, pacing rate, epinephrine, and intrinsic heart-rate control on the right ventricular evoked response. PACE 12:1115-1130
3. Plonsey RA (1979) A contemporary view of the ventricular gradient of Wilson. J Electrocardio 12:337-341
4. Steinhaus BM, Nappholz TA (1990) The information content of the cardiac electrogram at the stimulus site. Proc Ann Conf IEEE Eng Med Biol Soc 12:129-131
5. Rushmer RF, Smith OA Kr, Lasher EP (1960) Neural mechanisms of cardiac control during exertion. Physiol Rev 40 [Suppl 4]:27-34
6. Rushmer RF (1976) Cardiovascular dynamics, 4th edn. Saunders, Philadelphia
7. Sedney MI, Weyers E, Van Der Wall EE et al. (1989) Short-term and long-term changes of left ventricular volumes during rate-adaptive and single-rate pacing. PACE 12:1863-1868

8. Wallace AG (1963) Sympathetic influences on conduction in the intact heart. Fed Proc 22:578 (abstr)
9. Siebens AA, Hoffman BF, Enson Y et al. (1953) Effects of 1-epinephrine and 1-norepinephrine on cardiac excitability. Am J Physiol 175:1-7
10. Wallace AG, Sarnoff SJ (1964) Effects of cardiac sympathetic nerve stimulation on conduction in the heart. Circ Res 14:86-92
11. Randall WC, Priola DV (1965) Sympathetic influences on synchrony of myocardial contraction. In: Randall WC (ed) Nervous control of the heart. Williams and Wilkins, Baltimore, pp 214-244
12. Ross J Jr, Linhart JW, Braunwald E (1965) Effects of changing heart rate in man by electrical stimulation of the right atrium. Circulation XXXII:549-558
13. Benchimol A, Li Y, Diamond EG (1964) Cardiovascular dynamics in complete heart block at various heart rates. Circulation 30:542-553
14. Viersma JW, Bouman LN, Mater M (1968) Frequency, conduction velocity, and rate of depolarization in rabbit auricles. Nature 217:1176-1177
15. Cox RH (1972) Influence of pentobarbital anesthesia on cardiovascular function in trained dogs. Am J Physiol 223:651-659
16. Singer I, Olash J, Brennon AF et al. (1989) Initial clinical experience with a rate-responsive pacemaker. PACE 12:1458-1464
17. Paul V, Garratt C, Ward DE, Camm AJ (1989) Closed-loop control of rate-adaptive pacing: clinical assessment of a system analyzing the ventricular depolarization gradient. PACE 12:1896-1902
18. Singer I, Camm J, Brown R et al. (1990) Results with Prism-CL rate-modulating pacemaker. Rev Eur Technol Biomed 12:17
19. Singer I, Guinn V, Olash J et al. (1989) Effects of stress, experience and ß-blockade on the Prism-CL rate-modulating pacemaker. Clin Res 37:888A
20. Greenspan AM, Spielman SR, Horowitz LN et al. (1988) The electrophysiologic properties of esmolol, a short-acting beta-blocker. Int J Clin Pharmacol Ther Toxical 26:209-216
21. Curtis AB, Vance F, Shifrin K (1990) A successful method for minimizing stimulus polarization artifact for accurate evaluation of intracardiac evoked potentials. PACE 13:519
22. Curtis AB, Vance F, Miller-Shifrin K (1990) Characteristic variation in evoked potential amplitude with changes in pacing stimulus strength. Am J Cardiol 66:416-422
23. Livingston AR, Callaghan FJ, Byrd CL et al. (1988) Atrial capture detection with endocardial electrodes. PACE 11:1770-1776

Impedance-Derived Cardiac Signals: Preejection Interval, Stroke Volume and Ventricular Peak Ejection Rate for Rate – Adaptive Pacing and Antitachyarrhythmia Devices

R. CHIRIFE[1]

Introduction

Relative right ventricular volume changes can be detected by means of impedance techniques using conventional pacing electrodes. Therefore it is natural to think of it as a source of hemodynamic parameters applicable to sensor-driven rhythm control devices. The technique for obtaining a volume-related signal has been presented in depth by numerous authors [1–4] with significant differences on the number of electrodes employed and the hardware and software used for processing the signal.

Technical Considerations

The impedance method for blood-volume detection consists of driving an AC signal through a pair of intraventricular electrodes and measuring the resulting voltage from a different pair, also in the ventricular cavity. The measured voltage would thus be inversely proportional to the ventricular impedance. The impedance at the sensing pair of electrodes (Z) would consequently be a function of the blood volume (V), the distance between the electrodes (d), blood resistivity (r), and other factors. Likewise, blood volume between the sensing electrodes could be approximated by the formula [3] $V = rd^2/Z$.

For absolute volume measurements, several pairs of electrodes are used. If relative volume changes are sufficient, a standard bipolar and possibly even a unipolar lead configuration may be used. [5, 6]

A diagram of the circuitry generally employed for right ventricular volume detection for rate-adaptive pacing is shown in Fig. 1. A tripolar lead is used in order to improve the signal-to-noise ratio, since it is known that tieing the driving and sensing electrodes together intensifies unwanted local electrode-tissue interface motion artefacts. Using a tripolar lead, the driving of the AC signal is done between the case and the tip, and the sensing of the resulting impedance between the two rings. Volume

[1] Electrophysiology and Pacemaker Section, Institute of Cardiology, National Academy of Medicine, Buenos Aires, Argentina

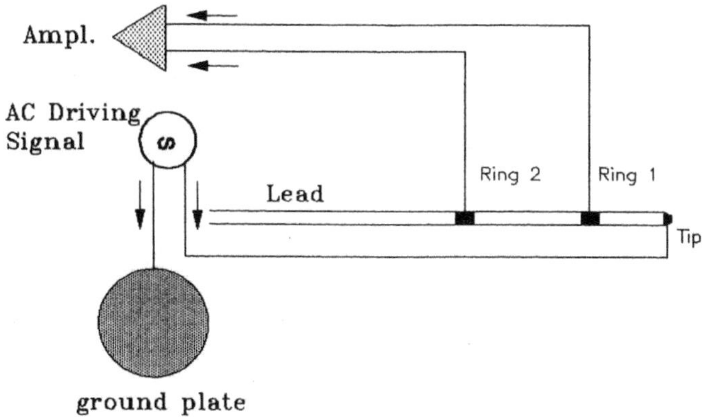

Fig.1. Connection diagram for impedance detection with a tripolar lead. The pacemaker can is the ground plate. Moving the proximal ring to the can, it is possible to use a standard bipolar lead

detection using a standard bipolar lead configuration has also been tested in previous investigations[5].

Generally, in order to obtain a suitable waveform for pacing and diagnostic purposes, it must be devoid of both motion artefacts and respiratory baseline drift. This can be easily achieved with multiring electrodes, but filtering and signal averaging are required for bipolar and unipolar lead configurations.

Cardiac Parameters Derived from Right Ventricular Impedance

The waveform obtained by the impedance method closely resembles the known physiologic volume changes throughout the cardiac cycle. Since for technical reasons current devices cannot be calibrated, the signal only provides information on relative changes. The time relationship between right ventricular stroke volume curve and other hemodynamic parameters is shown in Fig.2. Figure3 shows a typical right ventricular volume waveform during pacing and sinus rhythm. Atrial contraction causes a minor increase in ventricular volume. During isovolumetric contraction time there may be a minor upward deflection of the volume curve, possible due to motion or torsion of the heart and not related to a true volume change. Immediately after this deflection, ejection begins and a rapid downstroke is seen. The nadir of the curve corresponds to the end of ejection, as well as to the isovolumic relaxation phase. Rapid ventricular filling causes a return of the curve to the baseline.

While in Fig. 4 the shape of the impedance curve with a paced and an intrinsic beat is very similar, in individual cases this shape can be considerably different. Depending on the location of the electrode and on the pattern of the ventricular contraction, the impedance curve with spontaneous and paced beats can differ not only as far as the signal's amplitude is concerned, but also with regard to polarity, morphology, and timing.

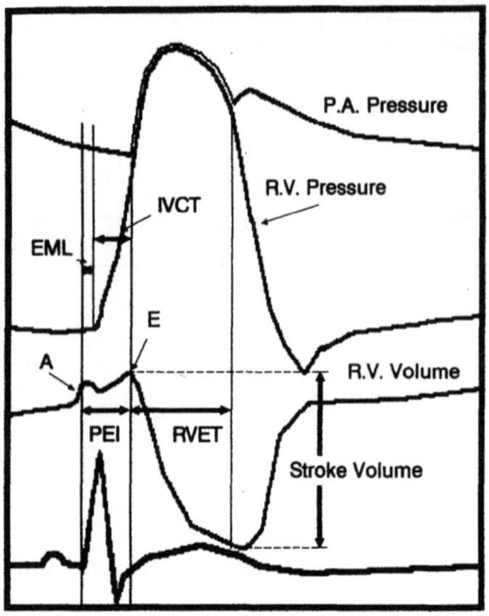

Fig. 2. Relationship between right ventricular (*RV*) volume waveform and right-sided pressure parameters. PEI is the sum of the electromechanical lag (*EML*) and isovolumetric contraction time (*IVCT*). *A* is the effect produced on the right ventricular volume by the atrial contraction, and *E* is the onset of ejection. The peak to nadir value is the relative stroke volume. *RVET*, right ventricular ejection time; *PA*, pulmonary artery

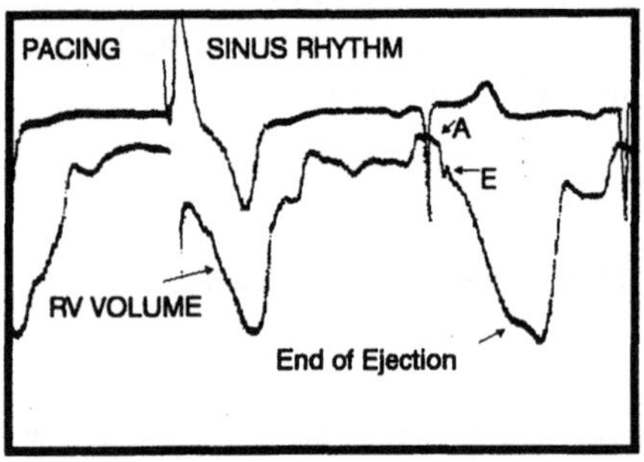

Fig. 3. Right ventricular (*RV*) volume during pacing and sinus rhythm. Impedance waveform was obtained with standard bipolar lead. *A*, effect produced on the right ventricular volume by the atrial contraction; *E*, onset of ejection

This constitutes a significant problem for data analysis, requiring intelligent data processing by means of different running averages for paced and intrinsic beats, currently not fully solved in implantable pacemakers. The ongoing description of impedance-derived cardiac signals does not enter this technical challenge and assumes these problems to be solved in the near future.

Right ventricular volume detection by the impedance technique allows at least three distinct applications: (1) rate-adaptive pacing using preejection interval, stroke volume or dV/dt, (2) evaluation of cardiac performance and (3) tachyarrhythmia discrimination.

From the relative stroke volume signal obtained with impedance techniques and the simultaneous intracardiac electrogram, the following cardiac parameters can be obtained:

1. Preejection interval (PEI)
2. Relative stroke volume (RSV) and cardiac output (RCO)

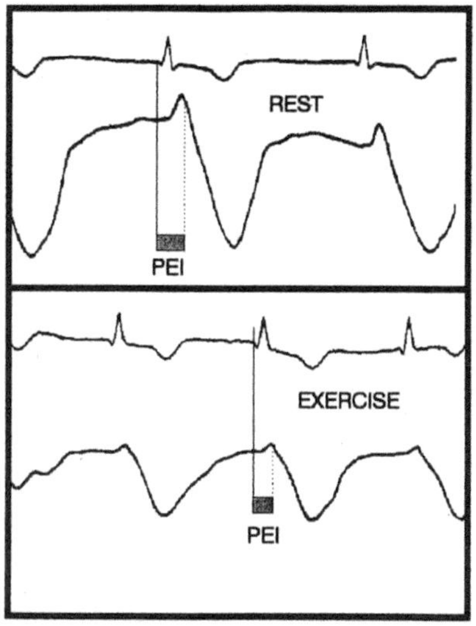

Fig. 4. PEI shortening with exercise. Tracing obtained with a standard bipolar lead

3. Relative right ventricular ejection rate (systolic dV/dt)
4. Right ventricular ejection time (RVET)
5. Electromechanical systole (EMS)
6. Relative right ventricular filling rate (diastolic dV/dt)

Published data are available only on stroke volume, dV/dt and PEI. The other variables are currently under evaluation and will not be considered here.

Preejection Interval

The PEI (or preejection period, PEP) is an electromechanical interval extending from the onset of QRS or pacing spike to the onset of ventricular ejection (Fig. 2).

PEI (PEP) is formed by two components: (1) the electromechanical lag, which is the interval from the onset of QRS or pacing spike to the onset of mechanical activation (this interval may be dependent on hormonal or neural influences, but its variability is minimal and directionally similar to that of PEI and (2) isovolumetric contraction time (IVCT), extending from the onset of mechanical activation to the onset of ejection. During this phase, ventricular pressure rises but there is no volume change as all cardiac valves remain closed. This interval is very important, since it determines the hemodynamic value of PEI. It is known that IVCT is influenced by sympathetic tone and catecholamines and thus is an indicator of the contractile state of the heart. It shortens in inverse proportion to increasing metabolic demands of exercise, paralleling the shortening of the atrial cycle length [7–9].

Left ventricular PEI can be easily measured with noninvasive techniques and was first suggested as a biosignal to control pacing rate in a previous communication [7].

Right ventricular PEI is measured from the onset of electrical depolarization (QRS or pacing spike) to the onset of right ventricular ejection. As was seen above, the onset of right ventricular ejection corresponds to the onset of rapid downward deflection of the ventricular volume curve (Fig. 2). Since ventricular volumes can be obtained by the impedance method using conventional pacing leads, right ventricular PEI seems ideal for implantable rhythm control devices [8, 10]. The shortening of PEI during exercise is depicted in Fig. 4.

But, as already mentioned, the natural difference in PEI between spontaneous and paced beats has to be considered by an appropriate algorithm. Additionally, in patients with AV block and dissociation between atrial contractions and ventricular-stimulated beats, the random occurance of AV synchronisation may affect the measurement of PEI.

Neurohormonal and Hemodynamic Influences on PEI

The autonomic nervous system causes very rapid cardiac responses in normal individuals [10] , whereas circulating catecholamines provide a more sustained action. A parallelism was observed between rapid atrial rate changes and PEI changes under increased sympathetic tone (such as handgrip test and emotional stress). It was also demonstrated that isoproterenol causes a parallel shortening of atrial cycle length and PEI, while keeping the ventricular-paced rate constant [7–9], suggesting that both (PEI and atrial rate) are influenced by the same reflexes and hormonal influences.

In the normal heart, adrenergic and cholinergic fibers have a chronotropic action on the heart. Both types of autonomic fibers innervate the atria and AV node, whereas mostly adrenergic fibers innervate the ventricles. In a PEI-controlled rate-adaptive pacemaker no significant vagal influence is thus expected. No change in PEI with carotid sinus massage (vagal stimulation) and no response of PEI to atropine injection has been observed [9]. Nonresponsiveness to vagal maneuvers may be a benefit rather than an inconvenience of PEI as a biosignal for rate control, particularly in patients who suffer from the hypersensitive carotid sinus syndrome.

It is known that in patients with AV block, who have normal sinus node function and who are paced at a fixed ventricular rate, the simultaneous atrial rate follows a nearly normal response pattern during exercise. In some patients, however, the atrial rate is faster than predicted for the workload. This is probably due to reflex mechanisms which cause a greater-than-normal stimulation of the SA node in the presence lower-than-needed heart rate. The reverse is true when the heart is paced at rest at rates faster than necessary. In this case the atrial rate slows down. This phenomenon has been described [9] and was manifested as a slight lenghtening of PEI with incremental pacing at rest, further demonstrating the physiological similarities between PEI and atrial rate. The extent of this negative feedback on the PEI does not appear to be of a sufficient magnitude to represent a true closed-loop mechanism, but it is felt that it may be beneficial in the operation of a rate-adaptive pacemaker.

The cause of PEI lengthening with increasing pacing rates at rest is not fully understood, but at least two mechanisms may be involved. One, PEI would shorten as a result of a neurohormonal feedback on the heart upon unnecessarily fast pacing rates, as is probably the case with the sinus node in patients with AV block and normal sinus function during incremental pacing [8]. The other, a simple hemodynamic effect, as pointed out recently [12]. In this latter situation, abbreviation of the diastole by pacing causes a rise in pulmonary artery diastolic pressure as a consequence of which PEI lengthens. In addition, a significant change in pulmonary artery diastolic pressure, such as that produced by Valsalva's maneuver, may also affect PEI (Fig. 5).

Two major applications of PEI in implantable rhythm control devices have been postulated: As a signal for driving rate-adaptive pacemakers [5–8] and to aid in the discrimination of tachyarrhythmias [13].

Use of PEI for Rate-Adaptive Pacing

The effects of hemodynamic challenges and pharmacologic interventions on PEI are well-known. [14–16] Of these, the following comprise the landmark features for the use of PEI in rate-adaptive pacing: (1) PEI shortening proportional to workload [5, 7, 9], (2) PEI shortening with inotropic agents [5, 7, 9, 14, 15], and (3) nondependence of PEI to incremental pacing at rest [5, 7, 9, 16].

The effect of betablockade, calcium channel-blocking agents, certain antiarrhythmic drugs, and cardiotonics are presently being investigated. Some of the subjects of the above studies were receiving beta-blocking agents, known to lengthen PEI, at the time of the cardiocirculatory challenges, but, still, shortening was noted with them. The same is true for patients with congestive heart failure, where it is known that PEI is prolonged at rest [14].

The use of PEI for rate-responsive pacing is thus considered promising and this biosignal seems very close to the ideal for the automatic control of heart rate with implantable pacemakers.

Clinical Studies on Implantable PEI-Controlled Devices. Results of the evaluation of the first PEI-controlled VVIR (ventricular paced, ventricular sensed, inhibited, rate adaptive) and DDDR (double pacing, double sensing, inhibited and triggering, rate adaptive) pacemakers are now available. The implanted units (CPI Precept VR and DR) offer the possibility of telemetry of measured sensor values which permits a noninvasive evaluation of PEI and SV during cardiocirculatory challenges.

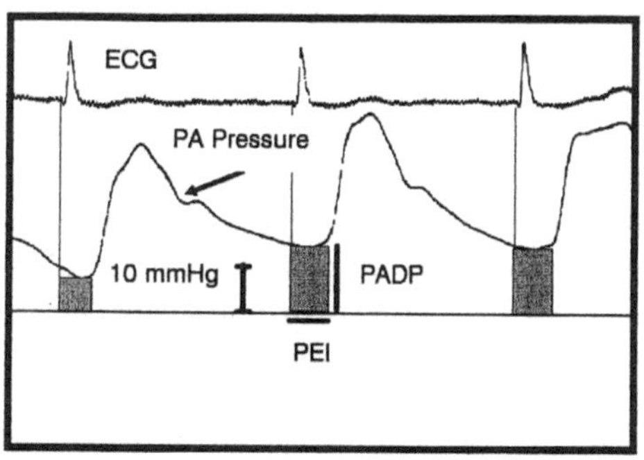

Fig. 5. Recording of the pulmonary artery (*PA*) pressure, just after the release of Valsalva's maneuver, when rapid pressure changes take place. PEI is measured from the onset of QRS to the upstroke of the PA pressure. The level of PA diastolic pressure (*PADP*), determines the duration of PEI. A lower pressure causes shorter PEI

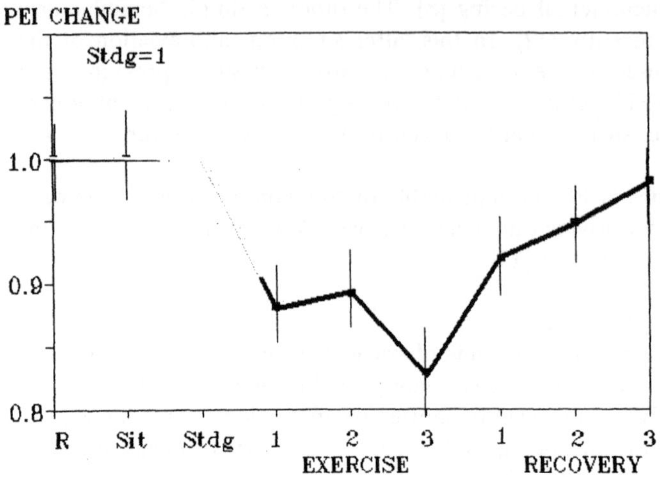

Fig. 6a. Effect of posture and exercise on PEI duration. PEI was measured by telemetry with CPI Precept pacemakers during exercise in nonrate-adaptive mode. Postural challenges preceded and followed 3 min of exercise. The patients were changed from the recumbent (*R*), to the sitting (*Sit*), and then to the standing (*Stdg*) position. This latter position was used as reference. *Vertical* lines represent the standard error of mean in a group of 25 patients. (Data cordially provided by CPI, St. Paul, MN, United States)

The patients were tested by: (1) postural changes (from recumbent to sitting to standing), (2) exercise in the VVI or DDD pacing modes, (3) exercise in VVIR or DDDR modes, and (4) incremental pacing.

During postural changes telemetry-measured PEI in each body position is depicted in Fig. 6a. It can be seen that postural changes are minimal. Postural maneuvers were done just before and right after exercise.

During exercise in nonrate-adaptive mode, PEI was measured by telemetry at rest and at each stage of exercise. Results are shown in Fig. 6a. PEI measured by the pacemaker from the right ventricular volume curve shortens as expected during exercise. The response is fast, similar to what was observed for left ventricular PEI [9].In adaptive-rate mode, the rate increment with exercise in each patient was dependent on slope and upper rate settings. An example is shown in Fig. 6b.

Incremental pacing caused no shortening of PEI. In some patients some lengthening was noted.

Use of PEI for Tachyarrhythmia Discrimination

Since PEI changes in close parallelism to changing metabolic demands and does not shorten (or lengthens slightly) with incremental pacing, it is reasonable to expect that it could be advantageous in discriminating sinus tachycardia from tachyarrhythmias. Physiologic sinus tachycardia could thus be defined as a rate increase accompanied by the shortening of PEI, whereas a tachyarrhythmia would be a fast rate with no shortening (or lengthening) of PEI. Preliminary studies in patients with spontaneous and simulated tachyarrhythmias have suggested that PEI may be efficaciously used in implantable rhythm control devices, particularly when the rate of the pathologic tachycardia is low and/or the physiologic tachycardia of exercise is high [13]. In these cases the rate cut-off of current implantable cardioverter-defibrillators may overlook

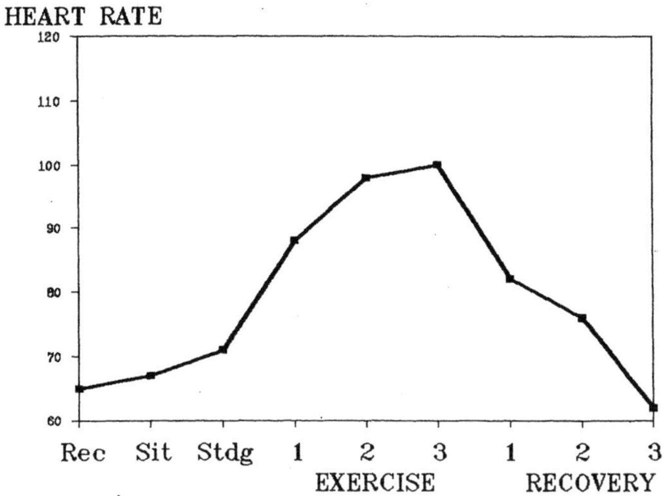

Fig. 6b. Example of one patient with VVIR Precept pacemaker during exercise in the rate-adaptive mode. Postural challenges were performed before and after the 3-min exercise test on a bicycle. *REC*, recumbent

a tachyarrhythmia, or produce a cardioversion shock during physiologic rate increase. A sensor-controlled cardioverter-defibrillator would thus have more sensitivity and specificity.

Relative Stroke Volume Changes

The difference between the maximum and minimum intracardiac impedance or peak-to-peak value is the stroke impedance. If the tracing is reversed (lower impedance shown as an upward deflection), the waveform resembles that of the ventricular volume. Peak-to-peak values would then be an indication of relative stroke volume (SV) changes (Fig. 2).

Use of Relative Stroke Volume for Rate-Adaptive Pacing

Since the effects of increased metabolic demands on SV are opposite to those of incremental pacing at rest, it seems natural that this variable may be suitable for automatic rate control. In a patient with complete heart block, an increase in SV due to an augmented metabolic demand would be sensed by the pacemaker. This larger sensed SV will, given the pacemaker algorithm, cause an increment in pacing rate, which in turn, will reduce SV back to resting levels. The endpoint of the device will then be the maintenance of a constant SV, which constitutes a true closed-loop system with negative feedback.

The above sequence of events will hold true only if there are no intercurrent causes for a change in SV. For example, if during exercise there are postural changes which affect SV, the pacemaker rate adaptation may be less predictable. Likewise, postural changes at rest may produce a rate response not mediated by metabolic demand. This behaviour of SV, albeit physiological, may be compensated for by position sensors which make the necessary corrections for body posture, preventing unnecessary pacemaker rate changes.

SV is known to be influenced by contractility, rate, venous return (preload), and afterload. The behavior of right ventricular impedance in patients with implanted CPI Precept pacemakers was done by means of the following challenges: (1) exercise (patients with and without AV block), (2) postural changes (recumbent – sitting – standing), and (3) incremental pacing.

Initial studies during *exercise* using an external computer to adjust pacing rate according to SV changes have shown a satisfactory performance [3]. More recently, permanently implanted devices incorporating a SV sensor (CPI Precept) have also shown adequate rate compensation with exercise (Cardiac Pacemakers Inc., personal communication). These devices permit telemetry of the waveform and numerical value of the relative SV signal. Using this, it was possible to observe SV response not only during exercise but also under postural challenges. Figure 7 shows the response of telemetered SV values during exercise in patients with complete heart block. Increased metabolic demands cause an increase in contractility leading to augmented SV. The testing protocol called for postural maneuvers just prior to and immediately following exercise.

The effects of *postural challenges* are depicted in Fig. 7. It shows telemetered SV values in a group of patients when going from the recumbent to the sitting to the upright position just before exercise and at the end of it.

Use of Relative Stroke Volume for Diagnostic Purposes

Telemetry of relative SV and cardiac output could conceivably be used in the clinical management of patients. Although with the current state of development of implantable devices an absolute cardiac output measurement is not feasible, it is very likely that relative measurements may serve. Since there is only a limited

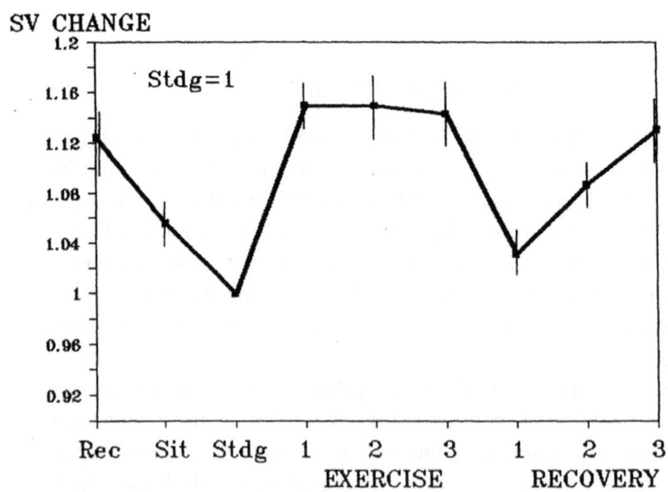

Fig. 7. Effect of posture and exercise on relative stroke volume (*SV*). Postural challenges are as described in Fig. 6. Standing values were used as a reference. *Vertical* lines show the standard error of mean for a group of 25 patients. (Data cordially provided by CPI, St. Maul, MN, United States)

number of implanted units under clinical investigation, no practical applications can be suggested yet.

Use of Relative Stroke Volume for Arrhythmia Discrimination

Although SV does not have the same value as PEI in distinguishing physiologic from pathologic tachycardia, it may serve a useful function in diagnosing severe hemodynamic deterioration during arrhythmia. For example, if during a tachyarrhythmia SV diminishes, it would indicate hemodynamic impairment and prompt action on it may be indicated.

Right Ventricular dV/dt

Although it is reasonable to assume that correlation exists between the ventricular rate of pressure rise (dP/dt) and ventricular peak ejection rate (dV/dt), not enough clinical information is available to ascertain the degree of reciprocal predictability. If indeed, dV/dt and dP/dt are equivalent, it may be possible to use dV/dt in place of dP/dt for rate control, although preload and rate compensation may be necessary. At present, the use of right ventricular dV/dt is under study, both for diagnostic and rate-adaptive purposes.

Conclusions

Impedance-derived cardiac volume measurements provide several hemodynamic parameters applicable for rate-adaptive pacing, tachyarrhythmia discrimination, and diagnostic purposes. All of these features may be obtained with conventional pacing leads, of known reliability and durability. It may be possible to combine them in a single implantable unit by the application of advanced algorithms to the sensor signal.

References

1. Geddes L, Hoff HE, Mello A, Palmer C (1966) Continuous measurement of ventricular stroke volume by electrical impedance. Cardiac Res Center Bull 4:118
2. McKay RG et al. (1984) Instantaneous measurement of left and right ventricular stroke volume and pressure – volume relationship with an impedance catheter. Circulation 69:703
3. Salo RW, Pederson BD, Olive AL et al. (1984) Continuous ventricular volume assessment for diagnosis and pacemaker control. PACE 7:1267
4. Boheim G (1988) Intrakardiale Impedanzmessung zur frequenzadaptiven Stimulation des Herzens. Doctoral thesis, Technical Faculty, University of Erlangen-Nuremberg
5. Chirife R, Shapland JE, Salo RW, Ortega DF, Olive AL, Pederson B (1987) Behavior of right pre-ejection interval under cardiocirculatory challenges. Possible use of this interval to drive closed-loop rate-responsive pacing systems. In: Belhassen B, Feldman S, Cooperman Y (eds) Cardiac pacing and electrophysiology. Creative Communications, Tel Aviv, p 143

6. Schaldach M (1989) PEP-gesteuerter Herzschrittmacher. Biomed Tech (Berlin) 34:177
7. Chirife R (1987) The pre-ejection period: an ideal physiologic variable for rate-responsive pacing. PACE 10:425 (abstr)
8. Chirife R, Pesce R, Valero de Pesce E, Favaloro M (1989) Initial studies on a new adaptive-rate pacemaker controlled by pre-ejection intreval on stroke volume. International congress on rate responsive pacing, 3 Sept, 1989, Vienna
9. Chirife R (1988) Physiological principles of a new method for rate-responsive pacing using the pre-ejection interval. PACE 11:1545
10. Klein H, Becht I, Siclari F, Kriva L, Mess J, Zimmer W, Costjens J (1989) First clinical experience with "Precept" – a new single- or dual-chamber adaptive-rate pacing system. PACE 12:656
11. Warner MR, Loeb JM: Beat by-beat modulation of A-V conduction: I. Heart rate and respiratory influences. Am J. Pysiol 251:1126
12. Chirife R, Ortega D (1989) Hemodynamic correlates of pre-ejection interval. Implications for adaptive-rate pacing. PACE 12:1297 (abstr)
13. Chirife R, Ortega DF (1989) Use of pre-ejection interval to discriminate physiologic from pathologic tachycardia. Symposium on rate responsive pacing, 27-29 Sept, 1989, Vienna
14. Harris WS, Schoenfeld CD, Weissler AM (1967) Effects of adrenergic receptor activation and blockade on the systolic pre-ejection period, heart rate and arterial blood pressure in man. J Clin Invest 46:1704
15. Martin CE, Shaver JA, Thompson ME et al. (1971) Direct correlation of external systolic time intervals with internal indices of left ventricular function in man. Circulation 44:419
16. Spodick DH, Doi YL, Bishop RL, Hashimoto T (1984) Systolic time intervals reconsidered. Reevaluation of the pre-ejection period: absence of relation to heart rate. Am J Cardiol 53:1667

Stroke Volume: A Hemodynamic Variable for Rate-Adaptive Pacing

R.W. SALO[1]

Introduction

The healthy human body is highly adaptable. Because of this fact, the clinical need for an artificially generated rate response in chronotropically incompetent, but otherwise healty patients was not generally acknowledged for years. Faced with greater than normal oxygen demand, the fixed-rate patient adapts by three mechanisms: an increase in stroke volume, an increase in the level of oxygen extraction from the blood and, if both of these prove insufficient, by a change in behavior. The latter usually involves, often subconsciously, removing the offending activity from his daily routine. The combination of these three mechanisms was effective enough in the majority of patients to mask the clinical need for a rate increase. However, since both the stroke volume and the percentage of oxygen which can be extracted from the blood are limited physiologically, there is always a loss of cardiac reserve in fixed-rate pacing.

The basis of a hemodynamically based rate-adaptive pacing system is to first sense the patient's physiological response to stress (i.e., his normal compensation mechanism) and based on this response provide the missing increase in heart rate. Since the measured variable is the body's substitute for a normal rate response, it is a high-level indicator which is a (biologically) processed summation of many low-level indicators (preload, afterload, contractiliy, pCO_2, etc.) and requires little additional processing to convert to an appropriate pacing rate. These systems inherently contain feedback, since the rate increase provided by the pacer will mediate the response of the compensation mechanism being monitored. Thus it is always possible to determine the appropriateness of the rate response from the behavior of the monitored variable.

Fixed-rate patients utilize both of the previously discussed physiological compensation mechanisms when accomodating to exercise. Generally, both the arteriovenous O_2 (AVO_2) difference and the stroke volume are observed to increase with workload. Since the oxygen level in the arterial blood remains approximately constant, it is possible to get an indication of the AVO_2 difference from the mixed-venous oxygen level in the right ventricle (RV). This is the basis of experimental rate-responsive pacing systems utilizing O_2saturation sensors.

[1] Cardiac Pacemakers, Inc., 4100 North Hamline Ave, St. Paul, MN 55112-5798, USA

Both stroke volume and O_2saturation are candidate physiological variables for rate response. When we approached this problem over 10 years ago, neither could be measured chronically with implantable sensors. For practical reasons, we chose to concentrate on the measurement of stroke volume by intracardiac impedance. This technique, although undeveloped at the time and applied only to external monitoring devices, provided the practical advantage of requiring only standard electrodes on the pacing lead. Thus concerns about the long-term viability and safety of the sensor were obviated.

Stroke Volume During Exercise

Although cardiac output may increase 500% or more during intense exercise, stroke volume in a healthy subject remains relatively constant. An early paper by Rushmer [1] demonstrated that cardiac output increases in healthy dogs during exercise were mediated almost exclusively by heart rate, with a minimal stroke volume increase. He stated in summary that his findings along with several others from the literature "document that increased stroke volume is neither an essential nor consistent feature of the cardiac response to exertion in either intact animals or normal humans." Controversy over the contribution of increased stroke volume to exercise response apparently arose from studies involving trained athletes, primarily marathon runners, who do show marked stroke-volume increases during exercise. Vatner and Boettcher [2] determined in the conscious dog that maximally tolerable volume loading, infusion of sympathomimetic amines and exercise did not affect or only modestly increased stroke volume, although cardiac output increases of more than 400% were observed.

In contrast to these studies, stroke-volume increases during exercise when the heart rate is constrained, as it is in patients paced at a fixed heart rate. Figure 1 [3] shows a typical increase during bicycle exercise at a fixed rate. Note that this patient, a well-trained individual with a healthy heart, is limited by maximum stroke volume to a cardiac output increase of 80% – 90%.

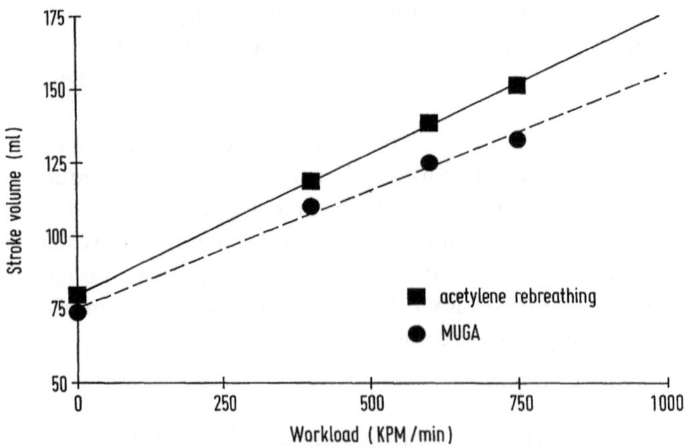

Fig. 1. Stroke volume measured by acetylene rebreathing and radioisotope imaging at rest and during bicycle exercise in a patient paced at a fixed rate of 70 ppm. *MUGA*, •

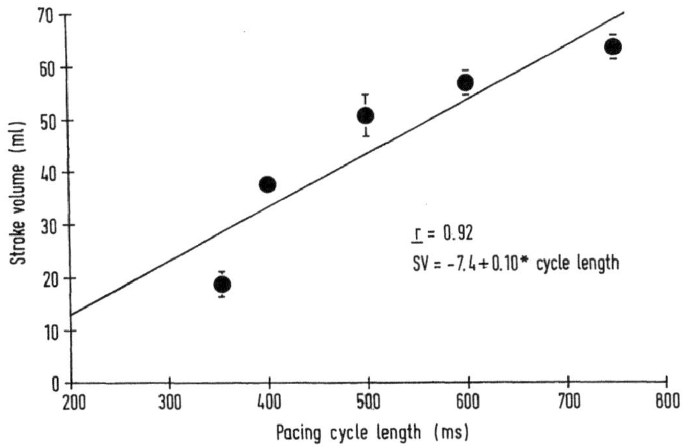

Fig. 2. Stroke volume (*SV*) measured by intracardiac impedance plotted as a function of pacing period. The measurements were made in a supine patient at rest. Note the rapid drop in stroke volume at the highest pacing rate (170 ppm)

There is a nearly linear relationship between stroke volume and cardiac period under steady-state conditions as shown in Fig. 2. Under constant venous return, the stroke volume is determined largely by the filling time available. At high-pacing rates (>170 at rest) without sympathetic stimulation, filling time becomes insufficient and the stroke volume and cardiac output drop precipitously, as is evident from the stroke volume at the shortest cycle length in Fig. 2. The fact that the stroke volume decreases with increased heart rate is significant. This sort of negative feedback is necessary for a stable closed-loop system.

Measurements of the stroke-volume response to exercise at a fixed heart rate and the stroke-volume response to heart rate at a fixed metabolic load (i.e., under steady-state conditions) provide the "open-loop" information necessary to set up the "closed-loop" system (i.e., modifying the heart rate based on stroke-volume information). Figure 3 is a diagram of a simplified closed-loop pacing system based on stroke-volume information. The goal of this pacing system is to maintain a constant stroke volume (indicated by *DESIRED* in the figure).

The normal physiological response to exercise or stress is an increase in circulating catecholamines, sympathetic stimulation, increased venous return (preload), and decreased vascular resistance (afterload). Any of these factors may alter the stroke volume in order to compensate for increased workload.

Intracardiac Impedance Measurement of Stroke Volume

The basis of the measurement of stroke volume by intracardiac impedance for pacing applications has been discussed previously [3] . A small (1-6 μA RMS) alternating current is driven between a distal electrode at the apex of the chamber and a proximal electrode, which is usually outside of the chamber. The electrical potentials generated by the flowing current are sensed by one or more (usually two) electrodes disposed between the current sources. The electrical impedance or resistance (since blood has

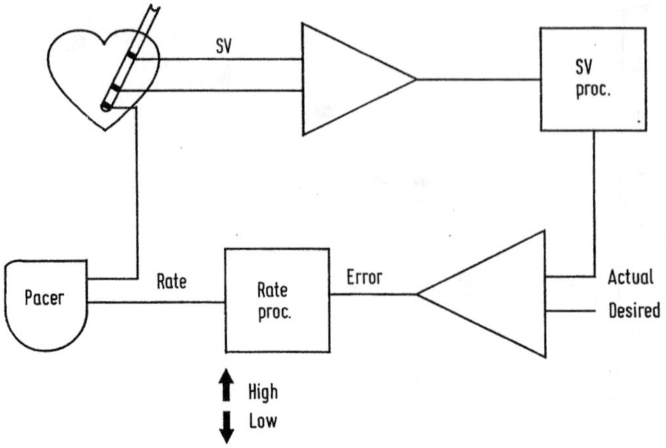

Fig. 3. Block diagram of a simplified closed-loop pacing system based on stroke-volume (*SV*) information measured by intracardiac impedance. This system attempts to maintain a constant stroke volume, indicated in the diagram by *DESIRED*

a very low capacitance, the two terms are interchangeable) between these sensing electrodes is computed by dividing the potential difference between the electrodes by the current. For a given distance L between the sensing electrodes and a blood resistivity ϱ the resistance R is related to the cross-sectional area A of the chamber or the chamber volume V by the equation $R = \varrho\,(L/A) = \varrho\,(L^2/V)$.

The stroke volume (SV) is related to end-diastolic resistance (EDR) and the change in resistance (ΔR) by the equation $SV = \Delta R/EDR\,(EDR + \Delta R)$.

Assuming the end-diastolic resistance remains relatively constant and that $EDR >> \Delta R$, then the stroke volume is proportional to ΔR. This relationship, although not entirely accurate, is generally usable as shown in Fig. 4 by the results of a typical animal experiment. The shortcomings of this simple mathematical approach and techniques for improving the accuracy of volume computations have been discussed at length [4, 5] .

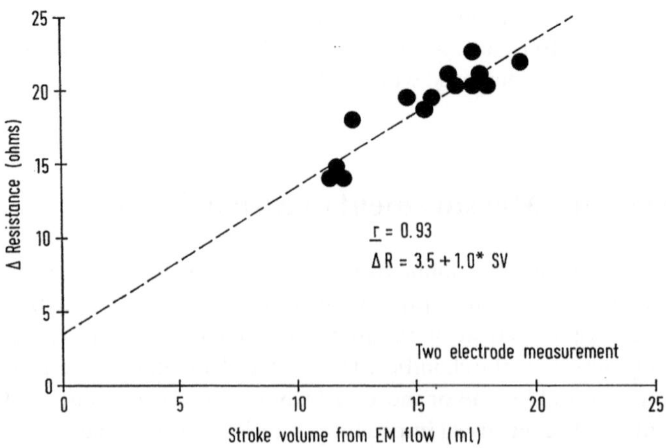

Fig. 4. The relationship between the change in resistance (ΔR), the peak-to-peak variation in measured impedance, and stroke volume (*SV*) measured by electromagnetic (*EM*) flow in a dog during infusion of dobutamine. Although the heart rate was not constant, the dobutamine was titrated to give a minimal heart rate increase

Rate Control by Stroke Volume

The continuous measurement of stroke volume and other volume parameters was not possible before the development of intracardiac impedance techniques and ambulatory beat-by-beat measurements were not practical before the advent of the PRECEPT pacemaker. Early studies were carried out exclusively on animals and usually with electromagnetic flow probes. These studies by Rushmer [1] and Vatner [2], proved conclusively that the body's primary means for increasing cardiac output is tachycardia. The first attempt to control pacing rate during exercise based on stroke volume information in a patient with complete AV block is shown in Fig. 5. In this case a proportion-integral controller was used in a closed-loop fashion to control the rate of a VVI pacemaker. Although this control was programmed with a very long time constant to guarantee stability, the rate response (although delayed) was entirely appropriate. At the peak exercise level of 750 kp m/min (≈ 76 W) there was a 23% increase in cardiac output and a 70% decrease in stroke volume with a rate response as compared to exercise at the same workload with a fixed rate of 70 ppm. The patient also reported reduced ventilatory drive and discomfort with the rate increase.

Practical Considerations

Although rate control based on stroke volume is a fundamentally simple concept, there are a number of practical aspects to be mastered in its application. An understanding of these considerations will aid the physician in his interpretation of clinical results.

The first step in the clinical application of the principle is the positioning of the impedance lead. Since the volume which most directly influences the measured impedance is bound vertically by planar surfaces perpendicular to the lead and passing

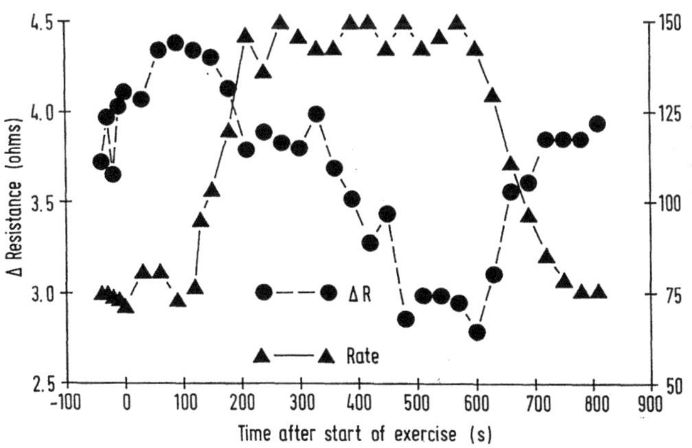

Fig. 5. Pacing rate and change in resistance (ΔR) during bicycle exercise. The pacing rate was controlled by a proportional-integral controller based on the stroke volume. The control algorithm attempted to maintain the stroke volume at the value measured at rest before the beginning of exercise. (Reproduced from [3].)

through the center of the sensing electrodes, and circumferentially by the walls of the ventricle, the lead is best positioned with the tip in the apex of the ventricle and the body of the lead extending along the longitudinal axis of the ventricle. Ideally, both sensing electrodes of a tripolar lead should remain in the ventricle to prevent contamination of the impedance signal by valve or atrial motion. Any impedance signal recorded at the time of implant may be contaminated by motion-related impedance artifacts. As the lead moves during a contraction, the measured impedance is affected by changes in lead position as well as by changes in volume. As the lead becomes encapsulated and fixed into position, this unwanted motion is reduced along with the "motion artifacts". This is evidenced, as shown in Fig. 6, by a large ΔR amplitude at implant, which decreases to a steady-state value within the next 2 weeks. Thus the impedance waveform at the time of implant is not a useful

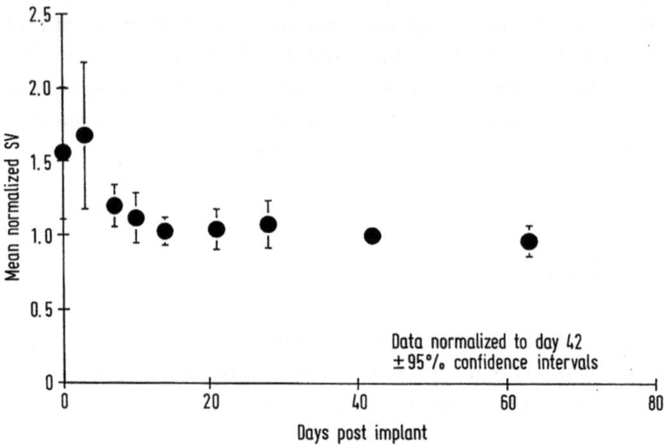

Fig. 6. Change in impedance, reflecting stroke volume (*SV*) as a function of time after implant of tripolar leads in twelve dogs. Mean values and 95% confidence intervals are indicated. The average impedance and change in impedance appear to reach a steady-state value after approximately 2 weeks

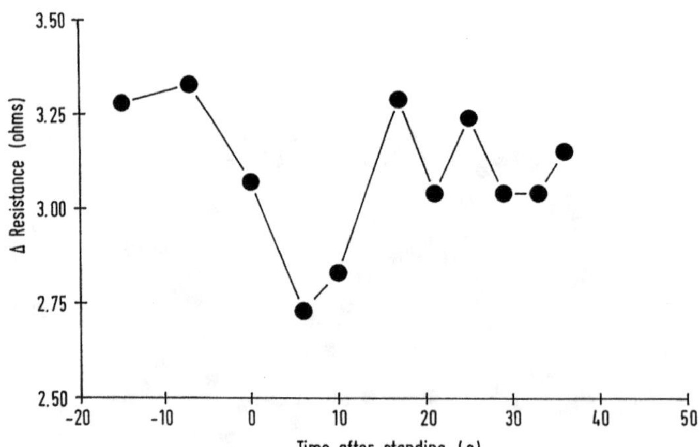

Fig. 7. The stroke volume as a function of time during the postural transition from supine to standing. Each point is the average of heart beats over a respiratory cycle. The patient reaches a steady-state stroke volume approximately 15 s after standing. Note the decrease in change in resistance immediately before standing up. The patient held his breath, performing an involuntary Valsalva's maneuver, while preparing to stand. A Valsavla's maneuver would be expected to reduce stroke volume. (Reproduced from [3].)

indicator of a good lead position. Fortunately, lead positions which look appropriate under fluoroscopy almost always result in good impedance signals after lead maturation.

Changes in posture are known to influence stroke volume. In the supine position, the average patient is at a maximum, or nearly maximum, stroke volume. The stroke volume drops when the patient sits and drops further still upon standing. In the normal individual, there is interplay between vascular resistance, heart rate and stroke volume to guarantee adequate tissue perfusion (i.e., cardiac output and pressure) for each posture. The fixed-rate patient must adjust vascular resistance to maintain a relatively constant cardiac output resulting in a stroke volume more or less independent of posture. Figure 7, which demonstrates the transient response of a fixed-rate patient's stroke volume during a postural change, exhibits the time course of the body's adjustment. Since it is expected that a patient in cardiac failure may not compensate as well or as quickly, this window into a physiological control system may someday prove useful in assessing cardiac function.

Summary

Realizing that human response to stress is complex and involves multiple parameters and control systems, it makes sense to use the body's inherent processing capabilities whenever possible and to concentrate only on high-level, preprocessed variables. Since a fixed-rate patient has only two mechanisms to accommodate increased workload, adjusting stroke volume and oxygen extraction, assessing these mechanisms gives a direct insight into metabolic demand at the highest level. Increased demand is always accompanied by increased stroke volume (within the limits of physiology) and the maintenance of a relatively constant stroke volume is indicative of meeting metabolic demand. A pacing system based on stroke volume measurements and attempting to maintain a relatively constant stroke volume should provide a pacing rate optimal for the body's needs at all times.

The development of the intracardiac impedance technique has made the long-term continuous measurement of stroke volume practical without the addition of sophisticated unproven sensors and has provided the basis for a pacemaker using stroke volume as a rate-control parameter.

References

1. Rushmer RF (1959) Constancy of stroke volume in ventricular reponses to exercise. Am J Physiol 196/4: 745
2. Vatner SF, Boettcher DH (1978) Regulation of cardiac output by stroke volume and heart rate in conscious dogs. Circ Res 42/4: 557
3. Salo RW, Pederson BD, Olive AL, Lincoln WA, Wallner TG (1984) Continuous ventricular volume assessment for diagnosis and pacemaker control. PACE 7: 1267
4. Salo RW, Wallner TG, Pederson BE (1986) Measurement of ventricular volume by intracardiac impedance: theoretical and empirical approaches. IEEE Trans Biomed Eng BME-33: 189
5. Salo RW (1989) The theoretical basis of a computational model for the determination of volume vy impedance. Automedica 11/4: 299

III. Electrocardiography of Rate-Adaptive Pacemakers

Electrocardiography of Rate-Adaptive Dual-Chamber (DDDR) Pacemakers: Lower Rate Behavior

S.S. BAROLD[1]

The lower rate interval (LRI) is the most basic and important interval of single- and dual-chamber pacemakers. Many manufacturers of DDD pulse generators utilize a V-V timing or ventricular-based timing system for control of the LRI of their devices. The LRI of a dual-chamber pulse generator is tradtitionally defined as the longest interval from a sensed or paced ventricular event to the succeeding ventricular stimulus [1]. The atrial escape (pacemaker VA) interval is defined as the interval from a ventricular paced or sensed event to the subsequent atrial paced event (provided there are no intervening atrial or ventricular sensed events). A ventricular sensed event either in the atrioventricular (AV) interval or atrial escape interval (AEI) resets both the LRI and the AEI so that both start again. Constancy of the atrial escape (pacemaker VA) interval is the cardinal feature of V-V lower rate timing (LRT). Hence, the term "V-V timing" is often used interchangeably with "VA timing" to emphasize constancy of the AEI in ventricular-based LRT [2].

In the DDDR mode, the LRI is variable and varies as the sensor-driven rate varies. At any given time, the duration of the LRI can be either the programmed LRI or the constantly changing sensor-driven LRI, whichever is shorter. The shortest sensor-driven LRI is equal to the programmed sensor-driven upper rate interval (URI).

Recently some pacemaker manufacturers introduced dual-chamber pulse generators with A-A timing. With an atrial-based timing system, the LRI is controlled by atrial rather than ventricular events. Other designs include modified V-V timing (pseudo A-A timing) and various hybrids of A-A and V-V timing. A-A timing was designed to avoid cycle-to cycle fluctuations or beat-to-beat oscillations.

Definitions

For this discussion, the following abbreviations are used: Ap, atrial paced event; Vp, ventricular paced event; As, atrial sensed event; Vs, ventricular sensed event. Thus AV intervals may assume one of the following combinations: As-Vs, As-Vp, Ap-Vs,

[1] Division of Cardiology, Department of Medicine, The Genesee Hospital, University of Rochester School of Medicine and Dentistry, 224 Alexander Street, Rochester, NY 14607, USA

and Ap-Vp. In V-V LRT, the LRI is the longest Vp-Vp or Vs-Vp interval. In A-A LRT, the LRI is the longest Ap-Ap or As-Ap interval. The definition of the AEI from Vp or Vs to the succeeding Ap is identical for all LRT mechanisms. AV delay as programmed refers only to the paced AV interval, i.e., Ap-Vp.

V-V and A-A Responses

For descriptive purposes, the behavior of a *single* pacemaker cycle initiated by any combination of atrial and ventricular events (As-Vs, As-Vp, Ap-Vs, Ap-Vp, or isolated Vs) can be considered in terms of one of two mechanisms.

1. *V-V response* in which the ventricular paced or sensed event determines the duration of the succeeding pacing cycle – Vp or Vs initiates a *constant* AEI (Vs-Ap or Vp-Ap) equal to its basic value in the free-running mode. If Ap terminating the AEI is followed by Vp, the Vs-Ap-Vp or Vp-Ap-Vp intervals will be constant and equal to the programmed LRI.
2. *A-A response* in which the atrial paced or sensed event determines the duration of the succeeding pacing cycle – As or Ap initiates a constant LRI (As-Ap or Ap-Ap) disregarding any Vs or Vp following As or Ap at the beginning of the pacing cycle (Fig. 1). Consequently the AEI adapts its duration (longer, shorter, or unchanged) to maintain a constant Ap-Ap or As-Ap relationship equal to the LRI.

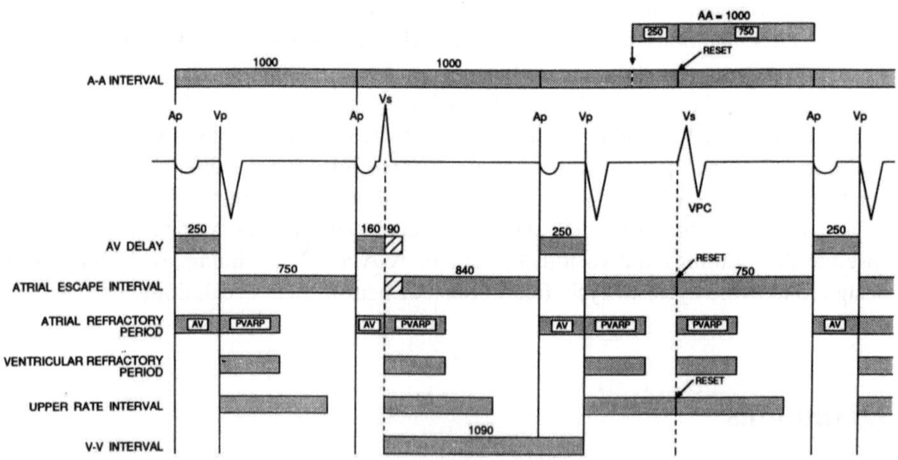

Fig. 1. Timing cycles of the Intermedics Cosmos II DDD pulse generator with A-A lower rate timing (LRT). Lower rate interval (LRI) = 1000 ms, AV = 250 ms (As-Vp = Ap-Vp), basic atrial escape interval (AEI) = 750 ms (during free-running pacing). The second Ap is followed by a conducted QRS complex Vs and Ap-Vs = 160 ms. Ap initiates an A-A (Ap-Ap) interval of 1090 ms. Consequently the AEI is equal to 750 + (250 – 160) = 840 ms. Note that the Vs-Vp interval = 1090 ms > atrial LRI. A ventricular extrasystole (*VPC*) beyond the AV interval initiates an AEI of 750 ms. *Solid vertical lines*, pace event time lines; *dashed vertical lines*, sense event time lines. (From [2])

3. *An isolated Vs*, e.g., ventricular extrasystole not preceded by an atrial event, uniformly initiates a V-V response in all contemporary types of LRT mechanisms.

Lower Rate Timing Vs Upper Rate Timing

Control of the LRI by either an A-A or V-V response should not be confused with behavior of the URI. All DDD and DDDR pacemakers possess a URI controlled and therefore initiated by a ventricular (paced or sensed) event. A DDDR device may function with either a common ventricular URI or two separate ventricular URIs as follows: (a) atrial-driven URI (sometimes known as the maximal tracking rate); and (b) sensor-driven URI.

The term "atrial-driven ventricular URI" is not contradictory because it refers to the shortest Vs-Vp or Vp-Vp where the second Vp is triggered by an As. The second Vp can only be released at the completion of the ventricular URI initiated by the preceding Vs or Vp. An atrial-based LRT does not mean that the URI is also atrial based because no DDD or DDDR pacemakers can function with a URI solely controlled by atrial events. Parenthetically, some DDD (Medtronic Symbios; Medtronic, Inc., Minneapolis, Minnesota, USA) and DDDR (Medtronic Synergyst II) pacemakers occasionally function with separate but linked atrial and ventricular URIs (i.e., each initiated by a paced or sensed event in its respective chamber and terminated by a *paced* event in the same chamber) that may become evident only under special circumstances [3]. The behavior of the Synergyst II DDDR atrial URI in response to a sensed ventricular extrasystole is discussed later.

V-V Lower Rate Timing

Rate Fluctuation Due to Ventricular Inhibition During Programmed AV Delay

During traditional DDD pacing with V-V LRT, when AV conduction is relatively normal, atrial capture (Ap) may give rise to a normally conducted QRS complex that may in turn inhibit the ventricular channel (Vs). In this situation, the QRS complex must occur before the completion of the programmed AV interval (Ap-Vp). Because the sensed QRS complex also starts a new LRI and AEI, this situation may lead to a fluctuation of the atrial pacing rate (faster than the lower rate for ventricular pacing) on a beat-to-beat basis or a constant atrial pacing rate faster than the lower (ventricular) rate [1, 3] (Fig. 2). With A-A LRT, the atrial pacing rate remains constant and independent of ventricular inhibition [4] .

In V-V pulse generators possessing a ventricular safety pacing (VSP) mechanism (to deal with crosstalk [5, 6], activation of VSP (by ventricular sensing of signals such as crosstalk) also causes an increase in the atrial pacing rate, but it is due to abbreviation of the Ap-Vp interval with the AEI (Vp-Ap) again remaining constant [1]. In pulse generators with V-V LRT, increase in the atrial rate due to ventricular inhibition is

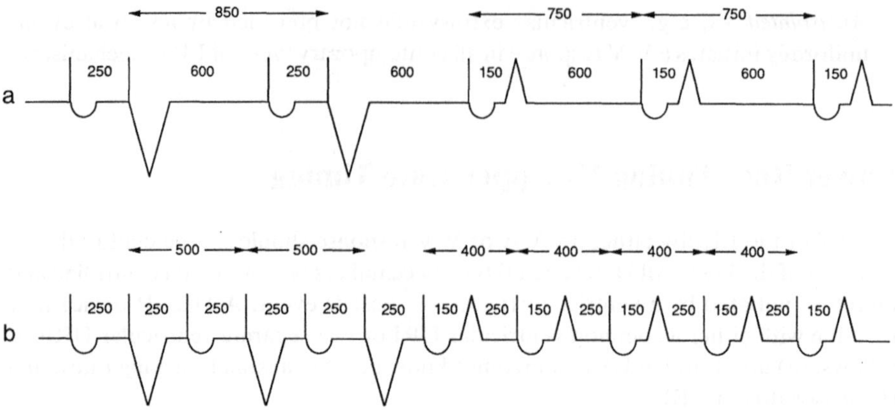

Fig. 2 a, b. Function of a DDDR pacemaker with V-V lower rate timing (LRT) showing the effect of ventricular inhibition. **a** DDD mode: lower rate interval (LRI) = 850 ms, AV = 250 ms, atrial escape interval (AEI) = 600 ms. On the *right*, when Ap is followed by a conducted QRS complex, the PR (Ap-Vs) interval shortens to 150 ms, but the AEI remains constant at 600 ms. Therefore the Ap-Ap interval decreases to 750 ms, i.e., the atrial pacing rate increases from 70 to 80 ppm. **b** DDDR mode: the programmed maximal sensor-driven rate is 120 ppm (500 ms). The AV interval remains at 250 ms so that the AEI shortens to 250 ms. On the *right*, when Ap is followed by a conducted QRS complex, the PR (Ap-Vs) interval shortens to 150 ms, but the AEI remains constant at 250 ms. Therefore the Ap-Ap interval decreases to 400 ms, i.e., the atrial pacing rate increases from 120 to 150 ppm. (From [2])

more pronounced at faster basic pacing rates [2, 4, 7], an important consideration in the design of rate-adaptive (DDDR) pulse generators because a programmed sensor- and atrial-driven upper rate (i.e., ventricular pacing rate) of 120 ppm might actually result in a faster atrial pacing rate of 150 ppm as shown in Fig. 2. Rate-adaptive shortening of the AV interval can effectively narrow or eliminate the difference between the faster atrial pacing rate (due to ventricular inhibition) and the programmed maximal rate, i.e., upper ventricular pacing rate (Fig. 3).

A-A Lower Rate Timing

The Intermedics Cosmos II (Intermedics, Freeport, Texas, USA) DDD and the ELA Chorus (ELA, Montrouge, France) DDD pulse generators are designed with a pure A-A or atrial-based LRT [8, 9]. When the atrial LRI of a DDD pacemaker with A-A timing is equal to the ventricular LRI of a DDD pacemaker with V-V timing, the basic AEI of both types of devices is identical during the free-running state with continuous atrial and ventricular pacing, i.e., DVI cycles terminating with an atrial stimulus (Ap) when there is no spontaneous activity. In a DDD pulse generator with A-A LRT, the duration of the AEI must be adapted to preserve constancy of the A-A interval (As-Vp, Ap-Ap). The actual AEI of a given pacing cycle will be equal to the sum of the basic AEI (as defined above) and an extension equal to the difference of the programmed AV delay (Ap-Vp) and the actual PR interval (Ap-Vs, As-Vs, As-Vp, or Ap-Vp) that immediately precedes the AEI. The AEI may therefore change by a positive value, zero, or even a negative value. This response assures that the A-A interval (As-Ap or Ap-Ap) remains constant under all circumstances, even when the sensed AV interval (As-Vp) and the paced AV interval (Ap-Vp) are different (Fig. 4).

Alternatively, the duration of the AEI may be calculated as the LRI less the AV interval immediately preceding the AEI.

Figures 1 and 4-6 illustrate the behavior of an atrial-based pulse generator under a variety of circumstances. When an A-A LRT pulse generator senses a late ventricular

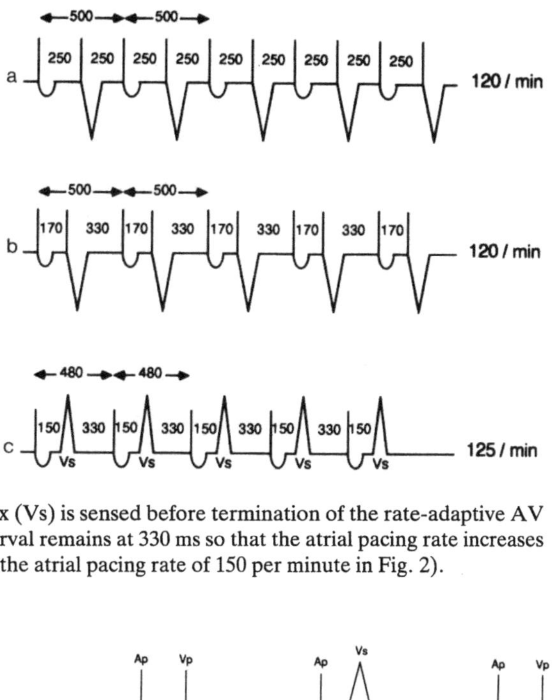

Fig. 3 a–c. Function of a DDDR pacemaker with V-V lower rate timing (LRT) showing the effect of a rate-adaptive AV delay that shortens on exercise. The maximal sensor-driven rate is 120 ppm (500 ms). The basic AV interval is 250 ms. **a** Maximal sensor-driven rate without rate-adaptive AV delay. **b** Maximal sensor-driven rate with rate adaptive AV delay. Note that the AV delay has shortened from 250 to 170 ms, and the sensor-driven atrial escape interval has lengthened from 250 ms (**a**) to 330 ms. **c** The maximal sensor-driven rate is 120 ppm (500 ms). The AV interval shortens to 150 ms because a conducted QRS complex (Vs) is sensed before termination of the rate-adaptive AV interval. As in **b**, the atrial escape interval remains at 330 ms so that the atrial pacing rate increases to only 125 per minute (compare with the atrial pacing rate of 150 per minute in Fig. 2).

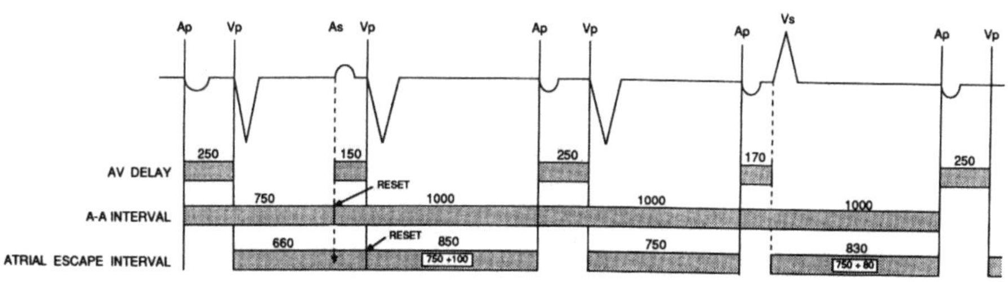

Fig. 4. Timing cycles of the Cosmos II DDD pulse generator with A-A lower rate timing (LRT) showing the effect of differential AV delays. The same parameters were programmed as in Fig. 1 except that As-Vp = 150 ms and Ap-Vp = 250 ms. The second Vp terminates the As-Vp interval = 150 ms and initiates an atrial escape interval (AEI) of 750 + (250 – 150) = 850 ms in order to maintain constancy of the A-A or Ap-Ap interval. On the *right*, the third Ap initiates an Ap-Vs interval = 170 ms. The corresponding AEI becomes 750 + (250 – 170) = 830 ms to maintain constancy of the A-A or Ap-Ap interval. (From [2])

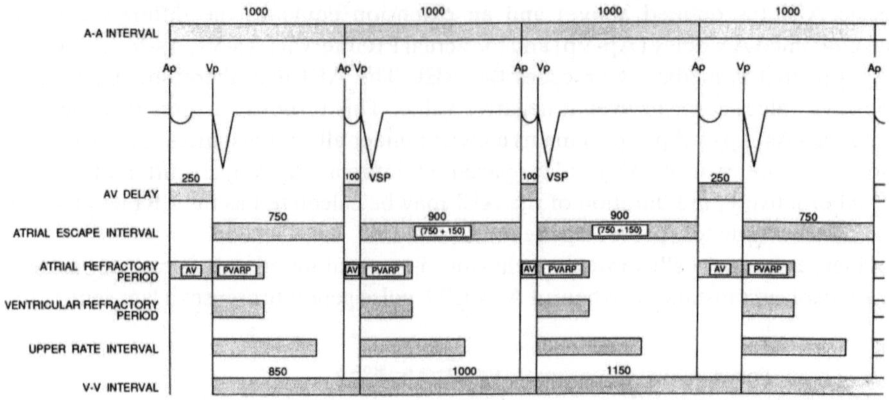

Fig. 5. Timing cycles of the Cosmos II DDD pulse generator with A-A lower rate timing (LRT) and the same parameters as in Fig. 1. Crosstalk induces ventricular safety pacing (*VSP*) with abbreviation of the Ap-Vp interval to 100 ms [5, 6] . The Ap-Ap interval remains constant so that the atrial escape interval (AEI) lengthens to 750 + (250 - 100) = 900 ms. During VSP, the pacing rate of a pulse generator with A-A LRT remains constant in contrast to an increase in the pacing rate in a DDD pulse generator with V-V LRT. At the termination of crosstalk, the Vp-Vp interval lengthens to 1150 ms > atrial lower rate interval (LRI). *Vertical lines*, pace event time lines. (From [2])

extrasystole (VE) preceded by a (nonconducted) P wave, it sees a short AV interval (i.e., Ap-Vs or As-Vs). Constancy of the A-A LRI mandates delay of the subsequent Ap and therefore lengthening of the AEI initiated by the VE. This causes hysteresis with regard to the interval between two ventricular events. Slowing of the ventricular rate may predispose to ventricular events. Slowing of the ventricular rate may predispose to ventricular bigeminy (rule of bigeminy) and may be undesirable in some patients [10].

Feasibility of DDI, DDIR, and DDDR Modes

A-A LRT is compatible with normal pacemaker function in the DVI and VDD modes, but incompatible with normal function in the DDI mode. A conventional DDI pulse generator is really a DDD pulse generator with V-V LRT in which the ventricular upper and lower rate intervals (rates) are identical [11, 12]. In the DDI mode with V-V LRT, an atrial extrasystole or sinus P wave (As) sensed beyond the PVARP will initiate a very long AV interval so that the pulse generator will release its ventricular stimulus (Vp) only at the completion of the (ventricular) URI (equal to the ventricular LRI). Thus a very early atrial extrasystole (As) may produce an extremely long As-Vp interval (Fig. 7).

The DDI mode with A-A LRT (controlling the LRI) creates a paradoxical situation where the LRI is an atrial interval controlled by atrial events, while the URI (which should be equal to the LRI) is a ventricular interval [2] . A DDI pacemaker with A-A

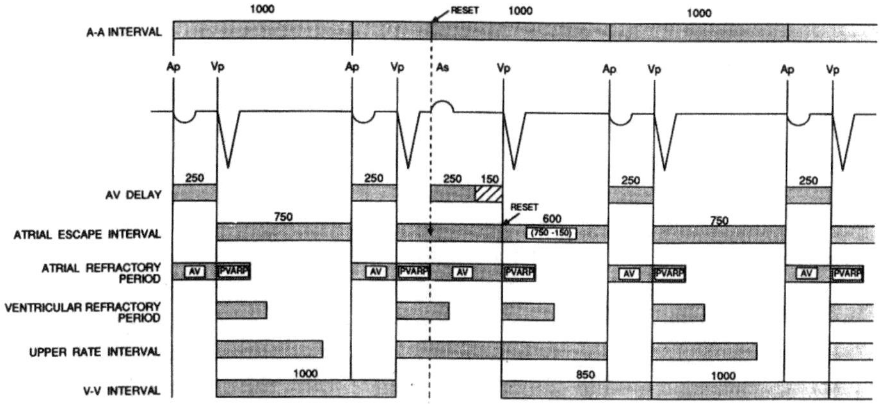

Fig. 6. Timing cycles of the Cosmos II DDD pulse generator with A-A lower rate timing (LRT) and the same parameters as in Figs. 1 and 5, except that the PVARP was shortened to allow for earlier atrial sensing. An atrial extrasystole (As) initiates an AV interval of 400 ms (As-Vp) to conform to the ventricular upper rate interval (URI) [10]. Therefore, the pulse generator emits Vp at the completion of the URI. Vp initiates an atrial escape interval (AEI) of 750 + (250 – 400) = 750 – 150 = 600 ms. The A-A interval remains constant at 1000 ms. *Solid vertical lines*, pace event time lines; *dashed vertical lines*, sense event time lines. (From [2])

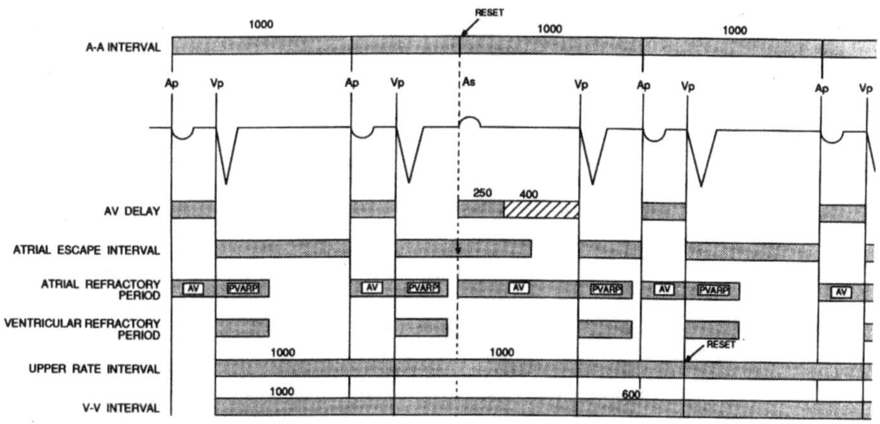

Fig. 7. DDI mode in the Cosmos II DDD pulse generator with A-A lower rate timing (LRT). In the DDD mode of this pulse generator, the lowest programmable upper rate is 80 ppm and the closest programmable lower rate is 78 ppm. For the sake of discussion it was assumed that both the upper rate and lower rate were programmable to 60 ppm in an attempt to obtain the DDI mode. AV = 250 ms. In the DDI mode, the ventricular upper rate interval (URI) should be equal to the lower rate interval (LRI), which in this case is atrial-based. An early As initiates a long As-Vp interval of 650 ms as in any DDD pulse generator (regardless of LRT) simply to conform to the ventricular URI (1000 ms and equal to LRI). With A-A LRT, because Vp terminates the As-Vp interval, Vp initiates an atrial escape interval (AEI) = 750 + (250 – 650) = 350 ms as shown. The As-Ap interval is, however, maintained at 1000 ms. The Vp-Ap-Vp = 350 + 250 = 600 ms in violation of the ventricular URI. This illustration demonstrates the incompatibility of A-A LRT with the DDI mode of pacing. *Solid vertical lines*, pace event time lines; *dashed vertical lines*, sense event time lines. (From [2])

LRT must, however, retain constancy of the atrial LRI (As-Ap or Ap-Ap). Preservation of the atrial LRI takes hierarchial precedence over any other intervals including the ventricular URI (equal to the atrial LRI). Thus, a DDD pulse generator with A-A LRT programmed with equal URI and LRI to produce the DDI mode will respond to a long (no. 1) As-Vp interval (initiated by a sensed early atrial extrasystole or even a sinus P wave) by reducing the subsequent AEI to maintain constancy of the atrial LRI or As-Ap interval. The subsequent AEI must therefore shorten by a value equal to the (long) As-Vp interval less the programmed Ap-Vp interval. This considerable shortening of the AEI will lead to the delivery of Ap (no. 2) close to the preceding Vp (no. 1) and the delivery of the succeeding Vp (no. 2) beyond but relatively close to the apex of the T wave generated by the preceding Vp (no. 1). In this way, by preserving the (atrial) LRI, the pacemaker violates the ventricular URI, which in the true DDI mode (V-V LRT) must necessarily be equal in duration to the LRI. In the conventional DDI mode with V-V LRT, the paced ventricular rate always remains constant, but this is impossible when the DDI mode is attempted with A-A LRT.

It appears from the above considerations that dual-chamber pulse generators need a ventricular-based LRI when functioning in the DDI or DDIR mode. This could be achieved automatically according to the programmed mode, or the type of LRT could itself be a programmable option avialable to match the desired pacing mode or circumstances. Alternatively, a pacemaker cycle could time out with either a V-V response or A-A response to avoid undesirable rate fluctuations as incorporated in recently designed hybrid DDDR systems (discussed later).

As with the DDI and DDIR modes, A-A LRT does not lend itself to smooth functioning of a DDDR pulse generator. Figure 8 shows how such a design to maintain the *atrial*-based LRI can force the pulse generator to violate its sensor-driven *ventricular* URI. An atrial-based DDDR system may violate its sensor-driven URI only when the atrial-driven URI is longer than the TARP. In other words, the potential for violating the sensor-driven URI exists whenever the As-Vp interval is extended by a Wenckebach upper rate response. The circumstances causing violation of the sensor-driven URI can be derived mathematically.

1. Violation of the sensor-driven URI can occur only when the maximal value of the so-called Wenckebach increment (W) of the AV interval [total atrial refractory period (TARP) – atrial-driven URI] exceeds the difference between the two URIs, i.e., W > (atrial-driven URI – sensor-driven URI). One should probably never program the atrial-driven URI < sensor-driven URI, i.e., atrial-driven upper rate faster than the sensor-driven upper rate.
2. The degree of violation (Δ) of the sensor driven URI (i.e., degree of shortening) is equal to the value of W less the difference between the sensor-driven URI and the sensor-driven interval (or sensor-driven LRI) provided the value of Δ is positive, i.e., Δ = W – (sensor-driven interval – sensor-driven URI). According to this formula, when the atrial-driven URI is > TARP, violation of the sensor-driven URI will occur when the sensor-driven interval (sensor-driven LRI) approaches the value of the atrial-driven URI. When the TARP is equal to the atrial-driven URI, the pacemaker cannot generate a Wenckebach upper rate response and therefore violation of the sensor-driven URI cannot occur.

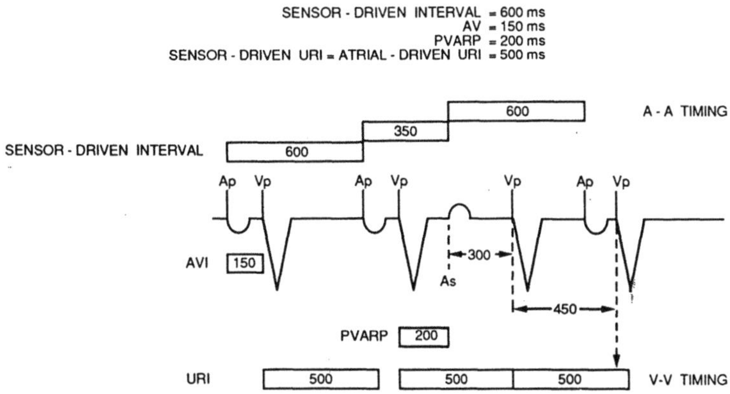

Fig. 8. Timing cycles of a hypothetical DDDR pulse generator with atrial-based lower rate timing. The sensor-driven URI is equal to the atrial-driven upper rate interval (URI) (500 ms). In the DDDR mode with a sensor-driven interval of 600 ms (effective sensor-driven lower rate interval [LRI] = 600 ms), a spontaneous P (As) initiates an AV interval, As-Vp, that is extended to conform to the atrial-driven ventricular URI (500 ms) initiated by the second Vp. The interval from the second Vp to the third Vp is equal to the atrial-driven ventricular URI. The sensed P wave, As, initiates a sensor-driven (atrial-based) LRI of 600 ms which by definition must terminate with Ap (i.e., last Ap). Since the programmed Ap-Vp interval is not allowed to lengthen (a response so far never used in pacemaker design), the last Vp is delivered according to the programmed Ap-Vp interval of 150 ms. Delivery of the last Vp violates the sensor-driven ventricular URI because the last Vp-Vp interval is 450 ms < 500 ms (duration of the common or sensor-driven URI). This example illustrates the two conditions required for violation of the sensor-driven URI by an atrial-based DDDR system: (a) atrial-driven URI is > total atrial refractory period (TARP) – this allows a Wenckebach upper rate response with extension of the As-Vp interval, W = maximal increment of the As-Vp interval (atrial-driven URI – TARP) – in this case the W interval = 500 – 350 = 150 ms; (b) violation of the sensor-driven URI occurs because Δ = W – (sensor-driven interval – sensor-driven URI) which is equal to 150 – (600 – 500) = 50 ms i.e. the value of Δ is greater than zero and represents the maximal degree of shortening or violation of the sensor-driven URI as shown in the diagram. (See text for details.)

Pseudo A-A Timing: Medtronic Synergyst I and Synergyst II DDDR Pulse Generators

The Medtronic Synergyst I and II DDD pulse generators are designed with a modified form of V-V LRT that superficially resembles A-A timing [13, 14]. The timing mechanism may be called pseudo A-A timing. In the Synergyst I and II pulse generators, the AV interval initiated by atrial sensing (As-Vp) is identical to that initiated by atrial pacing (Ap-Vp). In the Synergyst I and II design, constancy of the AEI controls the LRI as in V-V LRT. The pulse generator may be considered to initiate a constant AEI coincidentally with the generation of either an actual ventricular stimulus (Vp) or an implied one (Vpi) (Figs. 9, 10). A sensed ventricular event (Vs) during the programmed AV interval inhibits release of the ventricular stimulus (Vp). However, Vs during the programmed AV interval does not terminate the AV interval as occurs traditionally in pulse generators with V-V LRT. Rather, the pulse generator continues to time out the entire programmed AV interval. At the end of the programmed AV interval (As-Vp = Ap-Vp), the pulse generator behaves (in terms of its timing mechanism or cycles) as if a ventricular stimulus is actually generated (but does not reach the output terminals because of internal diversion within the circuitry), i.e., an implied ventricular stimulus (Vpi) is produced. The manufacturer has called this event the "impending or scheduled V-pace" [2, 14]. Vpi controls initiation of the AEI (and the LRI) precisely as if the ventricular stimulus had actually been released. This behavior may be conceptualized in terms of a "committed" AV interval as far as LRT is concerned [2] (Figs. 11–13). During VSP, the pulse generator delivers Vp prematurely, leading to abbreviation of the Ap-Vp interval. When Vp is triggered by VSP, it initiates a constant AEI and LRI, and the

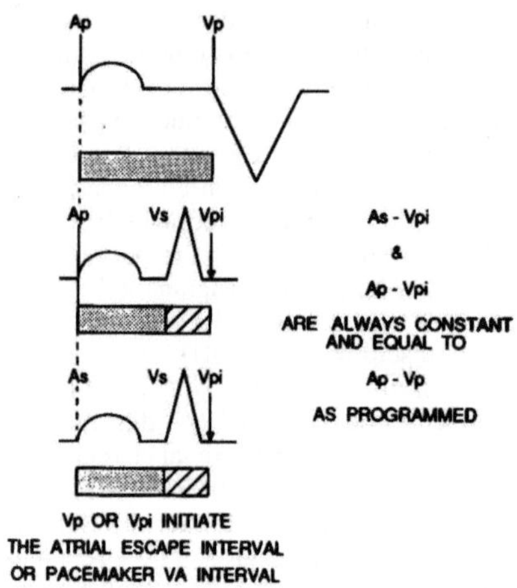

Fig. 9. Timing cycles of the Medtronic Synergyst I and II DDD and DDDR pulse generators with pseudo A-A lower rate timing (LRT) showing the function of the committed AV interval. Ap or As initiates a committed AV interval terminating with Vp or Vpi (i, implied). (See text for further details.) (From [2])

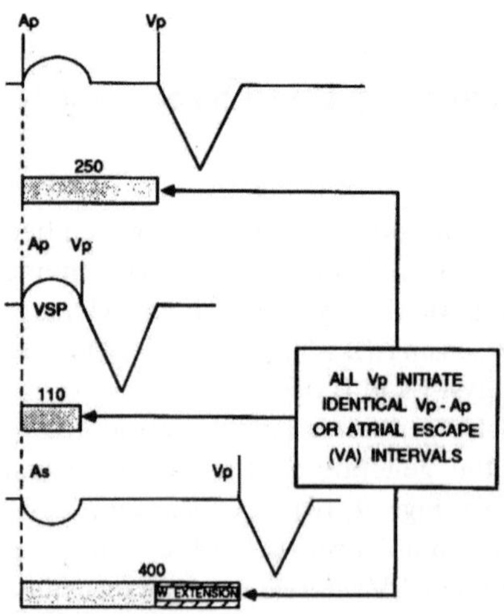

Fig. 10. Timing cycles of the Medtronic Synergyst I and II DDD and DDDR pulse generators with pseudo A-A lower rate timing (LRT) showing circumstances associated with a constant atrial escape interval (AEI) initiated by Vp. At the *bottom*, the As-Vp interval lengthens from the programmed value of 250 ms (*top*) to 400 ms because of upper rate limitation(URI > total atrial refractory period). The largest increment in the AV interval (or the Wenckebach extension, *W*) = 400 – 250 = 150 ms. (From [2])

timing mechanism does not wait for the committed Vpi (Fig. 12) scheduled to occur at the completion of the entire Ap-Vp interval as programmed. The response of the Synergyst I and II pacemakers to VSP differs from that of the Medtronic Elite units [15, 16] in the DDDR mode which responds to VSP with a truly committed AV interval where Vpi and not Vp (as in the Synergyst I and II design) actually starts the constant AEI.

The committed AV interval alway remains constant with Ap-Vpi always equal to the programmed Ap-Vp. Thus, when As-Vs is extended beyond the Ap-Vp interval to conform to the URI (Wenckebach upper rate response), extension of the AV interval beyond Vpi forces the pulse generator to initiate the LRI and AEI from Vs before completion of the atrial-driven URI. In other words, Vs usurps initiation of the LRI and AEI from the anticipated ventricular stimulus (Vp) that the pulse generator would have emitted at the completion of the atrial-driven URI had Vs not occurred. This response is identical to that of a traditional ventricular-based DDD pulse generator in the same circumstances.

In published literature concerning the Synergyst II DDDR pulse generator [17], Medtronic, Inc., has described the device as possessing atrial-based timing. Yet the same literature [17] also states that in the following three circumstances: (a) pacemaker Wenckebach operation; (b) ventricular safety pacing; or (c) pacemaker-defined ventricular extrasystole, there is an exception to A-A timing. Specifically the

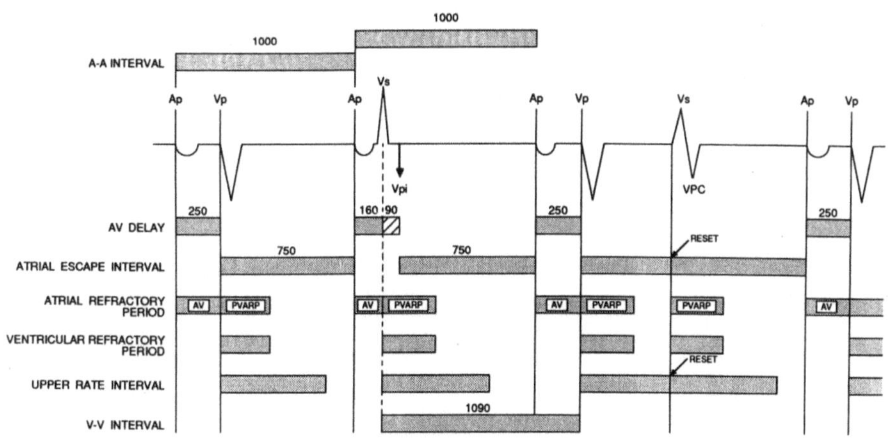

Fig. 11. Timing cycles of the Medtronic Synergyst II DDD pulse generator with pseudo A-A lower rate timing (LRT) in the DDD mode. Lower rate interval (LRI) = 1000 ms, AV = 250 ms, basic atrial escape interval (AEI) = 750 ms. The second Ap is followed by a conducted QRS complex, Vs; Ap-Vs = 160 ms. Ap initiates a committed AV interval of 250 ms, at the end of which an implied ventricular stimulus occurs (Vpi). Vs initiates the PVARP, Ventricular refractory period, upper rate interval (URI), but not the AEI. Vpi initiates the AEI of 750 ms (and therefore the LRI). Note that the Vs-Vp interval = 1090 ms > LRI. A ventricular extrasystole (VPC) beyond the AV interval initiates an AEI of 750 ms. Compare Fig. 11 with Fig. 1 and note that in certain circumstances the response of pulse generators with A-A and those with pseudo A-A LRT may be identical. *Solid vertical lines*, pace event time lines; *dashed vertical lines*, *sense event time lines*. (From [2])

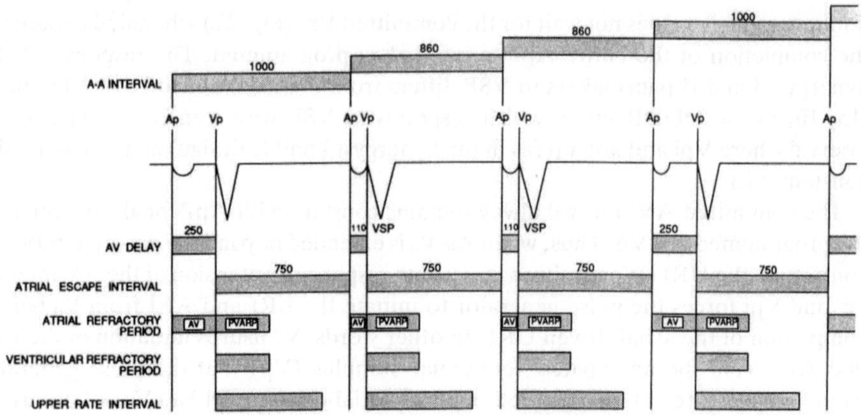

Fig. 12. Timing cycles of the Medtronic Synergyst II DDD pulse generator with pseudo A-A lower rate timing (LRT) with the same parameters as in Fig. 11. Crosstalk induces ventricular safety pacing (*VSP*) with abbreviation of the Ap-Vp interval to 110 ms. The atrial escape interval (AEI) remains constant, but the Ap-Ap interval shortens to 860 ms. The pacing rate therefore increases in contrast to a DDD pulse generator with A-A LRT where VSP activation does not increase the pacing rate (as shown in Fig. 5). *Vertical lines*, pace event time lines. (From [2])

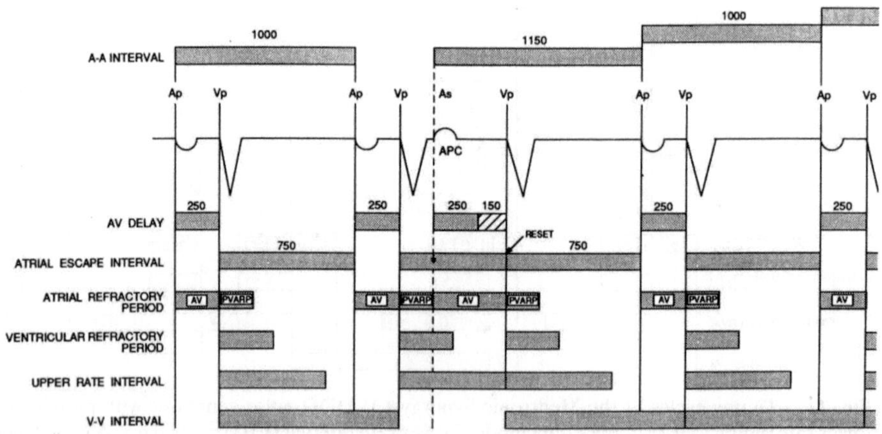

Fig. 13. Timing cycles of the Medtronic Synergyst II DDD pulse generator with pseudo A-A lower rate timing (LRT) with the same parameters as in Fig. 11 and 12 except that the PVARP was shortened to allow for earlier atrial sensing. An atrial extrasystole (As) initiates an AV interval of 400 ms to conform to the ventricular upper rate interval (URI). The pulse generator emits Vp at the completion of the URI. Vp initiates an atrial escape interval (AEI) of 750 ms. Consequently the As-Vp-Ap interval increases to 1150 ms– longer than the basic A-A interval (1000 ms) during continuous AV sequential pacing (Ap-Vp, Ap-Vp, etc.). *Solid vertical lines*, pace event time lines; *dashed vertical lines*, sense event time lines. (From [2])

literature states that "all three irregular occurrences restart the VA timer, effectively switching the pacemaker to a V-V timing mode for the cycle following the operation. These occurrences represent special situations that require the normal timing sequence to be altered by a sensed or paced ventricular event. Restarting the VA timer reestablishes A-A timing." We believe that this explanation of LRT pacemaker behavior switching back and forth from A-A to V-V timing according to circumstances may lead to confusion. The LRT mechanism of this particular pulse generator is really a modification of V-V LRT, and for this reason we believe that calling it pseudo A-A LRT is appropriate.

Hybrid LRT for DDDR Pacing

New designs of hybrid LRT for DDD pulse generators have incorporated some of the characteristics of both A-A and V-V LRT to avoid undesirable fluctuations of pacing rate (Fig. 14) produced by atrial-based and ventricular-based pulse generators under certain circumstances (Tables 1 and 2).

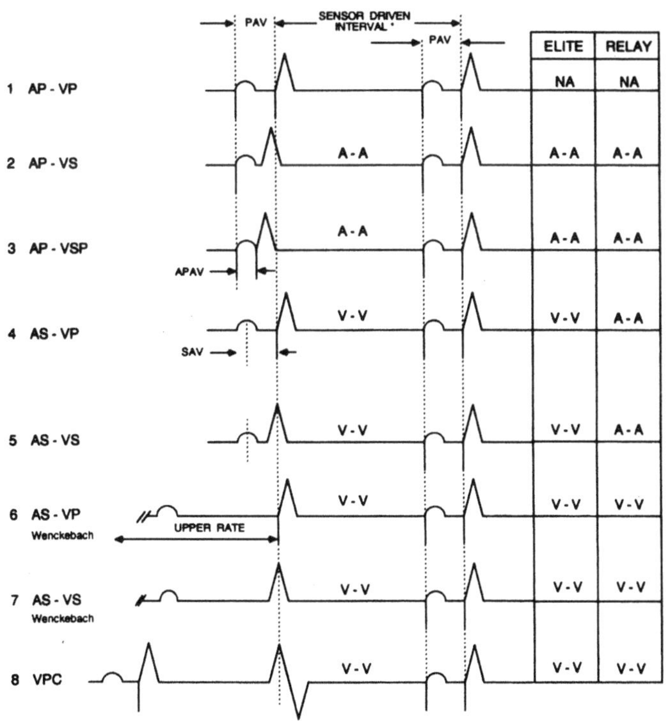

Fig. 14. Comparison of timing cycles of the Medtronic Elite and Intermedics Relay DDDR pulse generators. *AP*, atrial pace; *VP*, ventricular pace; *AS*, atrial sense; *VS*, ventricular sense; *VPC*, ventricular extrasystole; *VSP*, ventricular safety pace. AV interval: *SAV*, sensed; *PAV*, paced; *APAV*, abbreviated paced (VSP); *NA*, not applicable. Note that in *4*, the SAV is shorter than the PAV in *1*. In *6*, *upper rate* refers to the upper rate interval. The first *dotted vertical lines* on the *left* indicate the response of the atrial channel to either Ap or As. The *dotted vertical line beyond Ap or As* represents the beginning of the LRI. *Asterisk*, sensor-driven interval varies between lower rate interval and sensor-driven upper rate interval. (See text for details.)

Table 1. Lower Rate Behavior of Medtronic DDD and DDDR Pulse Generators: Committed AV Intervals

AV Interval	Symbios DDD Mode	Synergyst I and II DDD Mode	Synergyst II DDDR Mode	Elite* DDDR Mode	Elite* DDD Mode
1. Ap-Vs	V-V	Committed AV	Committed AV	Committed AV	V-V
2. Abbreviated Ap-Vp (VSP)	V-V	V-V	V-V	Committed AV	V-V
3. As-Vp < programmed Ap-Vp	NA	NA	NA	V-V	V-V
4. As-Vp > programmed Ap-Vp (as in Wenckebach response)	V-V	V-V	V-V	V-V	V-V
5. As-Vs < programmed Ap-Vp	V-V	Committed AV	Committed AV	V-V	V-V
6. As-Vs > programmed Ap-Vp (as in Wenckebach upper rate response)	V-V	V-V	V-V	V-V	V-V
7. VPC not preceded by As	V-V	V-V	V-V	V-V	V-V

The AV interval is uncommitted in all V-V cycles. VSP, ventricular safety pacing; VPC, ventricular premature contraction or extrasystole. NA = not applicable as As-Vp = Ap-Vp.

Table 2. Lower Rate Behavior of Intermedics DDD and DDDR Pulse Generator

AV Interval	Cosmos I DDD	Cosmos II DDD	Relay DDDR	Relay DDD
1. Ap-Vs	V-V	A-A	A-A	A-A
2. Abbreviated Ap-Vp (VSP)	V-V	A-A	A-A	A-A
3. As-Vp < programmed Ap-Vp	V-V	A-A	A-A	A-A
4. As-Vp > programmed Ap-Vp (prolongation in Wenckebach upper rate response)	V-V	A-A	V-V	V-V
5. As-Vs < programmed Ap-Vp	V-V	A-A	A-A	A-A
6. As-Vs > programmed Ap-Vp (as in Wenckebach upper rate response)	V-V	A-A	V-V	V-V
7. VPC not preceded by As	V-V	V-V	V-V	V-V

VSP, ventricular safety pacing.
* The behavior of the Elite II pulse generator is identical.

1. AV Interval Initiated by an Atrial-Paced Event

The Medtronic Elite DDDR pulse generator [15, 16] has two different sets of LRT according to the programmed mode (Fig. 14). In the non-sensor-driven DDD mode, the Elite functions as the Symbios DDD devices (but not Synergyst I and II) with pure V-V LRT, e.g., DDD, DDI, etc. (Table 1). In the DDDR mode, the LRT is based on the concept of a truly "committed AV interval" only when the pulse generator emits an atrial stimulus (Ap). Thus any abbreviated AV interval initiated by Ap ends either with a paced ventricular event, Vp on time according to the programmed Ap-Vp interval, or an impending or scheduled V-pace event as far as LRT control is concerned. The pulse generator behaves (in terms of its timing cycles) as if a ventricular stimulus is actually generated (but does not reach the output terminals), i.e., the pacemaker produces an implied ventricular stimulus (Vpi). The pulse generator uses the committed AV mechanism in only two situations associated with abbreviation of the AV interval initiated by Ap: (a) Ap-Vs (atrial pacing followed by a Vs); and (b) abbreviation of Ap-Vp due to VSP. The committed AV response keeps the interval between two atrial events constant. The committed AV response with VSP differs from that of the Synergyst I and II where the AEI begins with Vp and not Vpi as with the DDDR Elite pulse generator. The Elite device could therefore be described as a V-V unit with a truly committed AV interval (as far as the timing cycles are concerned) only when Ap initiates the AV interval. With the release of Ap, the Intermedics Relay DDDR pulse generator [18] functions exactly like the Medtronic Elite unit in the DDDR mode.

AV Interval Initiated by an As

The Medtronic Elite DDDR pulse generator will exhibit a V-V response to all situations that do not involve Ap, as follows: (a) As-Vp < Ap-Vp as programmed; (b) As-Vp > Ap-Vp as programmed (Wenckebach upper rate behavior; (c) As-Vs < Ap-Vp as programmed; and (d) As-Vs (Wenckebach equivalent) > Ap-Vp as programmed (Table 1).

The Intermedics Relay DDDR pulse generator will exhibit an A-A response following Ap and in the following situations that do not involve Ap: (a) As-Vp < Ap-Vp as programmed; and (b) As-As < Ap-Vp as programmed (Table 2). The Relay unit will exhibit a V-V response in the following situations: (a) As-Vp > Ap-Vp as programmed (Wenckebach upper rate behavior); and (b) As-Vs (Wenckebach equivalent) > Ap-Vp as programmed (Table 2).

Response to Sensed Ventricular Extrasystoles

A-A or V-V Response?

All ventricular extrasystoles (ventricular premature contractions, VPCs) not preceded by As initiate a V-V response regardless of the LRT mechanism (Figs. 1, 11). If As precedes Vs, the response will be V-V or A-A according to design. An A-A response will occur with the Synergyst I and II, Cosmos II, and Relay units, but not with the Elite pulse generator.

"DVI on VPC" and "+PVARP on VPC" Responses

In the Paragon DDD and the Synchrony DDDR devices (Pacesetter-Siemens, Sylmar, California, USA) [19, 20], automatic extension of the post-ventricular atrial refractory period (PVARP) after a VPC does not occur unless one of the above functions is specifically programmed. Without the PVARP extension function, a VPC merely initiates a basic AEI in the DDD mode or a sensor-driven AEI in the DDDR mode.

In the Paragon DDD and Synchrony I and II DDDR pulse generators programmed with the +PVARP on VPC feature, there is extension of the PVARP following a sensed VPC. The PVARP is extended to 480 ms. An unsensed P wave falling near the end of the extended PVARP may allow delivery of the subsequent atrial stimulus into the myocardial atrial refractory period related to the unsensed P wave (in the PVARP). Loss of atrial capture predisposes to retrograde ventriculoatrial conduction. To avoid such problems with the +PVARP on VPC feature, the pulse generator lengthens the AEI following a VPC to 830 ms (duration of PVARP at 480 ms plus an additional delay of 350 ms). In the DDDR mode, the +PVARP on VPC

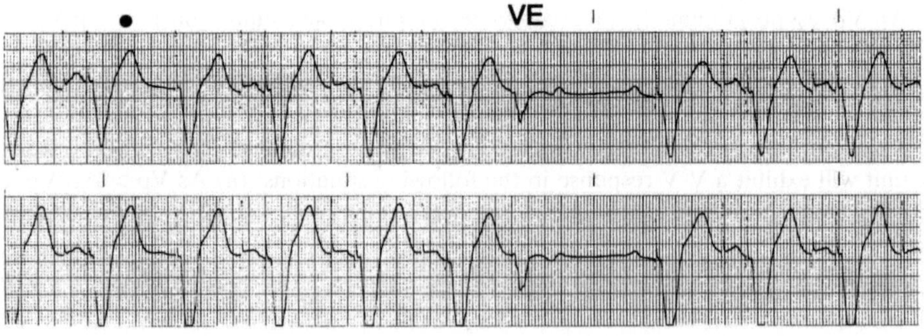

Fig. 15. Response of the Pacesetter-Siemens Synchrony DDDR pulse generator to a sensed ventricular premature contraction (VPC) (*VE*). Two ECG leads were recorded simultaneously at 50 mm/s. The *solid black circle* indicates sensing of a P wave beyond the PVARP. The sensed P wave inhibits release of the Ap at the termination of the sensor-driven atrial escape interval (AEI). The VPC (*VE*) disengages the AEI from the sensor drive for one cycle and the AEI initiated by the VPC lengthens to 830 ms. (See text for details.)

response disengages the AEI from the sensor drive for one cycle (Fig. 15). This response favors sensing of a spontaneous P wave by the atrial channel. If no sensed P wave occurs, the pacemaker releases an atrial stimulus 350 ms after the end of the PVARP ensuring atrial capture outside the atrial myocardial refractory period. When the +PVARP on VPC feature is programmed, one should probably not use this DDDR pulse generator with a high maximal sensor rate [7].

The DVI on VPC feature is similar to the DDX mode with the initiation of a DVI cycle (PVARP occupies the entire AEI). The AEI following sensing of a VPC in the DDD and DDDR modes is extended as in the +PVARP on VPC function, but only to its base value as programmed.

Prolongation of the AEI after automatic lengthening of PVARP regardless of the mechanism prevents the development of repetitive non-reentrant ventriculoatrial synchrony (AV desynchronization arrhythmia) by a VPC with retrograde conduction whenever the shorter sensor-driven AEI delivers Ap in the atrial myocardial refractory period related to the preceding retrograde depolarization linked to the VPC [21-23].

Pacemaker-defined VPC

In some DDD or DDDR pulse generators, a VPC (defined by the pulse generator as two consecutive ventricular events without an intervening sensed P wave) is accompanied by an automatic prolongation of the PVARP for one cycle, a response designed to prevent sensing of retrograde P waves. In the Elite, Cosmos II, and Relay pulse generators, if a refractory sensed atrial event occurs between two ventricular events (i.e., P wave detected in the terminal portion of the PVARP), the second ventricular event is also considered a pacemaker-defined VPC [15, 18]. This response (also seen in the DDIR mode) prevents a ventricular event resulting from an atrial extrasystole (with P wave in the PVARP) from being counted as a VPC and therefore avoids inappropriate automatic PVARP extension by an atrial extrasystole or sinus P wave falling in the terminal portion of the PVARP. Such an arrangement would also avoid atrial undersensing perpetuated by P waves continually falling within an automatically extended (and long) PVARP, e.g., as in relatively fast sinus rhythm associated with first-degree AV block [24–26] .

Response of Synergyst II DDDR Pulse Generator to a Sensed Ventricular Extrasystole

In the DDDR mode of the Synergyst II pulse generator (pseudo A-A LRT), a sensed VPC initiates an AEI equal to the programmed value, i.e., LRI – (Ap-Vp as programmed). In the DDDR mode, the sensor-driven LRI will shorten as the sensor-driven rate increases. A sensed VPC should therefore initiate an AEI = sensor-driven LRI – (Ap-Vp as programmed). In fact, this response occur up to a critical sensor-driven LRI, beyond which an additional AV interval (Ap-Vp) is added to the AEI, i.e., AEI = sensor-driven LRI – (Ap-Vp) + additional Ap-Vp interval = sensor-driven LRI

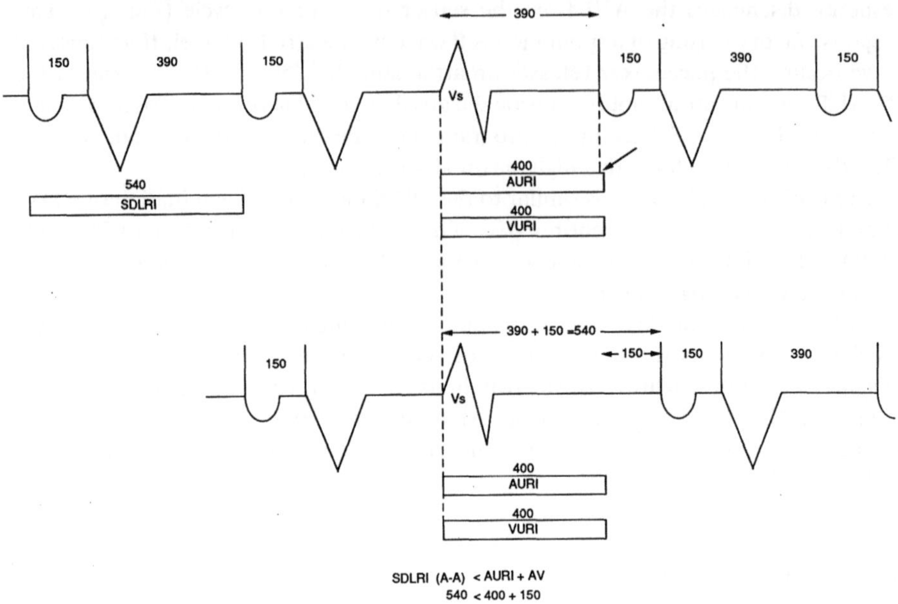

Fig. 16. Synergyst II DDDR response to a sensed ventricular extrasystole during sensor-driven (*SD*) pacing. SD lower rate interval (*SDLRI*) = 540 ms, SD atrial escape interval (*SDAEI*) = 390 ms, AV = 150 ms, upper rate = 150 ppm corresponding to upper rate interval (URI) = 400 ms. *Top*, a ventricular extrasystole (*Vs*) initiates an atrial URI (*AURI*) and a ventricular URI (*VURI*), both being 400 ms. Vs also initiates an SDAEI of 390 ms. Therefore, an atrial stimulus (Ap) released at the completion of the SDAEI (390 ms) would occur before the termination of the AURI. To avoid violation of the AURI, the pulse generator was designed to omit Ap at the end of the SDAEI as shown in the *lower diagram*. In this situation, the SDAEI is automatically lengthened by the duration of the AV delay (150 ms). Thus, the SDAEI initiated by Vs measures 390 + 150 = 540 ms. (From [2])

(Fig. 16). The mechanism of the AEI extension is related to the control of the atrial URI ([2, 17]; R McVenes, personal communication). In the DDDR mode, a VPC (diagnosed by the pacemaker as the second of two consecutive ventricular events with no intervening atrial event) initiates the following timing cycles: ventricular refractory period, sensor-driven AEI (and LRI), PVARP, PVARP extension, ventricular URI, and atrial URI (the last two intervals are equal).

Double Sensing of Ventricular Extrasystoles

The incidence of simultaneous or near-simultaneous sensing of ventricular extrasystoles (VPC) by the atrial and ventricular channels has not been investigated in detail in DDD pulse generators with V-V LRT. Although the depolarization emanating from a VPC may reach the ventricular lead before the atrial one, the VPC may actually be sensed by the atrial channel before the ventricular channel [2] (Fig. 17). This occurs because the smaller signal in the atrium may reach the very high sensitivity of the atrial channel before the larger signal in the ventricle attains the lower sensitivity of the ventricular channel, i.e., As-Vs = 0 or a very small positive value. During DDD pacing with V-V LRT, earlier or simultaneous atrial sensing of a VPC will go unnoticed because Vs immediately starts the AEI and the effect of As (atrial sensing of far-field ventricular signal) is negated. The consequences of this particular form of As could be documented with event markers by showing that a true atrial event (nearfield signal) cannot occur at this time (e.g., during the atrial myocardial refractory period or excluded by an esophageal electrocardiogram). However, in DDD pulse generators with pseudo A-A LRT, or a hybrid LRT with an A-A response following As, the effect of a VPC sensed by both atrial and ventricular channels will become evident, as shown in Figure 17. Prolongation of the AEI from double sensing of a VPC should not be misinterpreted as pacemaker malfunction, hysteresis, oversensing of the T wave, etc.

Ventricular Safety Pacing

A ventricular extrasystole sensed beyond the atrial stimulus and its succeeding ventricular blanking period can activate the ventricular safety pacing function of pulse

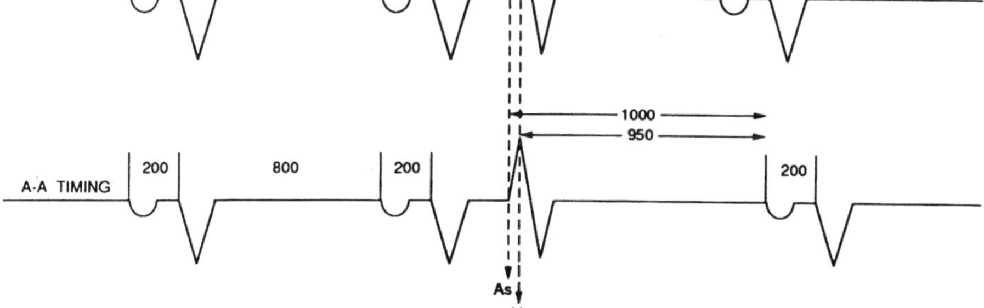

Fig. 17. Double sensing of ventricular extrasystole (*VE*) by DDD pulse generators. Farfield atrial sensing of the VE occurs before it is sensed by the ventricular channel. *Top*, DDD pulse generator with V-V lower rate timing (LRT). Early farfield atrial sensing does not interfere with the timing functions (except for omission of PVARP extension), and the VE initiates an atrial escape interval (AEI) of 800 ms. *Bottom*, DDD pulse generator with lower rate A-A response to As-Vs < programmed Ap-Vp. Early farfield sensing initiates a constant A-A interval (As-Ap) equal to the lower rate interval (LRI). As-Vs = 50 ms, so that the AEI initiated by the VE = 800 + (200 – 50) = 950 ms. (From [2])

generators with this characteristic resulting in Ap-Vp abbreviation. The duration of the AEI initiated by Vp will depend upon the designed lower rate behavior under these circumstances, i.e., either Ap initiates the LRI (A-A cycle) or Vp initiates the LRI (V-V cycle).

Compensatory Pause

In the old Siemens (Siemens-Elema, Solna, Sweden) 674 DDD pulse generator with atrial-based LRT, a VPC (not preceded by an atrial event) initiated an AEI equal to the LRI, i.e., base AEI + AV interval, producing a "compensatory pause" [2] . No contemporary LRT design produces such a response except the Synergyst II DDDR pulse generator under special circumstances as already discussed.

Conclusion

The various combinations of pacemaker LRI (A-A and V-V cycles) controlled by a variety of circumstances have rendered lower rate evaluation difficult. An easy way to remember the various responses is needed. First, the various types of AV intervals should be defined (Table 3).

Table 3. Types Of AV Intervals

	Shorter	Basic	Longer
Ap-Vp	+	+	–
Ap-Vs	+	+	–
As-Vp	+	+	+
As-Vs	+	+	+

Then one could assume that all LRT is *ventricular* based and that the presence of a *committed* AV interval (as far as the timing cycles are concerned) is the only variable to be considered in determining the type of lower rate response (Tables 1, 4). By knowing whether the AV interval is committed or not, the behavior of a given pacing cycle can be automatically predicted in terms of A-A or V-V response (Table 4). The termination of the committed AV interval indicates when the LRI and AEI begin. In other words, a V-V cycle begins with the implied ventricular stimulus (Vpi) terminating the committed AV interval. When the committed AV interval comes into play and Vpi initiates LRI and AEI, the pacing cycle will automatically adjust to provide the A-A interval (Ap-Ap or As-Ap) equal to the LRI. Thus, analysis of lower rate behavior requires knowledge of the circumstances in which the AV interval is truly committed (Table 4). When a committed AV interval does not come into play, the pulse generator functions with a traditional ventricular-based response. Thus by using the concept of the "committed AV interval," evaluation of LRI behavior can be determined under all circumstances without invoking a more complex (and unfamiliar) atrial-based LRT mechanism.

Table 4. Committed AV Interval

Pacemaker Model	Circumstances Associated With Committed AV Interval
Medtronic Elite I and II	After Ap Only
Intermedics Relay	After all AV intervals (initiated by Ap or As[a]) *shorter* than the programmed Ap-Vp interval
Medtronic Synergyst I and II	After all AV intervals (initiated by Ap or As[a]) *shorter* than the programmed Ap-Vp interval *except* when Ap-Vp is abbreviated due to ventricular safety pacing
Intermedics Cosmos II and Ela Chorus	After *all* AV intervals (initiated by Ap of As[a])

The following AV combinations do not occur during normal function: (a) Ap-Vs longer than programmed Ap-Vp; (b) Ap-Vp longer than programmed Ap-Vp.

[a] As-Vs may be shorter than, equal to, or longer than the programmed Ap-Vp during normal function when URI is > TARP that allows a pacemaker Wenckebach upper rate response.

References

1. Barold SS, Falkoff MD, Ong LS, Heinle RA (1988) Timing cycles of DDD pacemakers. In: Barold SS, Mugica J (eds) New perspectives in cardiac pacing. Futura, New York, p 69
2. Barold SS, Falkoff MD, Ong LS, Vaughan MJ, Heinle RA (1991) A-A and V-V lower rate timing of DDD and DDDR pulse generators. In: Barold SS, Mugica J (eds) New perspectives in cardiac pacing, vol 2. Futura, New York, p 203
3. Barold SS, Falkoff MD, Ong LS, Heinle RA (1988) Upper rate response of DDD pacemakers. In: Barold SS, Mugica J (eds) New perspectives in cardiac pacing. Futura, New York, p 121
4. Markowitz T, Prest-Berg K, Betzold R, Wibel F (1987) Clinical implications of dual chamber responsive rate pacing. In: Belhassen B, Feldman S, Copperman Y (eds) Cardiac pacing and electrophysiology. Proceedings of the VIIIth world symposium on cardiac pacing and electrophysiology. Keterpress, Jerusalem, p 165
5. Barold SS, Ong LS, Falkoff MD, Heinle RA (1985) Crosstalk or self-inhibition in dual-chambered pacemakers. In: Barold SS (ed) Modern cardiac pacing. Futura, New York, p 615
6. Barold SS, Belott PH (1987) Behavior of the ventricular triggerred period of DDD pacemakers. PACE 10:1237
7. Levine PA, Hayes DL, Wilkoff BL, Ohman AE (1990) Electrocardiography of rate-modulated pacemaker rhythms. Siemens-Pacesetter, Sylmar
8. Intermedics (1989) Cosmos II Models 283-03 and 284-05 cardiac pulse generators. Technical manual. Intermedics, Freeport
9. Ela Medical (1991) Physician manual, Chorus 6033 implantable dual chamber pulse generator, DDDMO. Ela Medical, Montrouge
10. Friedberg HD, Barold SS (1973) On hysteresis in pacing. J. Electrocardiol. 6:2
11. Barold SS (1987) The DDI mode of cardiac pacing. PACE 10:480
12. Barold SS, Falkoff MD, Ong LS, Heinle RA (1988) All dual chamber pacemakers function in the DDD mode. Am. Heart J. 115:1353
13. Medtronic (1989) Synergyst 7026/7027 dual chamber pacer with VVIR activity response and telemetry. Technical manual. Medtronic, Minneapolis
14. Medtronic (1989) Synergyst II 7070/7071 activity responsive dual chamber pacer with telemetry. Technical manual. Medtronic, Minneapolis

15. Medtronic (1991) Technical manual Elite 7074/75/76/77 activity responsive dual chamber pacemaker with telemetry. Medtronic, Minneapolis
16. Medtronic (1990) Elite user's guide. Medtronic, Minneapolis
17. Medtronic (1989) Synergystics, Synergyst II guidelines to operations and patient management. Medtronic, Minneapolis
18. Intermedics (1991) Physician manual. Relay DDDR pulse generator Model 293-03 and 294-04. Intermedics, Freeport
19. Pacesetter Systems (1988) Technical manual. Pacesetter Synchrony 2020T rate-modulated polarity programmable dual-chamber pacemaker. Pacesetter Systems, Sylmar
20. Pacesetter Systems (1988) Physician manual. Pacesetter Paragon bipolar/unipolar dual-chamber pacing systems Models 2010T and 2012T. Pacesetter Systems, Sylmar
21. Barold SS (1990) Repetitive non-reentrant ventriculoatrial synchrony in dual chamber pacing. In: Santini M, Pistolese M, Alliegro A (eds) Progress in clinical pacing. Excerpta Medica, Amsterdam p 451
22. Barold SS, Falkoff MD, Ong LS, Heinle RA (1988) Magnet unresponsive pacemaker endless loop tachycardia. Am. Heart J. 116:726
23. Barold SS, Falkoff MD, Ong LS, Heinle RA, Willis JE (1987) AV desynchronization arrhythmia during DDD pacing. In: Belhassen B, Feldman S, Copperman Y (eds) Cardiac pacing and electrophysiology. Proceedings of the VIIIth world symposium on cardiac pacing and electrophysiology. Keterpress, Jerusalem, p 177
24. Wilson JH, Lattner S (1989) Undersensing of P waves in the presence of an adequate P wave due to automatic postventricular atrial refractory period extension. PACE 12:1729
25. Greenspon AJ, Volosin KJ (1987) "Pseudo" loss of atrial sensing by a DDD pacemaker. PACE 10:943
26. Dodinot B, Costa AB, Godenir JP, Preiss MA (1991) "Functional" atrial sensing failures due to pacemaker tachycardia protection. PACE 14:656

Electrocardiography of Rate-Adaptive Dual-Chamber (DDDR) Pacemakers: Upper Rate Behavior

S.S. BAROLD[1]

The addition of non-atrial sensors such as activity, minute ventilation volume and the like to dual-chamber pulse generators has added a new dimension to the upper rate response. In fact, the incorporation of a sensor in a dual-chamber pulse generator necessitates two upper rates: one driven by atrial sensed events (sometimes called the maximal tracking rate) and the other driven by the sensor, not necessarily equal to the atrial-driven upper rate. The interplay of these two upper rates has created new complexity in the electrocardiographic interpretation of DDDR pacemaker function. [1–7].

This discussion of the upper rate behavior of DDDR pulse generators begins with a review of the upper rate behavior of the DDD mode because it forms the basis for the upper rate response of DDDR pulse generators.

Abbreviations and Definitions

The following abbreviations are used: Ap, atrial paced event; As, atrial sensed event; Vp, ventricular paced event; Vs, ventricular sensed event; P-P interval, the interval between two consecutive P waves in sinus rhythm; SD, sensor driven; SDI, sensor-driven interval. The definitions of the lower rate interval (LRI) and sensor-driven LRI are described in "Electrocardiography of Rate-Adaptive Dual-Chamber (DDDR) Pacemakers: Lower Rate Behavior" (this volume). The atrial escape interval (AEI) is the interval from a ventricular paced or sensed event to the succeeding atrial stimulus (Vp-Ap or Vs-Ap). The sensor-driven AEI decreases from the basic value of the AEI to the sensor-driven upper rate interval (URI) according to sensor activity.

Upper Rate Behavior

The *atrial*-driven URI refers to the shortest Vs-Vp or Vp-Vp where the second Vp is triggered by a sensed *atrial* event. The second Vp can only be released at the

[1] Division of Cardiology, Department of Medicine, The Genesee Hospital, University of Rochester School of Medicine and Dentistry, 224 Alexander Street, Rochester, NY 14607, USA

completion of the atrial-driven *ventricular* URI initiated by a preceding Vs or Vp. Obviously a DDD device possesses only one URI, i.e., the atrial-driven URI.

The *sensor-driven* URI refers to the shortest Vs-Vp or Vp-Vp where the second Vp is controlled by *sensor* activity. The second Vp can only be released at the completion of the sensor-driven *ventricular* URI initiated by a preceding Vs or Vp.

Upper Rate Response of DDD Pacemakers

In the DDD mode, URI always refers to the *atrial*-driven (ventricular) URI.

No Separately Programmable URI

The total atrial refractory period (TARP) is equal to the sum of the AV interval and the postventricular atrial refractory period (PVARP). In a DDD pacemaker without a separately programmable URI, the TARP is equal to the (ventricular) URI. Upper rate limitation governed solely by the duration of the TARP is a simple way of controlling the paced ventricular response to a fast atrial rate. An atrial rate faster than the programmed upper rate causes 2:1, 3:1, etc. fixed-ratio pacemaker AV block (n:1 block where n is a whole number). The AV interval (As-Vp) always remains fixed and equal to the programmed value. The (ventricular) upper rate of the pacemaker may be calculated by the formula: upper rate (ppm) = 60 000/TARP in milliseconds or 60/TARP in seconds. The TARP always defines the fastes atrial rate associated with 1:1 AV pacemaker response.

Separately Programmable URI

A pacemaker Wenckebach (or pseudo-Wenckebach, according to some authors) upper rate response during DDD pacing can occur only if the URI is longer than the TARP [8–10] (Fig. 1).

During the Wenckebach upper rate response, if W is equal to the increment of the AV interval per cycle, W = URI – (P-P interval). If W is equal to the maximal increment of the AV (As-Vp) interval, W = URI – TARP. Thus the AV interval will vary from the basic value of As-Vp (as programmed) to a value equal to (As-Vp) + (URI – TARP). For example, if URI = 600 ms, AV = 200 ms, PVARP = 200 ms, and P-P interval = 550 ms, the increment per cycle W = URI – (P-P interval) = 50 ms. The maximal increment of the AV interval, W = URI – TARP = 600 – 400 = 200 ms. The Wenckebach ratio can be calculated according to the formula of Higano and Hayes [11] as follows: $n = W/w = 4$. If N is the next integer above n, $N = 5$, Wenckebach ratio = $N + 1/N$ = 6/5. Thus, with the above parameters, a DDD pulse generator will exhibit 6:5 Wenckebach pacemaker AV block. The pacemaker will respond to an atrial rate faster than 100 ppm and less than 150 ppm with a Wenckebach upper rate response. The duration of the pause terminating the Wenckebach cycle may be

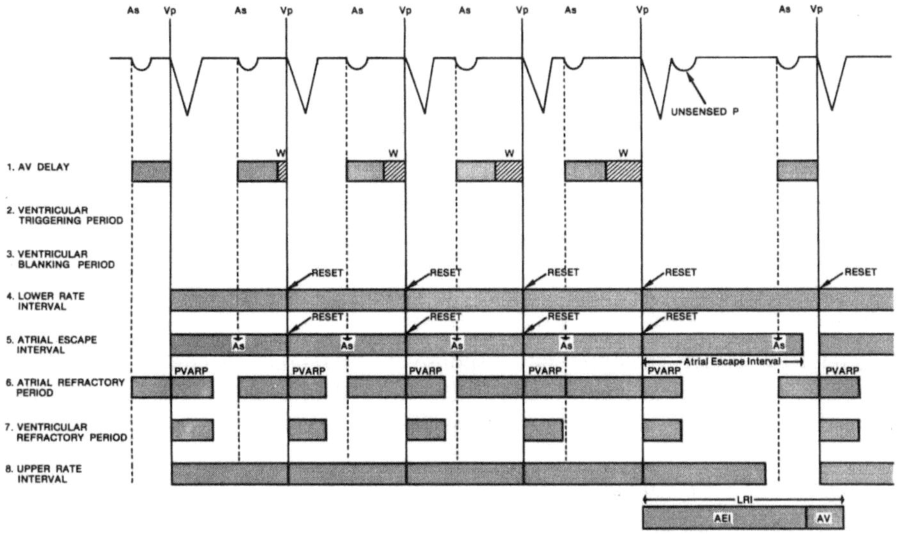

Fig. 1. DDD mode. Wenckebach upper rate response. The upper rate interval is longer than the total atrial refractory period (AV + PVARP) with AV at its programmed value. The P-P interval (As-As) is shorter than the upper rate interval, but longer than the total atrial refractory period. The As-Vp interval lengthens by a varying period (*W*) to conform to the upper rate limit interval. The maximal prolongation of the AV interval represents the difference between the upper rate interval and the total atrial refractory period, with AV at its programmed value. The As-Vp interval lengthens as long as the As-As interval (P-P) is longer than the total atrial refractory period. The sixth P wave falls within the PVARP and is unsensed and the cycle restarts. In the first four pacing cycles, the interval between ventricular stimuli (Vp-Vp) is constant and equal to the upper rate limit interval. When the P-P interval becomes shorter than the total atrial refractory period, a Wenckebach upper rate response cannot occur and fixed-ratio block (e.g., 2:1) will supervene. *Solid vertical lines*, pace event time lines; *dashed vertical lines*, sense event time lines. (From [31])

calculated by another formula published by Higano and Hayes [11] by knowing the atrial rate (P-P interval), TARP, and URI. When the P-P interval becomes shorter than TARP, i.e., less than 400 ms (corresponding to an atrial rate faster than 150 ppm), the Wenckebach upper rate response gives way to fixed ratio 2:1 pacemaker AV block.

URI Shorter than Total Atrial Refractory Period

When the URI is programmed to a shorter value than the TARP (despite the fact that the programmer and the pulse generators may seem to have accepted the command), the pacemaker obviously cannot exhibit Wenckebach pacemaker AV block.

The URI will be the longer of the two intervals, i.e., TARP and the programmer should alert the operator that such values are not acceptable in the DDD mode.

However, this paradoxical relationship may actually be programmable and clinically useful in some DDDR pacemakers, as discussed later.

URI Equal to the Total Atrial Refractory Period

If a separately programmable URI is equal to the TARP, a Wenckebach upper rate response cannot occur and the pulse generator will respond to fast atrial rates with only a fixed ratio pacemaker AV block.

URI Longer than TARP

When URI > TARP, the upper rate response of a DDD pulse generator depends on the duration of three variables: TARP, URI, and P-P intervals (corresponding to the atrial rate) and three situations may be considered.

P-P interval > URI. The pulse generator maintains 1:1 AV synchrony because the atrial rate is slower than the programmed upper rate.
P-P interval < URI. When the P-P interval becomes shorter than the URI but remains longer than the TARP, i.e., URI > P-P interval > TARP, the pulse generator responds with a Wenckebach pacemaker AV block.
P-P interval < TARP. When the P-P interval is shorter than TARP (and therefore also shorter than URI), a Wenckebach upper rate response cannot occur and the upper rate response consists of only a fixed-ratio pacemaker AV block regardless of the duration of the separately programmable URI.

Therefore, when the URI > TARP, a progressive increase in the atrial rate (shortening of the P-P interval) causes first a pacemaker Wenckebach upper rate response (when P-P < URI), and when the P-P interval becomes shorter than the TARP, the upper rate response switches from pacemaker Wenckebach AV block to 2:1 fixed-ratio pacemaker AV block (Table 1).

Table 1. DDD Mode: Upper Rate Response

Parameters	Response
1. P-P < TARP	Fixed ratio 2:1 AV block
2. P-P < TARP < atrial-driven URI	Fixed ratio 2:1 AV block
3. TARP < P-P < atrial-driven URI	Wenckebach upper rate response

Upper Rate and Duration of AV Interval

The AV interval initiated by As (As-Vp) and not the one initiated by Ap (either equal to or longer than the As-Vp interval) determines the point where fixed-ratio pacemaker AV block occurs, i.e., when P-P interval ≤ TARP, where TARP = (As-Vp) + PVARP. In some pulse generators, the TARP can shorten further on exercise by one of three mechanisms: (a) the As-Vp decreases with an increase of the sensed

LOWER RATE INTERVAL = 857 ms
ATRIAL D-URI = 600 ms
SENSOR D-URI = 400 ms
AV DELAY = 150 ms (rate-adaptive)
PVARP = 250 ms

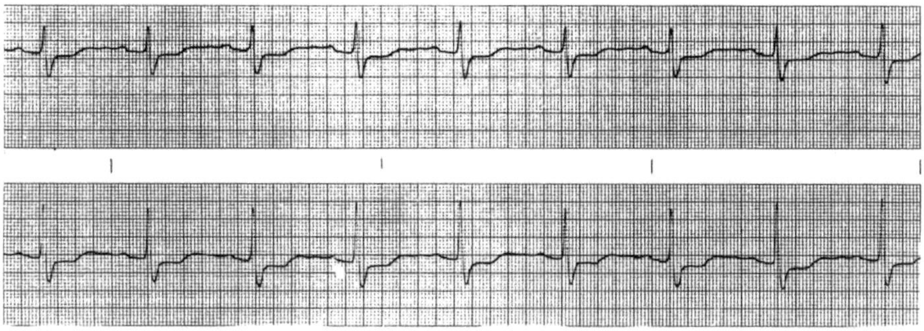

Fig. 2. Electrocardiogram showing a ventricular sensed repetitive aborted Wenckebach upper rate response during DDDR pacing on exercise. The PR interval (As-Vs) measures 160-180 ms. For this particular level of sensor activity, the rate-adaptive AV interval should be close to 100 ms (see Fig. 3). Therefore, the electrocardiogram shows apparent lack of atrial tracking (sensing). The sinus rate is faster than the atrial-driven upper rate, i.e., R-R interval is shorter than the atrial-driven upper rate interval (*ATRIAL D-URI*; 600 ms). The DDDR pacemaker senses the P waves beyond the post-ventricular atrial refractory period (PVARP) and initiates an extended AV interval to conform to the atrial-driven URI. The spontaneous QRS complex (Vs) occurs before completion of the atrial-driven URI. Vs repeatedly resets the atrial-driven URI. Two electrocardiographic leads were recorded simultaneously at paper speed = 50 mm/s

atrial rate and/or sensor activity; (b) PVARP shortens on exercise (adaptive PVARP); (c) both the As-Vp interval and PVARP shorten on exercise. In terms of the upper rate response, abbreviation of the AV interval initiated by atrial sensing (As-Vp < Ap-Vp) provides certain advantages: (a) there is a shorter TARP duration (As-Vp + PVARP) compared to the situation where As-Vp = Ap-Vp; (b) fixed-ratio pacemaker AV block begins at a faster sensed atrial rate when P-P interval < TARP; (c) with the separately programmable URI remaining constant, a shorter TARP widens the range of atrial rates associated with pacemaker Wenckebach AV block, i.e., the Wenckebach upper rate response begins at the same atrial rate, but fixed-ratio pacemaker AV block begins at a faster atrial rate; (d) a shorter TARP allows programming of a shorter URI (keeping URI > TARP) with preservation of the Wenckebach pacemaker AV block response.

Repetitive Aborted Wenckebach Upper Rate Response

In a Wenckebach sequence, the pulse generator extends the AV (As-Vp) interval so that Vp occurs only at the completion of the (atrial-driven) URI. An aborted Wenckebach sequence is defined as repetitive partial extension of the AV interval

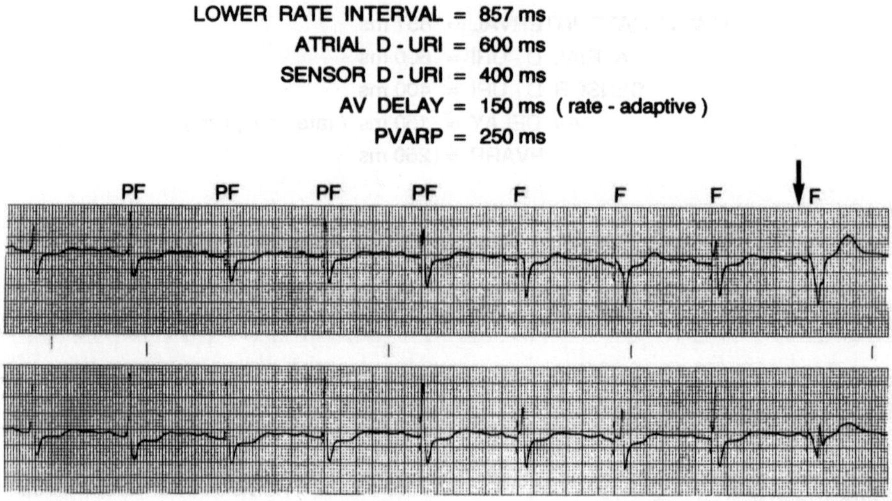

Fig. 3. Same patient as in Fig. 2. With slowing of the sinus rate, ventricular stimuli (Vp) begin to appear. Initially Vp falls within the QRS complex producing pseudofusion beats (*PF*). Then as the ventricular stimulus falls earlier in relation to the spontaneous QRS complex, Vp produces ventricular fusion beats (*F*). The PR interval (As-Vp) preceding the first two fusion beats is shorter than the PR intervals associated with pseudofusion beats and those in Fig. 2. The second-last beat (labeled *F*) could be a pseudofusion beat rather than a fusion beat. The pulse generator senses the last P wave (*arrow*) and initiates a short AV interval that represents the prevailing rate-adaptive AV interval at this particular level of exercise. Two electrocardiographic leads were recorded simultaneously at paper speed = 50 mm/s. *ATRIAL D-URI*, atrial driven upper rate interval; *SENSOR D-URI*, sensor-driven upper rate interval; *PVARP*, post-ventricular atrial refractory period

which, however, never attains its expected value in any given cycle according to the programmed URI because an earlier Vp or Vs event usurps control of the ventricular channel away from the atrial-driven URI. In other words, a premature Vp or Vs event prevents timing out of the URI which is therefore reset by the earlier Vp or Vs event. Therefore, the AV interval never completes its full extension according to the URI. There are two types of repetitive aborted Wenckebach upper rate responses: (a) initiated by Vs or a ventricular sensed repetitive aborted Wenckebach upper rate response; (b) initiated by Vp or a ventricular paced repetitive aborted Wenckebach upper rate response. Delivery of Vp before termination of the URI can only occur in the DDDR mode under certain circumstances that are discussed later.

Ventricular Sensed Repetitive Aborted Wenckebach Upper Rate Response

A DDD pacemaker with URI > TARP can produce a repetitive aborted Wenckebach upper rate response in the presence of sinus tachycardia with preserved AV conduction when the spontaneous ventricular rate is faster than the programmed upper rate (Figs. 2, 3). The ventricular sensed repetitive aborted Wenckebach upper rate response is characterized by an R-R or Vs-Vs interval < URI and a PR interval

(As-Vs) > longer than the programmed As-Vp interval. If TARP is < P-P < URI, sinus tachycardia without AV conduction produces a classic pacemaker Wenckebach upper rate response. However, the same sinus tachycardia associated with AV conduction forces the pulse generator to sense the conducted QRS (Vs) before the URI has timed out: Vs resets the URI, initiates a new URI, and the process repeats itself creating a self-perpetuating mechanism with Vs always preempting the expected ventricular stimulus Vp. The aborted Wenckebach response simulates atrial undersensing (lack of atrial tracking) because the partially extended As-Vs interval (to conform to the URI) is longer than the programmed As-Vp interval without extension. The pulse generator actually senses As beyond the PVARP but cannot emit Vp until completion of the URI. When a slower sinus rate lengthens the R-R interval to the point where it exceeds the URI, the pacemaker emits Vp after the programmed AV interval (As-Vp), now shorter than the partially extended AV interval during the aborted Wenckebach sequence (Fig. 3).

The aborted Wenckebach upper rate response has assumed greater importance in view of the increasing use of DDDR pulse generators and exercise testing (or other forms of activity) necessary to programm these complex devices appropriately.

So-Called Wenckebach Upper Rate Response in Single Cycles

In a DDD pulse generator with URI > TARP, an atrial extrasystole can prolong the As-Vp interval for a single cycle to conform to the URI. Some workers have attributed this response to Wenckebach upper rate behavior, creating potential confusion because a Wenckebach sequence does not actually occur. Rather, this response should be described in terms of the mechanism to conform to the URI being longer than the TARP or in terms of the same mechanism that produces Wenckebach upper rate response by virtue of the URI being longer than the TARP i.e. Av extension upper rate response.

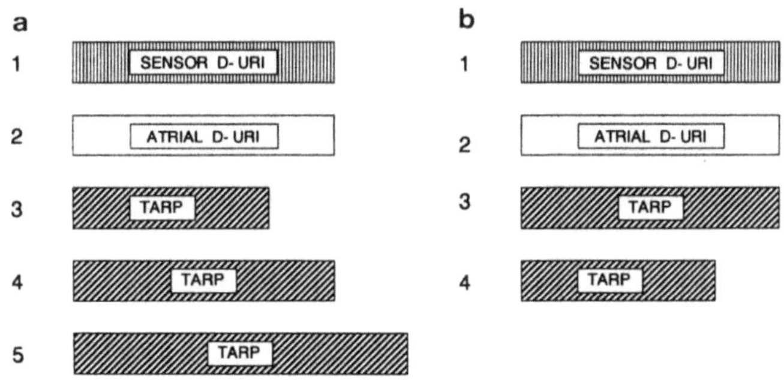

Fig. 4 a, b. DDDR upper rate intervals. The Intermedics Relay pulse generator (**b**) has a common upper rate interval (URI). The total atrial refractory period (TARP) can be programmed to a value shorter than or equal to but not longer than the atrial-driven URI. The Medtronic Synergyst II and Elite pulse generators (**a**) have a commen URI and the atrial-driven URI can be programmed to a value *shorter* or longer than the TARP or equal to it. When TARP is > URI, the atrial-driven URI (ATRIAL D-URI) becomes equal to the TARP and therefore functionally longer than the sensor-driven URI (SENSOR D-URI). (The Medtronic Elite II pulse generator allows programming of separate atrial-driven and sensor-driven upper rate intervals as well as TARP > atrial-driven URI like the Elite I device.)

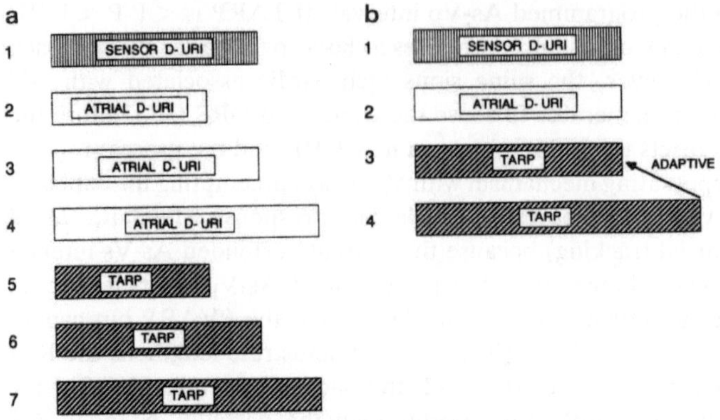

Fig. 5 a, b. DDDR upper rate intervals. The Synchrony (Pacesetter-Siemens) DDDR pulse generator (**a**) allows programming of the atrial-driven upper rate interval (*ATRIAL D-URI*) independently of the sensor-driven URI (*SENSOR D-URI*). The total atrial refractory period (*TARP*) cannot be programmed to a value *longer* than the atrial-driven URI, but it can of course be programmed to a value longer than the sensor-driven URI. In the Telectronics Meta DDDR pulse generator (**b**), the atrial-driven URI and sensor-driven URI are equal, and the TARP is adaptive and shortens with increasing sensor activity. When the sensor-driven interval (SDI) becomes equal to the common URI, the TARP also becomes equal to the common URI. Because TARP is ≥ atrial URI, no Wenckebach pacemaker AV block can occur. Furthermore, fixed-ratio pacemaker AV block cannot occur because when P-P is < TARP, the pulse generator is automatically converted to the VVIR mode

P-P Interval Equal to the URI but Longer than TARP

When the sinus rate is equal to the URI, the pulse generator continues to function with an extended As-Vp interval (longer than the programmed As-Vp) to conform to the URI. The ventricular pacing rate occurs at the programmed upper rate. This type of upper rate response should not be confused with a repetitive aborted Wenckebach response because the As-Vp interval and the URI both time out. Some pulse generators can interpret a sinus rate equal to the programmed upper rate as an endless loop tachycardia (at the upper rate) whereupon a single Vp is omitted automatically in an attempt to desynchronize ventricular and atrial activity [8] .

Upper Rate Response of DDDR Pulse Generators

Control of the upper rate involves (a) only two intervals (TARP and P-P intervals) with a simple DDD pacemaker; (b) three intervals (TARP, P-P interval, and URI) with a more complex DDD pacemaker with a separately programmable URI > TARP, and (c) four intervals (TARP, P-P interval, atrial-driven URI, and sensor-driven URI) in DDDR devices [3, 5, 12] (Figs. 4, 5).

The relationship between the sensor-driven URI and atrial-driven URI may take one of three forms: (a) sensor-driven URI > atrial-driven URI, i.e., the sensor-driven upper rate is slower than the atrial-driven upper rate; (b) sensor-driven URI = atrial-driven URI (common upper rates); and (c) sensor-driven URI < atrial-driven URI, i.e., sensor-driven upper rate faster than the atrial-driven upper rate.

Sensor-Driven URI Longer than Atria-Driven URI

There appears to be no real clinical use for a sensor-driven upper rate slower than an atrial-driven upper rate except perhaps to attenuate the effect of sudden deceleration of the sinus rate after effort [3]. As a rule, a sensor-driven URI > atrial-driven URI should not be programmed [3], and this combination will not be discussed further.

Sensor-Driven Upper Rate Equal to Atrial-Driven Upper Rate

When the sensor-driven URI is equal to the atrial-driven URI, three responses can occur: (a) Wenckebach pacemaker AV block if TARP < P-P interval < atrial-driven URI < SDI; (b) fixed-ratio pacemaker AV block if P-P interval < TARP < SDI; (c) AV sequential pacing if SDI < P-P interval with the AV sequential (Ap-Vp) pacing rate faster than the one that could be provided by atrial sensing with 1:1 AV synchrony. The maximal AV sequential pacing rate is equal to both the sensor-driven URI and the atrial-driven URI (Table 2).

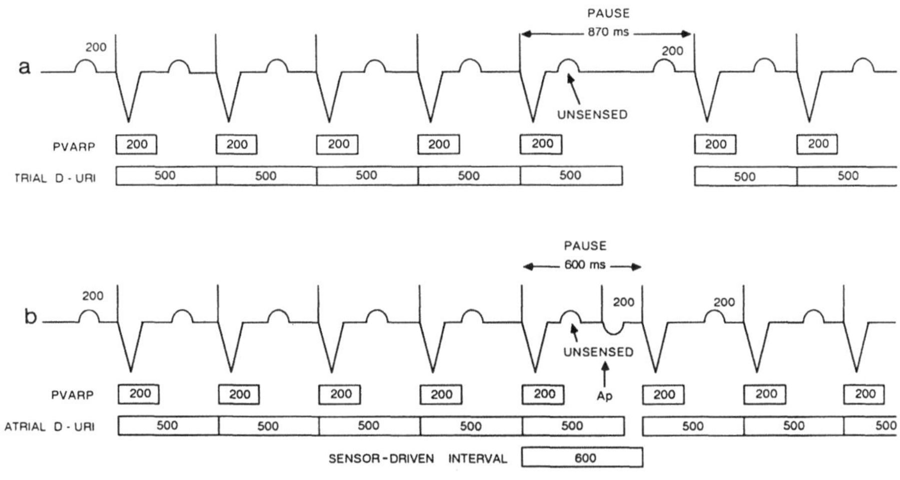

Fig. 6 a, b. DDD (**a**) and DDDR (**b**) pacing with pacemaker Wenckebach AV block. Lower rate interval = 1000 ms, atrial-driven upper rate interval (*ATRIAL D-URI*) = 500 ms, post-ventricular atrial refractory period (*PVARP*) = 200 ms, AV interval = 200 ms, (As-Vp = Ap-Vp in both the DDD and DDDR modes). A Wenckebach upper rate response occurs because the atrial-driven URI > total atrial refractory period (TARP). **a** DDD pacing with typical Wenckebach upper rate response. The pulse generator does not sense the sixth P wave in the PVARP, but senses the succeeding P wave so that the pause at the end of the Wenckebach cycle measures approximately 870 ms. **b** In the DDDR mode with the same basic parameters as in the DDD mode above Sensor driven interval (SDI) = 600 ms > atrial-driven URI. The pulse generator does not sense the sixth P wave in the PVARP. The pause at the end of the Wenckebach sequence is shorter than in the DDD mode above because the SDI equals 600 ms, and sensor-driven atrial escape interval (AEI) equals 400 ms. Thus, Ap occurs earlier (and closer to the preceding P wave in the PVARP) because its release is sensor controlled. The pause at the end of the Wenckebach sequence therefore shortens to the 600 ms SDI

Table 2. DDDR Upper Rate Response; atrial-driven URI equal to sensor-driven URI

Parameters	Response	Comments
1. P-P < TARP = atrial-driven URI < SDI	Fixed ratio 2:1 AV block with sensor-induced rate smoothing	
2. P-P < TARP < atrial-driven URI < SDI	As above	
3. P-P < TARP ≥ SDI	Atrial sensing cannot occur	Functions in DVIR mode
4. TARP < P-P < atrial-driven URI = sensor-driven URI < SDI	Wenckebach upper rate response with rate smoothing and pause at end of sequence	Atrial-driven URI times out. The pause at the end of Wenckebach sequence is equal to SDI.
5. TARP < P-P < atrial-driven URI = sensor-driven URI = SDI	Wenckebach upper rate response *without* a pause. Vp-Vp remains constant	Identical to DDIR mode; functionally equivalent to VVIR mode; atrial-driven URI times out

Pacemakers Wenckebach AV-block

A Wenckebach upper rate response occurs only when TARP < P-P interval < atrial-driven URI < SDI. During the Wenckebach upper rate response of a DDD pulse generator, when the P wave falls in the PVARP (and is unsensed), a pause occurs and the Wenckebach process repeats itself. The maximal duration of the pause (at the end of the Wenckebach sequence) measured between two consecutive ventricular stimuli (Vp-Vp interval) after a blocked or unsensed P wave is equal to the sum of the PVARP, P-P interval, and the programmed AV (As-Vp) interval provided the pulse generator senses the P wave that follows the unsensed one in the PVARP [8] If a P wave does not occur before the completion of the AEI, the pause will be equal to the LRI. During the Wenckebach upper rate response in the DDD mode, the atrial-driven URI times out with each constant Vp-Vp cycle (equal to URI) until a pause occurs, i.e., Vp-Vp lengthens only when a P wave falls in the PVARP. Thus the atrial-driven URI controls Vp release except in the pause terminating the Wenckebach sequence. In contrast to the DDD mode, DDDR pacing shortens the pause terminating the Wenckebach sequence to a value equal to the SDI (Fig. 6). Higano et al. [13] have called this effect "sensor-driven rate smoothing." Unlike true rate smoothing [8, 14] , sensor-driven rate smoothing occurs only at atrial rates faster than the atrial-driven upper rate (P-P < atrial-driven URI). In the DDDR mode, the pause terminating the Wenckebach cycle becomes progressively shorter as the SDI shortens, or as the sensor-driven rate increases.

A DDDR pulse generator working with a shorter sensor-driven AEI delivers Ap earlier in relation to the preceding ventricular event (Vs or Vp) than in the conventional DDD mode. The consequences of sensor-controlled earlier release of atrial stimuli (when the preceding P wave falls in the PVARP) is discussed below. The pause at the end of a Wenckebach cycle disappears when the SDI eventually becomes

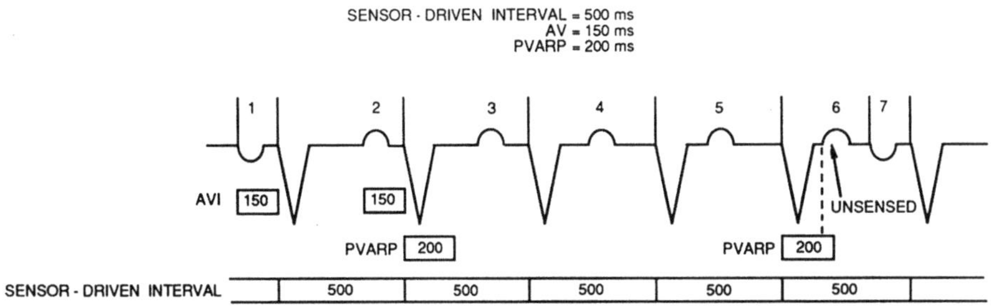

Fig. 7. DDIR mode. The sinus rate is faster than the sensor-driven rate, i.e., P-P interval < SDI (500 ms). In the DDI or DDIR mode, the ventricular paced rate (or the Vp-Vp interval) always remains constant and equal to the programmed lower rate interval or sensor-driven (lower rate) interval. The first atrial stimulus captures the atrium. The pulse generator senses the subsequent P waves (2 to 5). The P waves march through the pacing cycle with progressive prolongation of the AV interval. The sixth P wave falls in the 200 ms post-ventricular atrial refractory period (*PVARP*) and is therefore unsensed. The pacemaker delivers its next atrial stimulus (which captures the atrium and generates the seventh P wave) at the end of the sensor-driven atrial escape interval (AEI) (500 – 150 = 350 ms). Because the ventricular pacing rate (or Vp-Vp interval) remains constant, the DDIR mode is functionally equivalent to the VVIR mode (with AV dissociation) with the occasional occurrence of atrial extrasystoles (premature beats) when the pulse generator delivers Ap relatively close to the preceding (unsensed) P wave in the PVARP

equal to the sensor-driven URI. At that point, the pulse generator will continue to pace the ventricle regularly with constant Vp-Vp intervals at the sensor-driven URI (equal to the atrial-driven URI) and function as if it were in the DDIR mode (with a constant ventricular pacing rate and P waves marching through the cardiac cycle) (Fig. 7).

Pacemaker Fixed-Ratio AV Block

Fixed-ratio pacemake AV block occurs when the P-P interval < TARP < SDI. During DDD pacing, rapid acceleration of sinus rate may cause shortening of the P-P interval to a value less than the TARP, whereupon sudden 2:1 pacemaker AV block will occur. The abrupt fall in the paced ventricular rate seen in the DDD mode is attenuated in a DDDR system in the same way as the SDI abbreviates the pause at the end of Wenckebach cycles during DDDR pacing [7] (Fig. 8).

Sensor-Controlled Rate Smoothing and Atrial Competition

During DDDR pacing the shorter SDI and sensor-driven AEI generate Ap earlier than in the DDD mode (Ap can be relatively close to a preceding unsensed P wave in the PVARP). Ap occurs earlier in abbreviated pauses related to (a) fixed-ratio pacemaker AV block; and (b) the cycle terminating Wenckebach pacemaker AV block.

Sensor-controlled rate smoothing [13] can be useful in active patients that require a long PVARP for the prevention of endless loop tachycardia. For example, in the DDD mode a pulse generator with the following parameters – lower rate = 70 ppm,

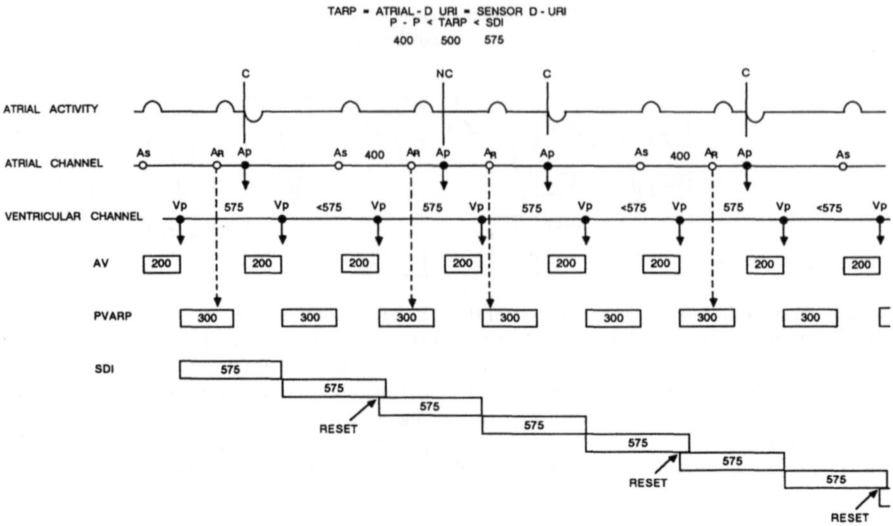

Fig. 8. Pacing by a DDDR pulse generator showing an upper rate response with fixed-ratio AV block. Atrial-driven upper rate interval (URI) = sensor-driven URI = total atrial refractory period (TARP). Fixed-ratio pacemaker AV block occurs because P-P interval (400 ms) is < TARP (500 ms). The Vp-Vp remains constant and equal to the sensor-driven interval (*SDI*) (575 ms). The second P (A_R) falls in the post-ventriuclar atrial refractory period (*PVARP*) and is therefore unsensed. The succeeding Ap is delivered at the end of the sensor-driven atrial escape interval (AEI) and captures the atrium (*C*) very close to the preceding spontaneous P (A_R). The fourth (As) P wave falls beyond the PVARP and initiates an AV interval of 200 ms. The Vp-Vp interval between the second Vp and the third Vp is shorter than 575 ms SDI (sensor-driven Vp-Vp interval) because the third Vp is controlled by As and not the sensor. The fifth P wave (A_R) falls in the PVARP. The pulse generator fires Ap at the end of the sensor-driven AEI, but Ap falls too close to the previous P wave (in the PVARP). Ap delivery within the atrial myocardial refractory period produces no capture (*NC*). Note that the SDI is reset whenever Vp occurs prematurely (earlier than the SDI of 575 ms) when triggered by As. Competitive atrial pacing produces complex electrocardiographic patterns

PVARP = 350 ms – if As-Vp shortens to 100 ms at the programmed (common) upper rate, a TARP of 450 ms will produce 2:1 fixed-ratio pacemaker AV block when the atrial rate exceeds 140 ppm. In this circumstance, in a DDDR device the sensor-driven rate and its corresponding SDI can reduce or even eliminate the abrupt drop in the paced ventricular rate produced by fixed-ratio pacemaker AV block in the DDD mode [7].

In the DDDR mode, fixed-ratio and Wenckebach pacemaker AV block can create complex electrocardiographic patterns [3, 7] (Fig. 8) with various combinations of (a) ineffectual Ap (no capture) when an early sensor-controlled Ap (delivered at the completion of sensor-driven AEI) falls in the atrial *myocardial* refractory period generated by the preceding unsensed P wave in the PVARP – loss of AV synchrony at a relatively high level of exercise is probably unimportant hemodynamically [7]; (b) effectual Ap with atrial capture but close to the previous P wave, i.e., atrial competition. Stimulation in the atrial vulnerable period (with the risk of inducing an atrial arrhythmia) represents at this time only a theoretical concern until more experience is obtained with these devices [15, 16]. Thus, at any one time, Vp may be preceded by one of the following: (a) ineffectual Ap; (b) effectual Ap close to the previous P wave; (c) sensed P wave triggering Vp. Furthermore, the pulse generator can release Ap either in the PVARP or beyond the PVARP (discussed later).

Atrial competition in the Wenckebach and fixed-ratio 2:1 pacemaker AV block can be reduced or minimized with correct selection of the pacing mode and programmable indices. On the other hand, during DDDR pacing, sensor-driven rate smoothing can be useful in active patients who do not tolerate the beat-to-beat variations in cycle length secondary to upper rate limitation in the DDD mode.

Total Atrial Refractory Period Longer than URI

Patients with atrial chronotropic incompetence and paroxysmal supraventricular tachyarrhythmias may benefit from a DDDR pulse generator programmed with a relatively slow atrial-driven upper rate to avoid tracking of fast unphysiologic atrial rates at rest and a faster sensor-driven upper rate to provide increase in the pacing rate on exercise. However, in some DDDR pulse generators with equal atrial-driven and sensor-driven upper rates, the two upper rate (intervals) cannot be dissociated (Fig. 4).

Obviously in the DDD mode, TARP > atrial-driven URI cannot exist because the atrial-driven URI becomes equal to the TARP. Consequently one could easily conclude that the two upper rates (atrial-driven and sensor-driven) in a DDDR device with a common upper rate are inextricably linked and cannot be dissociated. Indeed, as in the conventional DDD mode, some DDDR pulse generators with a common URI (e.g., Intermedics Relay; Intermedics, Angleton, Texas, USA) [17] permit programming of the TARP to a value equal to or shorter than, but not longer than the atrial-driven URI (equal to the sensor-driven URI) (Fig. 4). Yet, in any DDD or DDDR pulse generator it should be theoretically possible to program the TARP to a value equal to, shorter, or longer than the common URI. Indeed, in the Medtronic DDDR devices (Synergyst II and Elite; Medtronic, Inc., Minneapolis, Minnesota, USA) [18, 19] the TARP can be programmed to a value longer than the common URI (Fig. 4). Obviously if the TARP is ≥ common URI, no Wenckebach upper rate response with extension of the AV interval can occur. When TARP > common URI, the actual atrial-driven URI becomes equal to the duration of the TARP. This manipulation allows programming of a sensor-driven upper rate faster than the atrial-driven upper rate. The latter corresponds to the interval provided by the TARP and represents the rate at which fixed-ratio pacemaker AV block supervenes. Thus the atrial-driven URI can be *functionally* separated from the sensor-driven URI by programming a TARP longer than the common URI, i.e., atrial-driven URI = TARP > sensor-driven URI. In this way, fixed-ratio pacemaker AV block (e.g., 2:1) will occur at atrial rates slower than the programmed sensor-driven upper rate. This approach may be useful in limiting the atrial-driven upper rate in patients with paroxysmal supraventricular tachyarrhythmias (Table 3).

Table 3. DDDR Upper Rate Response

Parameters	Response	Comments
P-P < sensor-driven URI < TARP < SDI	Fixed ratio AV block with rate smoothing	Ap beyond PVARP
P-P[a] < sensor-driven URI < SDI < TARP	DVIR pacing	Ap in PVARP
P-P[a] < TARP = SDI	DVIR pacing	Ap at end of PVARP
P-P[a] > TARP = SDI	DVIR as above	As above

Atrial-driven URI = sensor-driven URI; capability of programming TARP > common URI; TARP > sensor-driven URI; functional atrial-driven URI (TARP) > sensor-driven URI.
[a] Duration of P-P interval is immaterial as pacer functions in DVIR mode, atrial sensing cannot occur because SDI is ≤ TARP.

Atrial Pacing in the PVARP

Atrial pacing can occur in the PVARP only when the sensor-driven URI < TARP, allowing an SDI < TARP (Figs. 9, 10). When the P-P interval shortens to a value less than the TARP, P waves fall in the terminal portion of the PVARP and are therefore unsensed. The DDDR pulse generator then takes over control of the atrial rhythm. Sensor-driven release of Ap may occur either in the PVARP or beyond it according to the SDI at any given time. An earlier Ap may result, as previously stated, in lack of capture (i.e., Ap in atrial *myocardial* refractory period generated by previous atrial depolarization) or capture with atrial competition. Note that it is possible for Ap to fall in the *myocardial* atrial refractory period generated by a preceding unsensed P wave within the *pacemaker* atrial refractory period (or PVARP). When the sensor-driven AEI is shorter than the PVARP (or SDI < TARP), Ap will fall consistently in the PVARP in the absence of sensed atrial activity.

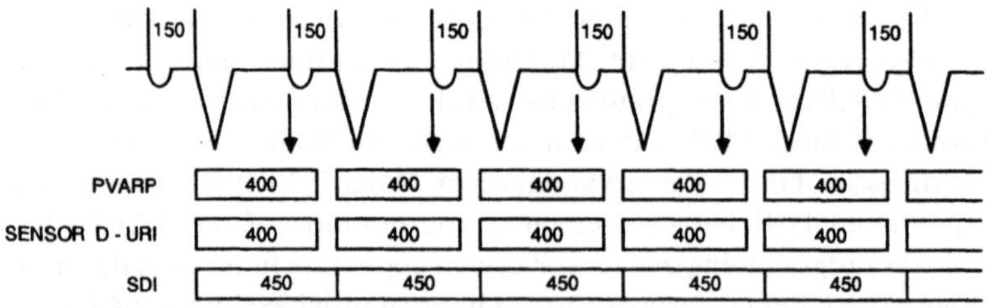

Fig. 9. Pacing by a DDDR pacemaker with total atrial refractory period (*TARP*) > common upper rate interval (*URI*). Ap-Vp = 150 ms. The atrial-driven URI and sensor-driven URI (*SENSOR D-URI*) should be equal (400 ms) according to pacemaker specifications when a 400-ms URI is programmed. However, TARP [AV + post-ventricular atrial refractory period (PVARP) = 550 ms (TARP > URI is allowed only in certain DDDR pulse generators)]. A 550-ms TARP actually represents an atrial-driven URI of the same duration and a Wenckebach upper rate response cannot occur. At that particular level of activity with an SDI = 450 ms, the sensor-driven atrial escape interval (AEI; 300 ms) is shorter than the 400-ms PVARP. Therefore the atrial stimulus is continually delivered within the PVARP

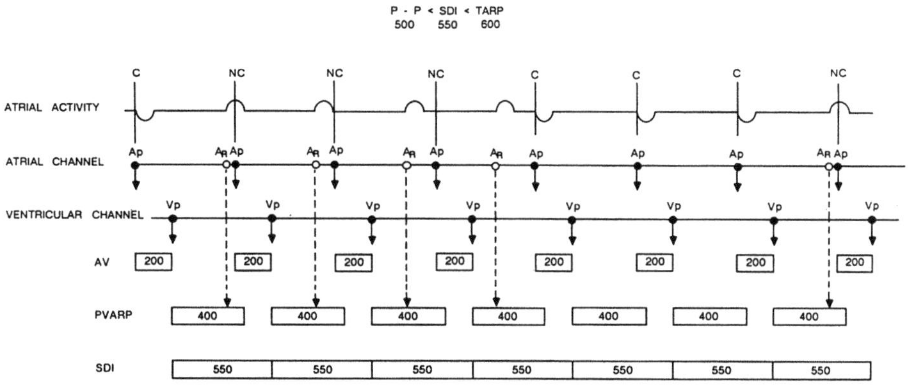

Fig. 10. Pacing in the DDDR mode with a common upper rate interval (URI) = 450 ms, AV = 200 ms, post-ventricular atrial refractory period (*PVARP*) = 400 ms, total atrial refractory period (*TARP*) = 600 ms, sensor-driven interval (*SDI*) = 550 ms. Provided the pulse generator allows programming TARP > common URI, these parameters indicate that atrial-driven URI (600 ms = TARP) > sensor-driven URI (450 ms = programmed common URI). There is an atrial sensing window beyond the PVARP, but it closes when SDI ≤ TARP. In this example, because SDI < TARP, the pulse generator cannot sense spontaneous atrial activity (A_R). Atrial pacing is asynchronous and Ap competes with A producing a response functionally equivalent to the DVIR mode. Therefore, both Ap-Ap and Vp-Vp intervals remain constant. *C*, capture; *NC* no capture (Ap in atrial myocardial refractory period)

Sensor-Driven Upper Rate Faster than Atrial-Driven Upper Rate

When sensor-driven URI is < atrial-driven URI, the upper rate response of a DDDR pulse generator depends on the interplay of four variables: P-P interval, TARP, atrial-driven URI, and sensor-driven URI [1, 5, 6, 12, 20]. The Pacesetter-Siemens Synchrony I and II DDDR devices (Pacesetter-Siemens, Sylmar, California, USA) provide all four separate intervals (Fig. 5). A sensor-driven upper rate faster than an atrial-driven upper rate may be useful in patients with paroxysmal supraventricular tachyarrhythmias and in patients requiring a very long PVARP to prevent endless loop tachycardia [12].

There are two basic situations where the sensor-driven URI is shorter than the atrial-driven URI:

1. As already outlined, when the pulse generator specifications indicate that the two upper rates are common, sensor-driven URI = atrial-driven URI, programming the TARP longer than the common URI (if possible according to design) in effect yields two different upper rates. Sensor-driven URI is less than TARP. The TARP now becomes the atrial-driven URI and allows only a fixed-ratio pacemaker AV block response to fast atrial rates. Obviously a Wenckebach upper rate response cannot occur.
2. Wenckebach upper rate response with extension of the AV interval: when TARP < atrial-driven URI, this relationship permits a modified Wenckebach upper rate response under appropriate circumstances, but no pause occurs at the end of the

Wenckebach sequence (in contrast to pauses seen with DDDR when atrial-driven URI = sensor-driven URI and SDI > atrial-driven URI) because SDI ≤ atrial-driven URI, as explained later. Extension of AV (As-Vp) interval beyond its programmed value can occur only when TARP < P-P interval (Table 4).

Atrial-Driven URI Longer than TARP

P-P Interval Longer than Sensor-Driven Interval Obviously when P-P interval > SDI, the pulse generator paces AV sequentially. Complexity occurs when the P-P interval is equal to or shorter than the SDI and sensor-driven URI.

Table 4. DDDR Upper Rate Response; sensor-driven URI < atrial-driven URI; TARP < atrial-driven URI[a]

Parameters	Response	Comments
1. P-P < SDI < atrial-driven URI		
Sensor-driven URI < TARP[a] < P-P < SDI < atrial-driven URI	Modified Wenckebach upper rate response with no pause; Vp-Vp = SDI	Functionally equivalent to DDIR mode; atrial-driven URI does not time out; Vp is sensor controlled; represents ventricular paced repetitive aborted Wenckebach upper rate response
TARP[a] < sensor-driven URI < P-P < SDI < atrial-driven URI	As above	As above
2. P-P < SDI = atrial-driven URI		
Sensor-driven URI < TARP[a] < P-P < SDI = atrial-driven URI	Wenckebach upper rate response with no pause; Vp-Vp = SDI = atrial-driven URI	Atrial-driven URI times out; resembles Wenckebach upper rate response with DDDR mode in which TARP < P-P < atrial-driven URI = sensor-driven URI = SDI
TARP[a] < sensor-driven URI < P-P < SDI = atrial-driven URI	As above	As above
3. P-P = SDI < atrial-driven URI		
Sensor-driven URI < TARP[a] < P-P = SDI < atrial-driven URI	Apparent P wave tracking with extended and constant As-Vp	Atrial-driven URI does not time out; Vp-Vp is controlled by SDI < atrial-driven URI
TARP[a] < sensor-driven URI < P-P = SDI < atrial-driven URI	As above	As above

[a] TARP < atrial-driven URI permits Wenckebach response with extension of As-Vp as programmed.

P-P Interval Shorter than Sensor-Driven Interval

When the atrial rate exceeds the sensor-driven rate (P-P interval < SDI), the SDI may also become shorter than the atrial-driven URI (i.e., P-P interval < SDI < atrial-driven URI), a relationship that cannot occur when the sensor-driven URI and atrial-driven URI are common and cannot be dissociated.

a) *Sensor-Driven Interval Shorter than Atrial-Driven URI.* In the absence of atrial activity, when SDI < atrial-driven URI, a pulse generator delivers an atrial stimulus (Ap) at the termination of the sensor-driven AEI and an accompanying ventricular stimulus (Vp) at the completion of the Ap-Vp interval. Vp occurs at the end of the SDI initiated by the preceding ventricular event, but before completion of the atrial-driven URI, also initiated by the same preceding ventricular event (Fig. 11). If a sensed P wave (As) occurs before the expected emission of Ap (controlled by the sensor-driven interval), the pulse generator inhibits the subsequent release of sensor controlled Ap (Fig. 11). Although the pulse generator omits Ap, it delivers Vp on time according to the SDI at that given time. Consequently the As-Vp interval extends beyond its programmed value, a response analogous to the classic pacemaker Wenckebach upper rate behavior (possible only if atrial-driven URI is > TARP). In this response, when the P-P interval < SDI < atrial-driven URI, P waves march through the pacing cycles and initiate As-Vp intervals of progressively longer duration until a P wave falls in the PVARP and is unsensed, a behavior resembling the classic pacemaker Wenckebach AV block upper rate response. However, there is no pause when the P wave is in the PVARP because release of the subsequent Ap and Vp is sensor controlled according to the SDI and the sensor-driven AEI (Fig. 11). The Vp-Vp interval therefore remains constant and equal to the prevailing SDI (either longer than the sensor-driven URI or equal to it) but shorter than the atrial-driven URI. The constant sensor-driven Vp-Vp interval with the occasional emission of Ap (when P is unsensed in the PVARP) resembles DDIR pacing (Fig. 7). In other words, when P-P < sensor-driven URI < atrial-driven URI, the atrial-driven URI does not time out because the SDI or the sensor-driven URI usurps control of the paced ventricular rate. The modified pacemaker Wenckebach upper rate response may be called a ventricular paced repetitive aborted Wenckebach upper rate response because the atrial-driven URI never times out. In this response, SDI obviously times out and, when SDI becomes equal to the sensor-driven URI, the latter also times out.

b) *Sensor-Driven Interval Equal to the Atrial-Driven URI.* When P-P < atrial-driven URI = SDI, a Wenckebach upper rate response will also occur with no pause at the end of the sequence in the cycle containing the unsensed P wave within the PVARP, as in Fig. 11. The Vp-Vp interval remains equal to the SDI and to the atrial-driven URI. Therefore, both SDI and atrial-driven URI time out, but not the sensor-driven URI. The effect is therefore identical to the situation where atrial-driven URI = sensor-driven URI = SDI, which also creates a classic Wenckebach upper rate response without a pause at the end of the sequence provided TARP < P-P < SDI. In the latter situation, alle three intervals (atrial-driven URI, sensor-driven URI, and SDI) time out at the end of every Vp-Vp cycle (Figs. 6, 7).

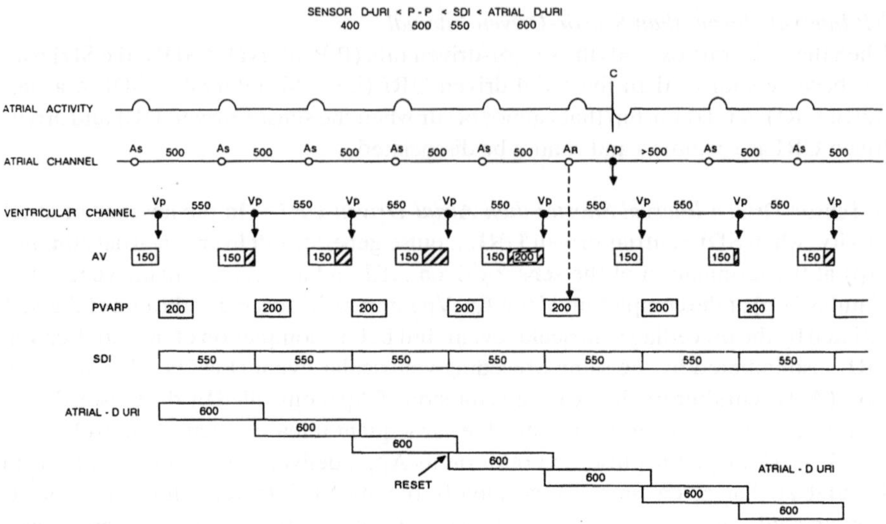

Fig. 11. Pacing by a DDDR pulse generator with the sensor-driven upper rate interval (*URI*) (400 ms) < atrial-driven URI (*ATRIAL D-URI*) (600 ms). Sensor-driven URI (*SENSOR D-URI*) (400 ms) < P-P interval (500 ms) < sensor-driven interval (*SDI*) (550 ms) < atrial-driven URI (600 ms). As-Vp = Ap-Vp = 150 ms, post-ventricular atrial refractory period (*PVARP*) = 200 ms, total atrial refractory period (*TARP*) = 350 ms. TARP < P-P < atrial-driven URI. The maximal increment of the AV interval during the Wenckebach upper rate response is 600 – 350 = 250 ms. The first P wave initiates an AV interval of 150 ms. The second P wave initiates an AV interval extended beyond 150 ms to conform to the atrial-driven URI. The atrial-driven URI does not time out because the SDI is shorter than the atrial-driven URI. Thus, the delivery of Vp is sensor controlled and the Vp-Vp interval is controlled by the sensor or the SDI. The AV interval cannot fully extend to the completion of the atrial-driven URI because an earlier Vp (sensor controlled) terminates the AV interval. This response may be called a ventricular paced repetitive aborted Wenckebach upper rate response. The sixth P wave falls in the PVARP and is therefore unsensed (A_R). The next Ap released at the end of the sensor-driven atrial escape interval (AEI) (550 – 150 = 400 ms) occurs 400 ms from the previous Vp, close to the sixth P wave, but capable of atrial capture. There is no pause at the end of the Wenckebach sequence because Vp-Vp interval is controlled by sensor activity or the SDI and not by atrial-driven URI which is therefore continually reset by the earlier Vp. On the *right*, the process then repeats itself

P-P Interval Equal to the Sensor-Driven Interval

If atrial sensing produces sustained inhibition of Ap, pacemaker behavior resembles P wave tracking seen in DDD pulse generators, a situation called "apparent tracking" by Higano and Hayes [5] . When TARP < P-P = SDI < atrial-driven URI, sustained apparent P wave tracking occurs with an extended As-Vp interval that remains constant (Fig. 12).

When SDI < atrial-driven URI, the P waves start AV interval but, unlike the Wenckebach response in the DDD mode, the pulse generator never completes the AV interval (though it is extended to some extent) because the pulse generator emits Vp at the completion of the SDI causing continual reset of the atrial-driven URI by the

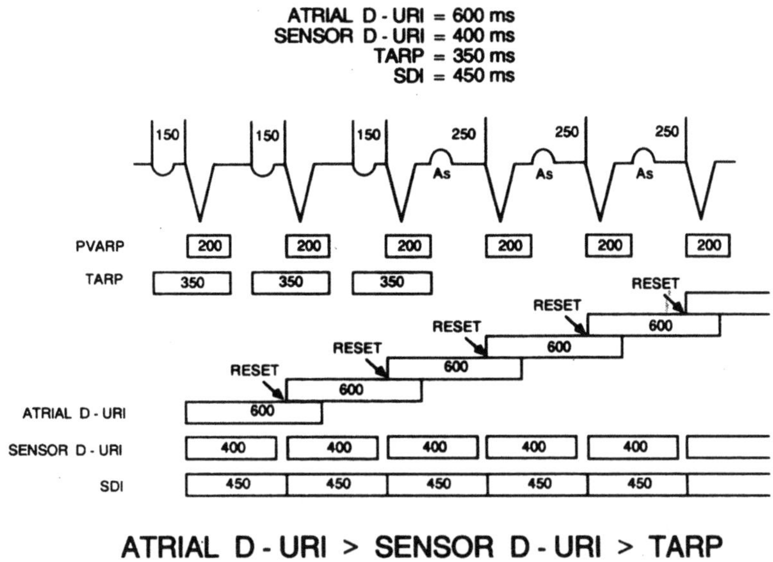

Fig. 12. Pacing with a DDDR pulse generator showing apparent P wave tracking. Atrial-driven upper rate interval (*ATRIAL D-URI*) > sensor-driven URI (*SENSOR D-URI*). As-Vp = Ap-Vp = 150 ms. The sinus rate is equal to the sensor-driven rate (P-P interval = sensor-driven interval (*SDI*) = 450 ms). The pulse generator senses the last three spontaneous P waves (As). A sensed P wave initiates an AV interval of 150 ms, but at the completion of the 150-ms AV interval, the atrial-driven URI (600 ms) has not yet timed out. Consequently the pacemaker extends the AV interval to conform to the atrial-driven URI (600 ms). The latter does not time out because the pulse generator emits Vp at the termination of the 450-ms SDI initiated by the preceding ventricular event. The As-Vp interval is stretched to 250 ms. (In the absence of sensor activity or SDI, the As-Vp interval would have stretched to 400 ms to conform to the atrial-driven URI.) Delivery of the last three ventricular stimuli is sensor controlled. The atrial-driven URI is repeatedly reset by the early delivery of sensor-controlled Vp, producing apparent P wave tracking at a rate faster than the programmed atrial-driven upper rate. Although this form of apparent P wave tracking resembles that shown in Fig. 13, the mechanism is different. In this example, delivery of Vp is sensor controlled while in Fig. 13 delivery of Vp is controlled by the atrial-driven URI. In Fig. 13 the sinus rate is equal to the common URI while in Fig. 12, P-P = SDI. *TARP*, total atrial refractory period; *PVARP*, post-ventricular atrial refractory period

sensor-controlled Vp (Figs. 11, 12). The Vp-Vp interval is sensor driven and the atrial-driven URI does not time out. This response with AV interval prolongation resembles other situations where the atrial-driven URI actually times out: e.g. DDDR mode with TARP < P-P DDDR mode with TARP < P-P interval = atrial-driven URI = sensor-driven URI (Fig. 13).

In summary, when sensor-driven URI < atrial-driven URI, the response of a DDDR pulse generator depends on the relationship of the P-P interval to SDI, and there are four possibilities provided P-P > TARP, making AV extension possible: (a) P-P > SDI: AV sequential pacing; (b) P-P < SDI < atrial-driven URI: modified Wenckebach upper rate response with P waves marching through the pacing cycle and

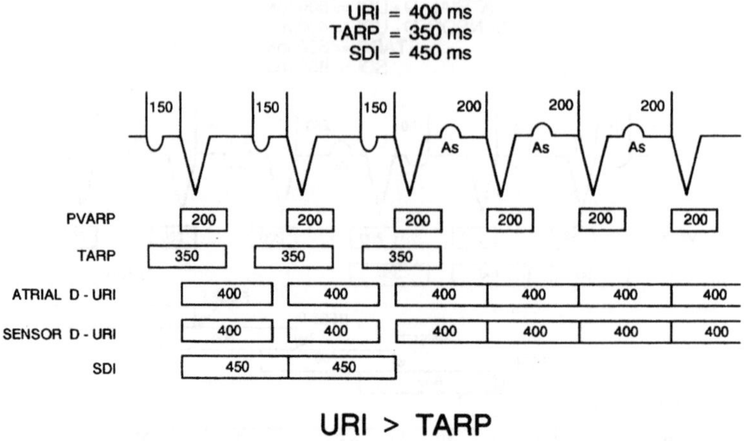

Fig. 13. Pacing by a DDDR pulse generator with a common upper rate interval (*URI*) (atrial-driven URI (*ATRIAL D-URI*)) = sensor-driven URI (*SENSOR D-URI*). As-Vp = Ap-Vp = 150 ms. The sinus rate is equal to the programmed upper rate, i.e., P-P interval = atrial-driven URI = sensor-driven URI = 400 ms. On the *right* the As-Vp interval remains constant but extended (by 50 ms) to conform to the atrial-driven URI. The sensor-driven interval (*SDI*; 450 ms) is longer than the common URI (400 ms). Therefore the pulse generator releases Vp at the completion of the atrial-driven URI. Delivery of the Vp is not sensor controlled. Although this response resembles that in Fig. 12, the timing cycles and control of Vp are different. *PVARP*, post-ventricular atrial refractory period; *TARP*, total atrial refractory period

no pauses (Fig. 11) – a similar response occurs when P-P < SDI = atrial-driven URI when the atrial-driven URI also times out; (c) P-P = SDI < atrial-driven URI: sustained apparent P wave tracking with a fixed but extended As-Vp interval (Fig. 12); (d) fluctuations of P-P interval to a value equal to, longer, or shorter than the SDI leads to irregular patterns with intermittent inhibition of Ap creating complex electrocardiograms as shown in Fig. 14. In all these situations, apparent P wave tracking should not be misinterpreted as pacemaker malfunction.

Pauses During Wenckebach Upper Rate Behavior

A pause during pacemaker Wenckebach upper rate response (possible only when TARP < atrial-driven URI) with rate-smoothing effect occurs only when P-P < atrial-driven URI = sensor-driven URI < SDI (Fig. 6). In the related situation where P-P < atrial-driven URI = sensor-driven URI = SDI, no pause occurs in the Wenckebach sequence. In the modified forms of Wenckebach upper rate response (ventricular paced repetitive aborted Wenckebach upper rate response), when P-P < SDI < atrial-driven URI or P-P < SDI = atrial-driven URI, no pause follows an unsensed P wave in the PVARP at the termination of the Wenckebach sequence (Fig. 11). Without a pause, the DDDR mode functions essentialy in the DDIR mode or as a pseudo-VVIR device with occasional “atrial premature beats” or “atrial extrasystolles” due to atrial capture from the release of Ap whenever a P wave falls in the PVARP and is unsensed.

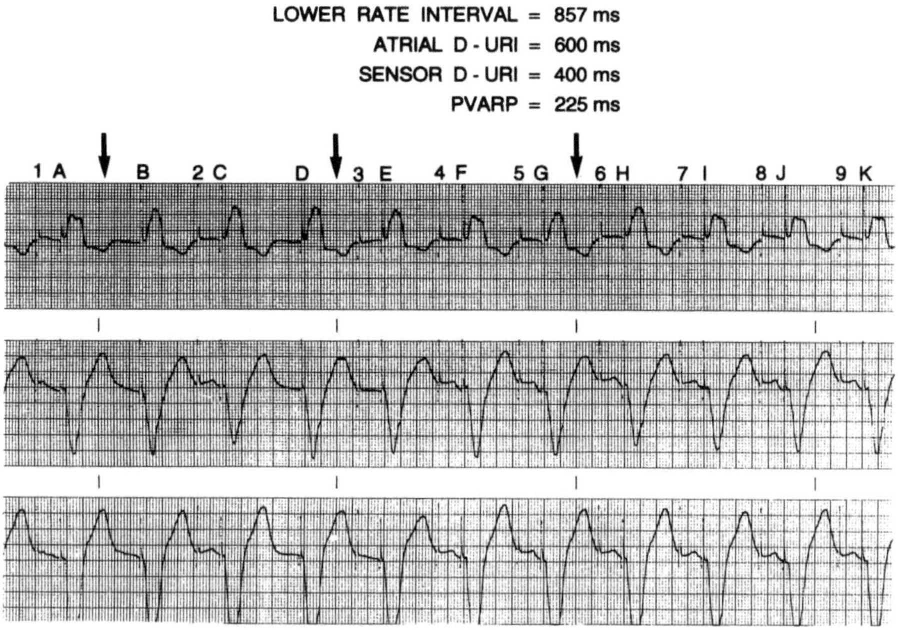

Fig. 14. Electrocardiogram showing complex arrhythmia during DDDR pacing with a Pacesetter-Siemens Synchrony pulse generator. The electrocardiogram was taken at double speed (50 mm/s) with three simultaneous leads during exercise in a patient with atrial extrasystoles, but no retrograde ventriculoatrial conduction. The first Ap captures the atrium and Vp follows the first Ap. The *arrow* between *A* and *B* points to an atrial extrasystole (not seen because it lies within the ST segment) sensed by the atrial channel which therefore inhibits release of Ap. Delivery of Vp (*B*) is sensor controlled and the (*A-B*) interval (Vp-Vp) = sensor-driven interval (SDI) = 500 ms approximately. Depolarization due to Ap is isoelectric in the *upper strip* except for the first Ap which may be an atrial fusion beat. The second Ap (*2*) also causes atrial capture. The pulse generator senses another atrial extrasystole between *C* and *D*, beyond the post-ventricular atrial refractory period (*PVARP*), and again inhibits Ap at the completion of the sensor-driven atrial escape interval (AEI) initiated by Vp (*C*). The (*C-D*) interval (Vp-Vp) = SDI = 500 ms. The *second arrow* (between *D* and *E*) points to an atrial extrasystole falling within the 225-ms PVARP. The succeeding Ap (*3*) does not capture the atrium because it is too close to the previous atrial depolarization and therefore in the atrial myocardial refractory period. Subsequent Ap events (*4-9*) capture the atrium. The *third arrow* points to another atrial extrasystole (between *G* and *H*) that occurs earlier than the one between *D* and *E* (within the PVARP). However, the sixth Ap (*6*) occurs beyond the atrial myocardial refractory period and therefore captures the atrium. *ATRIAL D-URI*, atrial-driven upper rate interval

Upper Rate Response with Automatic Switching of Pacing Mode

The DDDR mode of the Telectronics (Denver, Colorado, USA) Meta DDDR pulse generator possesses a common URI (sensor-driven URI = atrial-driven URI) [21] . A pacemaker Wenckebach AV block upper rate response cannot occur because the

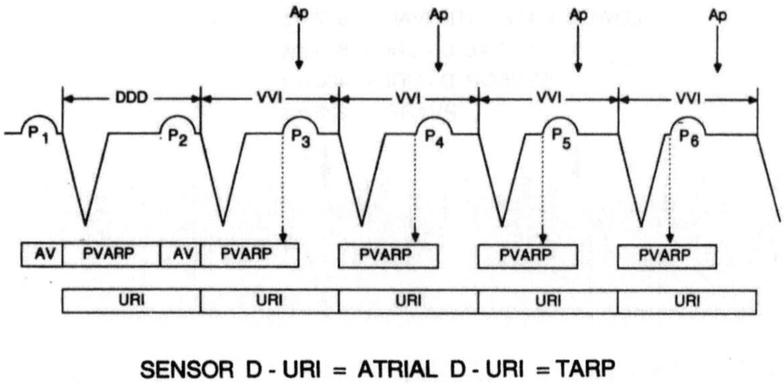

Fig. 15. DDDR pacing with the Telectronics (minute ventilation) Meta DDDR pulse generator showing the upper rate response. The pulse generator has a common upper rate [atrial-driven upper rate interval (*ATRIAL D-URI*) = sensor driven URI (*SENSOR D-URI*)]. (*TARP*) gradually shortens with exercise (increased sensor activity) so that when sensor-driven interval (SDI) = URI, TARP = URI. The first and second P waves are sensed outside the post-ventricular atrial refractory period (*PVARP*), and both initiate an AV interval as programmed. The third P wave (*P3*) occurs in the PVARP, but is sensed by the atrial channel whereupon the pulse generator inhibits release of the next Ap, producing a modified VVIR cycle. The VVIR cycle is sensor driven and in this particular case the VVIR cycles are equal to the URI, i.e., SDI = URI. The fourth, fifth, and sixth P waves fall in the PVARP and also inhibit release of Ap

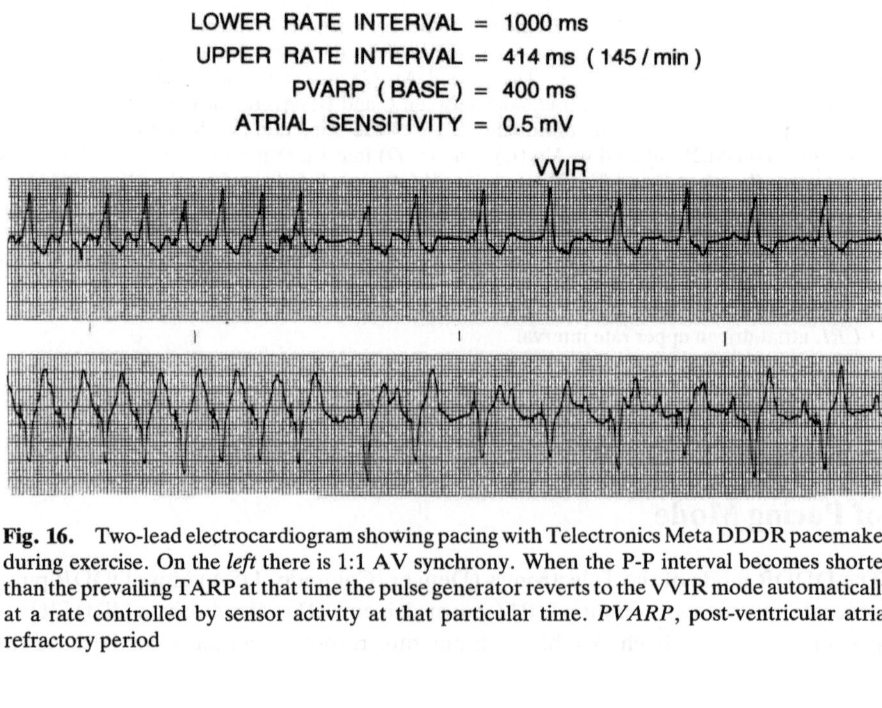

Fig. 16. Two-lead electrocardiogram showing pacing with Telectronics Meta DDDR pacemaker during exercise. On the *left* there is 1:1 AV synchrony. When the P-P interval becomes shorter than the prevailing TARP at that time the pulse generator reverts to the VVIR mode automatically at a rate controlled by sensor activity at that particular time. *PVARP*, post-ventricular atrial refractory period

upper rate interval (common sensor and atrial driven) is shorter than the TARP. During exercise the pulse generator shortens both the AV interval and the PVARP according to sensor input. The TARP always remains longer than the sensor-driven or atrial-driven URI except when the pulse generator paces at the URI, whereupon the TARP becomes equal to the common URI. The Telectronics Meta DDDR pulse generator (now released in the United States), when programmed to the DDDR mode, reverts to the VVIR mode whenever the atrial channel detects supraventricular tachycardia (or sinus tachycardia) with a cycle length shorter than the prevailing TARP [21] . In the Meta DDDR pulse generator, a P wave sensed in the terminal portion of the PVARP (relative refractory period) inhibits release of the subsequent atrial stimulus providing a modified VVIR cycle (Figs. 15, 16) This design prevents competitive atrial pacing between the spontaneous atrial and paced atrial rhythms. However, the pulse generator cannot detect an extremely premature P wave very close to the preceding QRS complex (atrial extrasystole or retrograde P wave) because it falls in the initial portion of the PVARP functioning as an absolute atrial refractory period. In such a case, competitive atrial pacing would occur, a rare situation with appropriate pacemaker programming. In the modified VVIR mode, a ventricular event continues to initiate a PVARP in the atrial channel so that atrial events continually sensed within the PVARP perpetuate the modified VVIR (or VDIR) mode. Preliminary experience with the Meta DDDR in patients with paroxysmal atrial tachyarrhythmias is encouraging [22–28].

Disadvantages of the present device include response with VVIR cycles to sinus tachycardia (a physiologic rhythm) and single atrial extrasystoles and the risk of farfield oversensing (especially in the unipolar mode) during the terminal portion of the PVARP (relative refractory period) because the absolute refractory period portion of the PVARP is relatively short (100 ms). Conversion to the VVIR mode may lead to repetitive retrograde VA conduction with P waves falling within the PVARP. When such retrograde P waves are sensed by the pulse generator, release of the atrial stimulus is inhibited, thereby perpetuating retrograde conduction. For this reason, in the Meta DDDR, after sensing eight consecutive P waves (not necessarily retrograde) within the PVARP, the duration of a single pacing cycle is automatically lengthened. In this way, without a P wave beyond the PVARP, the pulse generator is committed to deliver a delayed atrial stimulus sufficiently removed from the previous retrograde P wave to avoid stimulation within the atrial myocardial refractory period generated by the preceding atrial depolarization [29, 30]. Future generations of the Meta DDDR and other pulse generators will eventually possess a more refined and efficient mode-switching mechanism and more extensive programmability, e.g., number of cycles before mode switching goes into effect.

Functional Mode Versus Programmed Mode

During DDDR pacing, a particular programmed pacing mode may effectively function in another mode according to circumstances. A DDDR pacemaker can switch its functional pacing mode in the following situations.

DDDR to DVIR Mode

When SDI ≤ TARP, the atrial channel paces asynchronously and the DDDR mode functions as a DVIR mode. For example, if AV = 200 ms, PVARP = 400 ms, TARP = 600 ms. When the SDI reaches 600 ms, or less, the pacemaker functions in the DVIR mode because these parameters obliterate the atrial sensing window (Fig. 10).

DDIR to DVIR Mode

In the DDIR mode with AV = 150 ms, PVARP = 350 ms, and LRI = 1000 ms, the atrial sensing window is equal to LRI – TARP = 500 ms. As the sensor-driven LRI shortens with exercise, the atrial sensing window also shortens. Eventually when the SDI reaches 500 ms (corresponding to a rate of 120 per minute), the programmed indices obliterate the atrial sensing window and the pacemaker then functions in the DVIR mode.

DDDR to DDIR Mode

1. Any Wenckebach upper rate response without a pause at the termination of the cycle (when the P wave falls within the PVARP) is functionally equivalent to the DDIR mode. In a pulse generator with equal atrial-driven URI and sensor-driven URI, shortening of the SDI (i.e., sensor-driven LRI) on exercise brings it closer to the atrial-driven or common URI. The pacing mode begins to resemble the DDIR mode. When the difference between the URI and the SDI becomes small, the Wenckebach pause becomes inconspicuous so that the pacing mode looks like the DDIR mode (constant rate of ventricular pacing) with an occasional, hardly discernible, slight prolongation of the Vp-Vp interval at the end of the Wenckebach sequence. When the SDI = atrial-driven URI = sensor-driven URI, no pauses occur at the end of the Wenckebach cycle and the pacing mode becomes effectively DDIR. In this situation, the Vp-Vp interval becomes equal to the atrial-driven URI.
2. A Wenckebach upper rate response without pauses (functionally equivalent to the DDIR mode) can also occur when P-P < SDI < atrial-driven URI provided TARP < atrial-driven URI. The SDI becomes the Vp-Vp interval when SDI < atrial-driven URI. This response may be called a ventricular paced repetitive aborted Wenckebach upper rate response (Fig. 11). When SDI equals atrial-driven URI, the Vp-Vp becomes equal to the SDI and the atrial-driven URI, also producing a modified pacemaker Wenckebach AV block response (without a pause at the end of the sequence).

Table 5. Characteristics of DDD and DDDR Pulse Generators

	URI > TARP Wenckebach upper rate response	Fixed rate AV block	Sensor-driven URI > atrial-driven URI	Sensor-driven URI < atrial-driven URI	Sensor-driven URI independent of TARP; TARP > common URI	Competitive pacing outside PVARP	Atrial pacing in PVARP	Adaptive PVARP with exercise
Cordis DDD[a]	No	Yes	NA	NA	NA	NA	No	No
Standard DDD	Yes	Yes	NA	NA	NA	NA	No	No
Medtronic Synergyst I and II[b] and Elite*	Yes	Yes	No	No	Yes	Yes	Yes	No
Pacesetter-Siemens Synchrony I and II[c]	Yes	Yes	Yes	Yes	Prolongation of TARP automatically lengthens atrial-driven URI	Yes	Yes	No
Intermedics Relay[d]	Yes	Yes	No	No	No	Yes	No (as TARP never > SDI)	No
Telectronics Meta DDDR[e]	No	No	No	No	No	No, as atrial stimulus is inhibited by P wave sensed in PVARP	No	Yes
Telectronics Meta DDDR programmed to DDD mode[e]	Yes	Yes	NA	NA	NA	NA	No	No

NA, not applicable.

[a] Cordis Inc., Miami, FL, USA.
[b] Medtronic Inc., Minneapolis, MN, USA.
[c] Pacesetter-Siemens, Sylmar, CA, USA.
[d] Intermedics Inc., Angleton, TX, USA.
[e] Telectronics Inc,, Denver, CO, USA.

The Medtronic Elite II DDDR is similar to the Elite I device execpt that the sensor-driven upper rate interval can be programmed independently of the atrial-driven upper rate interval in the Elite II.

DDIR Mode to VVIR Mode

As discussed above, in the DDIR mode when the atrial rate is faster than the sensor-driven interval, P waves march through the pacing cycle until one falls in the PVARP and is unsensed. The pulse generator then emits an atrial stimulus at the end of the sensor-driven AEI, a situation functionally equivalent to the VVIR mode with AV dissociation and occasional atrial extrasystoles, the latter being due to occasional atrial stimulation [3] (Fig. 7.).

Conclusion

Table 5 outlines the characteristics pertaining to the upper rate behavior of a number of DDDR pacemakers. The interpretation of DDDR pacemaker electrocardiograms can be difficult and requires a thorough knowledge of pacemaker specifications and timing cycles. In this respect, telemetered event markers and pacemaker/programmer-generated diagnostic diagrams depicting timing cycles and their precise duration will undoubtedly prove invaluable.

References

1. Levine PA, Hayes DL, Wilkoff BL, Ohman AE (1990) Electrocardiography of rate-modulated pacemaker rhythms. Siemens-Pacesetter, Sylmar
2. Vey G, Werner K (1989) Interaction of sensor-driven pacing and intrinsic atrial activity in dual chamber rate-responsive pacemakers. PACE 12:1577
3. Ritter P (1990) La stimulation DDDR définitive: aspects techniques. Stimucoeur 18:29
4. Hayes DL, Higano ST (1991) DDDR pacing. Follow-up and complications. In: Barold SS, Mugica J (eds) New perspectives in cardiac pacing. Futura, Mt Kisco, p 473
5. Higano ST, Hayes DL (1989) P wave tracking above the maximum tracking rate in a DDDR pacemaker. PACE 12:1044
6. Hayes DL, Higano ST, Eisinger G (1989) Electrocardiographic manifestations of a dual-chamber, rate-modulated (DDDR) pacemaker. PACE 12:555
7. Hanich RF, Midei MG, McElroy BP, Brinker JA (1989) Circumvention of maximum tracking limitations with a rate-modulated dual chamber pacemaker. PACE 12:392
8. Barold SS, Falkoff MD, Ong LS, Heinle RA (1988) Upper rate response of DDD pacemaker. In: Barold SS, Mugica J (eds) New perspectives in cardiac pacing. Futura, Mt Kisco, p 69
9. Furman S (1985) Dual chamber pacemakers. Upper rate behavior. PACE 8:197
10. Stroobrandt R, Willems R, Holvoet G, Bakers J, Sinnaeve A (1986) Prediction of Wenckebach behavior and block response in DDD pacemakers. PACE 9:1040
11. Higano ST, Hayes DL (1990) Quantitative analysis of Wenckebach behavior in DDD pacemakers. PACE 13:1456
12. Higano ST, Hayes DL, Eisinger G (1989) Advantage of discrepant upper rate limits in a DDDR pacemaker. Mayo Clin Proc 64:932
13. Higano ST, Hayes DL, Eisinger G (1989) Sensor-driven rate smoothing in a DDDR pacemaker. PACE 12:922
14. VanMechelen R, Ruiter J, DeBoer H, Hagemeijer F (1985) Pacemaker electrocardiography of rate smoothing during DDD pacing. PACE 8:684
15. Fuer JM, Shandling AH, Ellstad MH (1990) Sensor-modulated dual-chamber cardiac pacing. Too much of a good thing too fast? PACE 13:816

16. Spencer WH, Markowitz T, Alagona P (1990) Rate augmentation and atrial arrhythmias in DDDR pacing. PACE 13:1847
17. Intermedics (1991) Physician manual. Relay DDDR pulse generator model 293-03 and 294-04. Intermedics, Freeport
18. Medtronic (1989) Synergyst II 7070/7071 activity responsive dual chamber pacer with telemetry. Technical manual. Medtronic, Minneapolis
19. Medtronic (1991) Technical manual. Elite 7074/75/76/77 activity responsive dual chamber pacemaker with telemetry. Medtronic, Minneapolis
20. Pacesetter Systems (1988) Physician manual. Pacesetter Synchrony 2020T rate-modulated polarity programmable dual-chamber pacemaker. Pacesetter Systems, Sylmar
21. Mugica J, Barold SS, Ripart A (1991) The smart pacemaker. In: Barold SS, Mugica J (eds) New perspectives in cardiac pacing, vol 2. Futura, Mt Kisco, p 545
22. Ilvento J, Fee JA, Shewmaker AA (1990) Automatic mode switching from DDDR to VVIR. A management algorithm for atrial arrhythmias in patients with dual chamber pacemakers. PACE 13:1199
23. Lau CP, Tai YT, Fong PC, Li JB, Chung FL (1990) Clinical experience with a minute ventilation sensing DDDR pacemaker. Upper rate behavior and the adaptation of PVARP. PACE 13:1201
24. Gibson S, Paul V, Ward D, Camm AJ (1990) Differentiation of atrial arrhythmias from sinus rhythm by DDDR pacemakers. Eur Heart J 11:313
25. Brinker J, Simmons T, Kay N, Sheehy P, Love C, Ilvento J, Batey R, Wolff L, Wilber D, Trantham JL, Damiano R (1991) Initial experience with a minute ventilation based dual chamber rate adaptive pacemaker. PACE 14:663
26. Vanerio G, Patel S, Ching E, Simmons T, Troham R, Wilkoff B, Castle L, Maloney J (1991) Early clinical experience with a minute ventilation sensor DDDR pacemaker. PACE 14:664
27. Davis M, Pitney M, May C (1991) Automatic mode switching and program selection in a rate adaptive dual chamber pacemaker. PACE 14:664
28. Sweesy M, Batey R, Forney R, Holland J (1991) Automatic mode change in a DDDR pacemaker for supraventricular tachyarrhythmias. PACE 14:737
29. Barold SS, Falkoff MD, Ong LS, Heinle RA (1988) Magnet unresponsive pacemaker endless loop tachycardia. Am Heart J 116:726
30. Barold SS (1990) Repetitive non-reentrant ventriculoatrial synchrony in dual chamber pacing. In: Santini M, Pistolese M, Alliegro A (eds) Progress in clinical pacing 1990. Excerpta Medica, Amsterdam, p 451
31. Barold SS et al. (1988) All dual chamber pacemakers function in the DDD mode. Am Heart J 115:1353

IV. Clinical and Practical Aspects of Rate-Adaptive Pacing

Is Rate-Adaptive Ventricular Pacing Already Obsolete?

M. ROSENQUIST, C. EDELSTAM, and R. NORDLANDER[1]

Introduction

Pacing from the right ventricular apex was first introduced into clinical practice in 1958. Since then, a tremendous technological development has been introduced, leading to the use of more physiological pacing systems including single pacing units with rate-responsive function and atrial synchronous pacing systems with or without rate-responsive mode.

Ventricular pacing is today the most commonly used pacing mode, worldwide. Ventricular rate-responsive pacing (VVI-R) is a simple and an elegant method for achieving protection against bradycardia while providing the patient with an increased heart rate during physical stress. In addition, some sensors will also react to changes in metabolic demands, thus increasing the heart rate not only during physical, but also during mental stress.

The aim of this presentation is to review possible advantages and disadvantages with ventricular rate-responsive pacing in comparison to other more physiological pacing modes.

Physiological Consideration

Normal heart activity is characterized by different mechanisms such as:

1. The ability to increase the heart rate during physical exercise
2. Synchronization between atrial and ventricular contraction
3. A normal ventricular activation pattern utilizing the intact AV conduction system
4. A shortening of the AV delay during an increase in heart rate

Ventricular rate-responsive pacing will provide the patient with a rise in heart rate during physical exercise. VVI-R pacing, however, will not allow for AV synchrony nor a normal ventricular activation pattern or rate-adaptive AV delay (Table 1).

The presence of AV synchrony provides an improvement in cardiac output due to

[1] Department of Cardiology, Karolinska Hospital, 104 0 1 Stockholm, Sweden

Table 1. Physiological Pacing – Does It Exist?

	VVI(R)	AAI(R)	DDD(R)
AV synchrony	–	+	+
Rate response	+	+	+
Normal activation	–	+	–[a]
Rate-adaptive AV delay	–	–	+

[a] Unless the AV delay is prolonged to allow for a normal antegrade conduction.

an increased stroke volume. This seems to be especially important at rest and so far no clear hemodynamic benefit of AV synchrony has been shown during exercise. Another advantage of AV synchrony is that the risk for retrograde conduction causing symptoms of dizziness and hypotension ("the pacemaker syndrome") is reduced.

Clinical data evaluating the possible importance of a normal ventricular activation pattern are scarce. However, animal data and recently published clinical investigations indicate that the preservation of a normal ventricular activation seems to result in an improved left-ventricular performance during both rest and exercise [1, 2]. Both ventricular and atrial synchronous pacing cause an abnormal ventricular activation sequence when stimulating from the right-ventricular apex. It has been suggested that a more normalized activation pattern could be achieved, if the right ventricle was stimulated from the proximal septum [3].

As there is normally in healthy subjects a decrease in the PR interval during physical exercise, it has been anticipated that a rate-dependent AV delay in patients with atrial synchronous pacemakers might improve exercise capacity. Despite the fact, that six different studies have addressed this question [4–9], no consensus exists regarding its effect on exercise capacity. Another potential advantage with rate-adaptive delay is, however, that it allows a higher upper heart rate in patients with AV synchronous pacing and pacemaker-mediated arrhythmias.

Are Artificial Sensors as Good as the Sinus Node?

It is today well accepted that single-lead rate-responsive pacemakers will improve the exercise capacity as compared to fixed ventricular pacing. Furthermore, all commercially available artificial sensors show an adequate heart rate response to exercise when compard with healthy controls. However, recently published data by Sulke et al. [10] emphasizes, that artificial sensors are inferior to the sinus node in mimicking the heart rate response during various standardized everday activities. These activities included, in addition to a graded treadmill exercise test, posture changes, mental stress, suitcase lifting, changes in walking speed, and staircase ascent and descent. It has been suggested, that some of these problems might be resolved by combining various types of sensors, thus fine-tuning the heart rate response to various types of mental and physical stress. So far, however, the sinus node seems to give the best form of rate-responsive pacing during everyday activities.

Optimal Cardiac Pacing in Sinus Node Disease

Sinus node disease is today the most common indication for cardiac pacing in both Europe and the United States, accounting for about 40% – 55% of the pacemaker population [11, 12]. Previous studies on patients with sinus node disease indicated that the natural course was characterized by a higher incidence of new chronic atrial fibrillation and stroke. However, the prognosis of sinus node disease was earlier not considered to be influenced by cardiac pacing [13].

Studies utilizing more physiological pacing modes in patients with sinus node disease indicated that patients provided either with atrial or AV-synchronous pacemakers showed an improved hemodynamic performance, when AV synchronization and/or a normal ventricular activation pattern was preserved [14]. Furthermore, patients utilizing AV synchronization had fewer symptoms of pacemaker syndrome due to the absence of retrograde conduction [15].

Despite the absence of prospective studies comparing atrial or AV-synchronous pacing with ventricular pacing, data have accumulated over the last few years, indicating the beneficial long-term effects of physiological pacing modes in patients with sinus node disease [16–21]. These studies indicate that patients provided with physiological pacing systems (AAI or DDD) seem to have a significantly more favorable natural course than patients provided with ventricular pacing systems. These favorable results include a decreased risk in the development of chronic atrial fibrillation and also suggest a tendency towards a lower incidence of congestive heart failure, stroke, and mortality (Table 2).

In addition, the presence of atrial pacing has been suggested [22] to reduce attacks of paroxysmal atrial arrhythmias in patients with the tachycardia bradycardia syndrome which accounts for about 40% of the patients with sinus node disease.

It is, however, important to emphasize that these studies are retrospective comparative studies and, despite the fact that they all seem to reach the same conclusion, there is still a need for prospective randomized studies to definitely establish the advantage of physiological pacing systems over ventricular pacing in patients with sinus node disease.

The Need for Rate-Response in Sinus Node Disease

It could, of course, be argued that patients with sinus node disease would still benefit more from a ventricular rate-responsive pacing system allowing for an adequate increase in heart rate during physical stress which could not be achieved in patients provided with AAI or DDD pacemakers.

However, in this context it is important to remember that only about 40% of patients with sinus node disease are unable to achieve an adequate maximal heart rate during physical exercise [23]. In addition, the average heart rate over 24 h in patients with sinus node disease seems not to differ from that of healthy controls [24]. If a rate-responsive pacing system should be provided in patients with sinus node disease, it should exclusively be for patients who do not exhibit an adequate rise in heart rate during physical exercise and who, in addition, have a decreased exercise performance.

Table 2. Comparative studies: AAI/DDD versus VVI in sinus node disease

Study	Patients (*n*)	Follow up months	CAF (%)	Stroke (%)	CHF (%)	Deaths (%)
Rosenqvist et al. [17]						
AAI	89	44	6.7	12	15	8
			***	NS	***	*
VVI	79	47	47	15	37	23
Sasaki et al [18]						
AAI/DDD	24	20	0	0	4	12.5
			**	*	NS	NS
VVI	25	35	36	20	28	24
Bianconi et al. [19]						
AAI/DDD	153	44	18	4	NA	14
			*	NS		NS (p=0.08)
VVI	150	59	39	10	NA	31
Santini et al. [20]						
AAI	135	>60	12	2[a]	NA	3[b]
			**			**
VVI	125	>60	44	8[a]	NA	14[b]
Kallryd et al. [21]						
AAI	66	32	8	5	3	19
			*	NS	NS	NS (p=0.09)
VVI	37	26	30	11	11	35

[a] Data refer to cerebrovascular mortality. [b] Data refer to cardiac mortality.
AAI, atrial inhibited pacing; DDD, AV sequential pacing; CAF, chronic atrial fibrillation, CHF, congestive heart failure; VVI, ventricular inhibited pacing; NA, data not given; NS, non-significant.
* $p<0.05$ ** $p<0.01$ *** $p<0.005$

Furthermore, if a patient with sinus node disease exhibits chronotropic insufficiency, rate-responsive function can be achieved by AAI-R or DDD-R systems. Recently published data indicate an improved exercise capacity in patients with sinus node disease and chronotropic insufficiency using AAI-R as compared to AAI systems [25].

Atrial or AV-Synchronous Pacing in Sinus Node Disease?

A possible disadvantage with atrial pacing in sinus node disease is the possibility of impending high-grade AV block. A recent review examining the prevalence of high-grade AV block among patients paced with atrial inhibiting systems indicates that the risk for development of clinically significant high-grade AV block over the long term seems to be low, approximately 1% annually [26]. Provided that patients with sinus node disease are examined with respect to associated AV conduction disorders during intraoperative testing [23], the risk for development of high-grade AV block is probably limited. In patients with associated conduction disorders it is therefore more rational to use AV-sequential pacing systems with or without a rate-responsive function than to use ventricular pacing modes.

Another possible disadvantage with atrial pacing is the lack of control of the AV delay, especially during exercise. Whether or not this is important for patients with sinus node disease and chronotropic incompetence is at present unclear. The potential benefits of a rate-adaptive AV delay should, however, also be balanced against the potential drawback of including an altered ventricular activation sequence caused by ventricular stimulation [2].

In conclusion, considerable data in the literature indicate that patients with sinus node disease should be primarily provided with pacing systems allowing for AV synchronization and a normal ventricular activation pattern. In patients with chronotropic insufficiency these systems should be combined with possibilities of rate response. Ventricular pacing in sinus node disease should thus be avoided and prescribed only to patients with atrial stand-still or where atrial lead implantation is not possible for surgical reasons.

VVI-R Vs DDD or DDD-R Pacing in High-Grade AV Block

During the last decade numerous publications have shown that atrial synchronous pacing is superior to ventricular pacing with respect to left-ventricular performance, exercise capacity, and well-being [27–33].

Short-Term Effects

Hemodynamic changes: At rest a properly timed atrial contribution to stroke volume provides a higher cardiac output compared to fixed-rate ventricular pacing [27, 28]. Exercise studies have clearly shown that the ability to increase heart rate is of greatest importance, increasing cardiac output and exercise tolerance and is not further influenced by the preservation of AV synchrony [27, 29, 30]. In Karlöfs early report from 1975 [27], comparing atrial synchronous pacing to ventricular pacing matched to the same ventricular rate, AV synchrony caused only a moderately (8%) higher cardiac output than rate-matched ventricular pacing when moderate workloads were used. Kristensson et al. [29], in a similar study using heavier workloads, found no significant difference in cardiac output and exercise capacity by adding AV synchronization to increased ventricular rate, suggesting that the atria might have different actions at rest and during exercise. At rest they mainly serve as booster pumps, whereas during exercise they mainly act as conduits for venous blood. It is therefore reasonable to conclude that the importance of atrial contribution to cardiac output is greatest at rest, whereas atrial contribution to left-ventricular filling diminishes during exercise.

Metabolic Effects: VVI Vs VDD, VVI Vs VVI-R. Results from our institution have shown that the myocardial oxygen consumption is the same in fixed-rate ventricular pacing compared to atrial synchronous pacing [34, 35] and to QT-sensor-driven VVI-R pacing [36]. That is to say, for the same cost in myocardial oxygen consumption one achieves a higher cardiac output with rate-adaptive pacing. Hence rate-adaptive pacing offers a more economic cardiac function than fixed-rate pacing. Norepinephrine overflow from the heart is greater in fixed-rate ventricular pacing compared to that of atrial synchronous pacing or VVI-R pacing both at rest and especially during exercise [35, 36] (Table 3).

VDD Vs VVI-R. Linde-Edelstam et al. [37] compared rate-adaptive ventricular pacing to atrial synchronous pacing at rest and during exercise in 18 patients with DDDR pacemakers in an acute invasive study. As expected, cardiac output at rest was significantly higher in the VDD mode due to the higher stroke volume. There were no significant differences between VDD and VVI-R regarding cardiac output during exercise, nor with respect to central pressures, myocardial oxygen consumption, or cardiac sympathetic activity either at rest or during exercise. There are thus no data indicating that there are any significant differences with respect to central hemodynamics or cardiac metabolism in patients paced either with VVI-R pacing or DDD.

Long-Term Effects

The increased norepinephrine overflow in patients with VVI pacemakers may have negative long-term effects. Thus it has been suggested that prolonged increase in cardiac sympathetic activity over time might cause or accelerate heart failure due to a reduction of cardiac beta receptor sensitivity [38]. Furthermore, patients with left-ventricular failure have been shown to have higher levels of norepinephrine [39]. Support for this hypothesis is given in two retrospective long-term studies [40, 41] comparing the survival of patients paced with fixed-rate compared to atrial synchronous pacing. Both studies found that atrial synchronous pacing seems to improve survival in patients with preexisting congestive heart failure.

It is today not possible to establish whether these unfavorable long-term effects seen from fixed ventricular pacing can be avoided by rate-adaptive ventricular pacing or whether AV synchrony is also a necessary prerequisite. Faerestrand et al. [42], in a

Table 3. Previous Comparisons: exercise studies

	VVI/VDD Pehrsson et al. [35]	VVI/VVI-R Hedman et al. [36]	VVI-R/VDD Edelstam et al. [37]
Heart rate	↗	↗	=
Cardiac output	↗	↗	=
MVO2	=	=	=
Norepinephrine	↘	↘	=

Symbols denote changes compared to VVI.

long-term study regarding valvular function assessed by serial Doppler echocardiographic measurements in patients treated with VVI-R compared to patients treated with atrial synchronous pacing, found that patients with VVI-R pacing developed valvular insufficiency to a significantly greater extent (50%) than patients treated with DDD pacing (15%). Although these findings might have important implications, they need to be confirmed by others before any general statements with respect to long-term effects of VVI-R pacing can be made.

Differences in Wellbeing. Despite the fact that several studies seem to demonstrate an improved feeling of wellbeing among patients provided with DDD or VVIR pacemakers as compared to fixed ventricular pacing, studies comparing the effects of VVI-R and DDD pacing are scarce. One recent study by Bubien et al. [43] compared exercise capacity and quality of life in eight patients in a prospective randomized single-blind cross-over design over a 12-week time period. Despite the fact that there were no significant differences with respect to exercise capacity, functional capacity, wellbeing, and cardiac symptoms, seven of eight patients preferred the DDD mode. In a randomized cross-over study comparing four rate-responsive modes VVI-R, DDD, DDI-R and DDD-R in patients with complete heart block and chronotropic incompetence, Sulke et al. [44] actually found a similar difference in wellbeing between VVI-R and DDD/DDD-R. There are thus at least two studies which indicate a better quality of life with the preservation of AV synchrony. In addition, three studies [45–47] claim improved submaximal or maximal exercise capacity using DDD-R as compared to VVI-R.

Although AV-synchronous pacing has several theoretical advantages over VVI-R pacing, there is a lack of data that strongly argues that VVI-R pacing is obsolete in patients wiht high-grade AV block. Further studies have to be undertaken comparing the natural course with respect to late development of cardiovascular complications before any certain recommendations can be made regarding the optimal choice of pacing mode.

Are There Individual Patients That Will Benefit More from Atrial Synchronous than VVI-R Pacing? How Should They Be Selected? Patients with intact VA conduction clearly benefit from atrial synchronous pacing since the development of the pacemaker syndrome is reduced. Left-ventricular compliance has been shown to decrease with age, which means that elderly patients may become more dependent on atrial systole for left-ventricular filling [48]. Furthermore, patients with left-ventricular hypertrophy caused by pressure overload benefit from atrial synchronous pacing, as do patients with hypertrophic cardiomyopathy or in acute stress, e.g., postoperative cardiovascular surgery patients or patients with myocardial ischemia [49–51].

General Conclusions

1. The sinus node, nature's own sensor, is still the best and should be retained whenever possible.
2. Ventricular pacing should be avoided in sinus node disease.
3. In patients with high-grade AV block, DDD/DDD-R is superior to VVI-R with

respect to left-ventricular function at rest, submaximal exercise and well-being. Prospective long-term studies are still warranted to demonstrate possible differences in cardiovascular complication rates.

4. Ventricular rate-responsive pacing is not obsolete, but its prescription should be limited to patients in whom AV-synchronous pacemakers cannot be implanted.

References

1. Park RC, Little WC, O'Rourke RA (1985) Effect of alteration of left ventricular activaton sequence on the left ventricular end systolic pressure-volume relationship in closed-chest dogs. Circ Res 57:706-717
2. Rosenqvist M, Isaac K, Botvinick EH, Dae MW, Cockrell J, Abott JA, Schiller NB, Griffin JC (1991) Relative importance of activation sequence compared to AV synchrony in left ventricular function. Am J Cardiol 67:148-156
3. Karpawich PP, Chang CH, Kukus LR, Justice CD (1991) Initial histologic comparison between apical and a new septal ventricular pacing method in immature canines. PACE 67:148-156
4. Rydén L, Karlsson O, Kristensson BE (1988) The importance of different atrioventricular intervals for exercise capacity. PACE 11:1051-1062
5. Mehta D, Gilmour S, Ward DE, Camm AJ (1989) Optimal atrioventricular delay at rest and during exercise in patients with dual chamber pacemakers. Br Heart J 61:161-166
6. Haskell RJ, French WJ (1989) Physiological importance of different atrioventricular intervals to improved exercise performance in patients with dual chamber pacemakers. Br Heart J 61:46-51
7. Ritter P, Daubert C, Mabo P, Descaves C, Gouffault J (1989) Hemodynamic benefit of a rate adapted AV delay in dual chamber pacing. Eur Heart J 7:637-647
8. Eugene M, Lascault G, Frank R, Fontaine G, Grosgogeat Y, Teillac A (1989) Assessment of the optimal atrioventricular delay in DDD paced patients by impedance pletysmography. Eur Heart J 3:250-256
9. Landzberg JS, Franklin JO, Mahawar SK, Himelman RB (1990) Benefits of atrioventricular synchronization for pacing with an exercise rate response. Am J Cardiol 66:193-197
10. Sulke N, Pilips A, Henderson RA, Bucknall CA, Sowton E (1990) Comparison of the normal sinus node with seven types of rate responsive pacemaker during everyday activity. Br Heart J 64:25-31
11. Feruglio GA, Richards AF, Steinbach K, Feldman S, Parsonnet V (1987) Cardiac pacing in the world. A survey of the state of the art. PACE 10:768-777
12. Parsonnet V, Bernstein AD, Galasso D (1988) Cardiac pacing practices in the United States 1985. Am J Cardiol 62:71-77
13. Shaw DB, Holman RR, Gowers JI (1980) Survival in sinoatrial disease. Br Med J 280:139-134
14. Wirtzfeld A, Schmidt G, Klein G, Worzewski W (1981) Long-term effect of atrial pacing in patients with sick sinus syndrome. PACE 4:A77
15. Stone JM, Bhakta RD, Lutgen J (1982) Dual chamber sequential pacing management of sinus node disease dysfunction. Advantages over single chamber pacing. Am Heart J 104:1319
16. Sutton R, Kenny RA (1986) The natural history of sinus node disease. PACE 9/II:1110-1114
17. Rosenqvist M, Brandt J, Schüller H (1988) Long-term pacing in sinus node disease. Effects of stimulation mode in cardiovascular morbidity and mortality. Am Heart J 116:16-22
18. Sasaki Y, Shimotori M, Akahane K, Yonekura H, Hirano K, Endoh R, Koike S, Kawa S, Furuta S, Homma T (1988) Long-term follow-up of patients with sick sinus syndrome: comparison of clinical aspects among unpaced, ventricular inhibited paced, and physiological paced groups. PACE 11:1575-1583
19. Bianconi L, Boccadamo R, Di Florio A, Carpino A, Catalano A, Stella C, Distolese H (1989)

Atrial versus ventricular stimulation in sick sinus syndrome: effects on morbidity and mortality. PACE 12:1236
20. Santini M, Alexidou G, Ansalone G, Cacciatore G, Cini R, Turitto G (1990) Relation of prognosis in sick sinus syndrome to age, conduction defects and modes of permanent cardiac pacing. Am J Cardiol 65:729-735
21. Kallryd A (1990) Atrial versus ventricular pacing in sinus node disease. Clinical experience. Presented at the 6th Nordic symposium on cardiac pacing, Århus
22. Denjoy I, Leclerq JF, Druelles P, Daubert C, Coumel P (1989) Comparative efficacy of permanent atrial pacing in vagal atrial arrhythmias and in bradycardia-tachycardia syndrome. PACE 12:1236
23. Rosenqvist M, (1990) Atrial pacing for sick sinus syndrome. Clin Cardiol 13:43-47
24. Kallryd A, Kruse I, Ryden L (1989) Atrial inhibited pacing in the sick sinus node syndrome: clinical value and the demand for rate responsiveness. PACE 12:954-961
25. Rosenquist M, Arén C, Kristensson BE, Nordlander R, Schüller H (1990) Atrial rate responsive pacing. Effect on exercise capacity. Eur Heart J 11:537-542
26. Rosenqvist M, Obel IW (1989) Atrial pacing and the risk for AV block: time for a change in attitude? PACE 12:97-101
27. Karlöf I (1975) Hemodynamic effect of atrial triggered versus fixed rate pacing at rest and during exercise in complete heart block. Acta Med Scand 197:195-206
28. Kruse I, Arnman K, Conradsson TB, Rydeú L (1982) A comparison of acute and long term hemodynamic effects of ventricular inhibited and atrial synchronous ventricular inhibited pacing. Circulation 65:846-855
29. Kristensson BE, Arnman K, Rydén L (1985) The haemodynamic importance of atrioventricular synchrony and rate increase at rest and during exercise. Eur Heart J 6:773-778
30. Fananapazir L, Bennett HD, Monks P (1983) Atrial synchronized ventricular pacing: contribution of the chronotropic response to improved exercise performance. PACE 5:601-608
31. Heldman A, Nordlander R (1988) QT sensing rate adaptive pacing compared to fixed rate ventricular inhibited pacing. A controlled clinical study. PACE 12:374-385
32. Pehrsson SK (1983) Influence of heart rate and atrioventricular synchronization on maximal work load tolerance in patients treated with artificial pacemakers. Acta Med Scand 214:311-315
33. Pehrsson SK, Nordlander R, Hedman A (1989) Rate responsive pacing and exercise capacity. PACE 12:749-751
34. Karlsson J, Nordlander R, Pehrsson SK, Åström H (1987) Myocardial oxygen demands of atrial triggered versus fixed rate ventricular pacing in patients with complete heart block. PACE 10:1154-1159
35. Pehrsson SK, Hjemdahl P, Nordlander R, Åström H (1988) Sympathoadrenal activity and cardiac performance at rest and during exercise in patients with ventricular demand compared to atrial synchronous pacing. Br Heart J 60:212-220
36. Hedman A, Hjemdahl P, Nordlander R, Åström H (1990) Effects of mental and physical stress on central hemodynamics and cardiac sympathetic nerve activity during QT interval sensing rate responsive and fixed rate ventricular inhibited pacing. Eur Heart J 11:903-915
37. Linde-Edelstam C, Hjemdahl P, Pehrsson K, Åström H, Nordlander R (1990) Is DDD pacing superior to VVI-R? Effects on myocardial sympathetic activity and myocardial oxygen consumption. PACE 15:425-434.
38. Bristow MR, Ginsburg R, Minobe W, Cubiciotti RS, Sageman WS, Lurie K, Billingham HE, Harrison DC, Stinson EB (1982) Decreased catecholamineamine sensitivity and beta-adrenergireceptor density in failing human hearts. N Engl J Med 307:205-211
39. Cohn JN, Levine B, Olivari MT, Gaiberg V, Lura D, Francis GS, Simon AB, Rector T (1984) plasma norepinephrine as a guide to prognosis in patients with chronic congestive heart failure. N Engl J Med 311:819-823
40. Alpert MA, Curtis JJ, Sanfelippo JF, Flaker GC, Walls JT, Mukerji V, Villarreal SK, Madigan NP, Kroll RB (1986) Comparative survival after permanent ventricular and dual chamber pacing for patients with high degree atrioventricular block with and without preexistent congestive heart failure. J Am Coll Cardiol 7:925-932
41. Linde-Edelstam C, Güllberg B, Nordlander R, Pehrson JK, Rosenquist M, Rydeú L (1992) Longevity in patients with high degree atrioventricular block paced in the atrioventricular synchronous or the fixed rate ventricular mode. PACE 15: 304-313

42. Faerestrand S, Ohm OJ (1988) Dual chamber pacing (DDD) and activity sensing rate-responsive ventricular pacing (PRP): long-term effect on AV valvular function. PACE 11:851 (abstr)
43. Bubien RS, Kay GN (1990) A randomised comparison of quality of life and exercise capacity with DDD and VVIR pacing modes. PACE 13:524 (abstr.)
44. Sulke N, Dritsas A, Chambers J, Sowton E (1990) A randomized cross over study of four rate responsive modes. PACE 13:534 (abstr)
45. Higano ST (1990) Hemodynamic importance of atrioventricular synchrony during low levels of exercise. Cardiostim Rev Eur Technol Biomed 12:35:93
46. Alagona P (1990) Improved exercise tolerance with dual chamber versus single chamber rate adaptive pacing. Cardiostim Rev Eur Technol Biomed 12:57:181
47. Jutzy RV, Florio J, Isaeff DM, Marsa RJ, Bausal RC, Jutzy KR (1990) Comparative evaluation of rate modulated dual chamber pacing and VVIR pacing. Cardiostim Rev Eur Technol Biomed 12:57:182
48. Myreng Y, Nitter-Hause S (1989) Age-dependency of left ventricular filling dynamics and relaxation as assessed by pulsed Doppler-echocardiography. Clin Physiol 9:99-106
49. Pearson AC, Labowitz AJ, Mrosek D, Williams GA, Kennedy HL (1987) Assessment of diastolic function in normal and hypertensive hearts: comparison of Doppler echocardiography and M-mode echocardiography. Am Heart J 113:1417-1425
50. Murakami T, Hess OM, Gage JE, Grimm J, Krayenbühl HP (1986) Diastolic filling dynamics in patients with aortic stenosis. Circulation 73:1162-1172
51. Ilecito S, Amico A, Marangelli V, D'Ambrosio G, Rizzon P (1988) Doppler Echocardiographic evaluation of the effect of atrial pacing-induced ischemia on left ventricular filling in patients with coronary artery disease. J Am Coll Cardiol 11:953-961

AAI and AAI-R Pacing: Clinical and Technical Aspects

H. Schüller, J. Brandt, and T. Fåhraeus[1]

Permanent atrial pacing in sinus node disease was first successfully applied in 1964 [1]. Despite the fact that sinus node disease is today a common indication for permanent pacemaker treatment, the overall rate of atrial pacemaker implantations has remained low. Nevertheless, considerable experience has been gathered with permanent atrial stimulation. This is a review of aspects of atrial pacing that are relevant to the clinician.

Hemodynamic Aspects

The negative hemodynamic consequences resulting from ventricular pacing in patients with a preserved sinus node activity have been repeatedly demonstrated [2–4] and are especially pronounced when there is ventriculo-atrial conduction. In addition to the hemodynamic benefits of a properly timed atrial contraction, there is accumulating evidence that a physiological ventricular activation sequence is of significant importance in terms of cardiac output, regional myocardial function, cardiac efficiency, and diastolic function [5–9]. From a strictly hemodynamic point of view, atrial pacing is thus superior to ventricular pacing as well as to atrioventricular synchronous stimulation.

Several clinical studies have indicated a superiority of atrial pacing as compared to ventricular pacing in sinus node disease. During long-term follow up, atrial stimulation has been shown to result in lower incidences of permanent atrial fibrillation, congestive heart failure, and arterial thromboemoblism [10–13]. No prospective and randomized study has been published, but atrial stimulation appears to result in a lower mortality than ventricular pacing in patients with sinus node disease [11, 14].

[1] Department of Cardiothoracic Surgery, University Hospital, Lund, Sweden

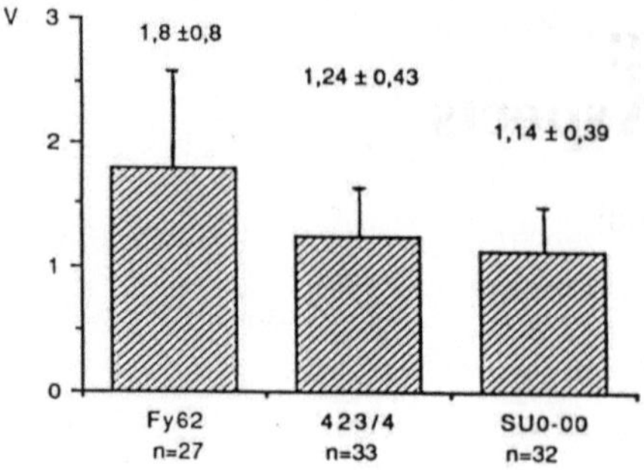

Fig. 1. Noninvasively determined chronic pacing thresholds in patients with three different atrial pacing leads: Osypka FY 62 (platinum tip, screw-in), Siemens 423/424 (carbon tip, passive fixation) and Stöckert SU0-00 (carbon-coated tip, screw-in). Chronic thresholds ar higher with the platinum screw-in lead, but the two leads with carbon tips show comparable, low thresholds despite the different fixation principles

Atrial Lead

Early applications of permanent atrial pacing employed epicardial electrodes [1] or coronary sinus leads [15, 16]. Presently, several transvenous lead models for endocardial atrial pacing are available, and both passive-fixation and active-fixation leads have been shown to perform satisfactorily (Figs. 1 + 2). Dislodgement rates are acceptable with current lead models [17, 18]. The stimulation thresholds are somewhat higher in the atrium than in the ventricle at lead implantation, but chronic thresholds do not differ significantly [19, 20]. The presence of sinus node disease, as well as increased age, has been shown to result in lower acute P wave amplitudes [21] ; there appear to be some differences between active- and passive-fixation atrial leads regarding the post-implant evolution of the atrial endocardial electrogram [22], but permanent P wave undersensing is rare with modern pulse generators [21].

The possibility of far-field sensing of the ventricular complex must be considered. This is frequently demonstrable with unipolar atrial leads [23], and the phenomena of "inappropriate pacemaker bradycardia" [23, 24], "pseudo P wave undersensing" [23], and impaired rate responsiveness with rate adaptive pacing [25] have all been described in this setting. However, when pulse generators with a wide range of sensitivity and refractory period settings are used, far-field QRS complex sensing can be dealt with efficiently [26].

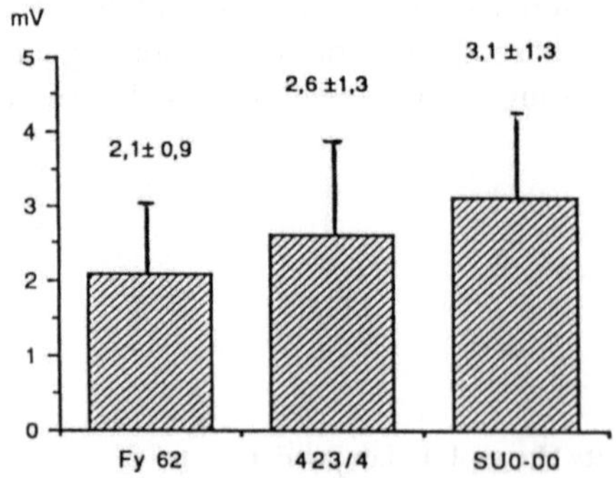

Fig. 2. Noninvasively determined chronic sensing thresholds in patients with the same atrial lead types as in Fig. 1. Sensing thresholds are acceptable with all three lead types. Study time was longer than 3 months

Atrioventricular Conduction

In patients with sinus node disease, abnormalities of the atrioventricular conduction can often be demonstrated by invasive electrophysiology [27, 28]. This has resulted in some reluctance to implant AAI pacemakers. Howeveer, there is now ample evidence that the risk of developing second- to third-degree atrioventricular block during long-term follow up in AAI patients is indeed low. A recent review covered 28 publications reporting on a total of 1878 patients, with a median annual incidence of 0.6% [29]. This firmly supports the view that routine implantation of dual-chamber pacemakers is not indicated in sinus node disease. Commonly, the occurrence of second-degree atrioventricular block at an atrial pacing rate of below 130 or 140 per minute is considered a contraindication for single-chamber atrial stimulation, but there is little scientific evidence of the prognostic value of the Wenckebach point. It remains to be determined whether patients at risk for subsequent development of high-degree atrioventricular block can be identified at the time of pacemaker implantation.

Carotid Sinus Syndrome

Owing to the risk of atrioventricular conduction disturbances, single-chamber atrial pacing cannot be considered appropriate in carotid sinus syndrome [30].

Chronotropic Incompetence

Patients with sinus node disease commonly show an inability to raise the sinus rate adequately in response to exercise. There is no universally accepted definition of chronotropic incompetence, but the prevalence thereof ranges between 24% and 64% in different studies of sinus node disease [31–37]. For this subgroup of patients, rate adaptive atrial pacing (AAI-R) appears an attractive treatment. AAI-R pacing has been shown to result in increased exercise capacity [38, 39] and lower blood lactate levels during exercise [40] as compared to standard atrial stimulation. Rate-adaptive pacemakers with a motion sensor [39–41], respiratory-dependent pulse generators [38], and temperature-guided units [42] have been used on the atrial level. Successful AAI-R pacing requires the patient to have an adequate adaptation of the atrioventricular conduction when the atrial rate is increased during exercise [43]. A few cases with atrioventricular block at increased pacing rates during physical stress have been reported in conjunction with antiarrhythmic medication [44–46], but in the vast majority of cases atrioventricular conduction is sufficiently enhanced in response to exercise [41]. It is important to carefully match the response of the activity sensor to the degree of physical activity in order to avoid "overpacing" of the atrium with a subsequent risk of atrioventricular block. The clinical feasibility of AAI-R pacing in selected cases of sinus node disease, including bradycardia-tachycardia syndrome, has recently been demonstrated [39–41].

Economic Aspects

Comparisons between the total cost of different pacemaker treatment modalities are necessarily complex. In addition to the price of the pacemaker system and the expense of the primary implantation with hospitalization, the overall cost effectiveness is influenced by follow-up costs, pulse generator and lead life span, and complications occurring during the treatment. Dual-chamber pacing has been shown to result in significantly higher costs than single-chamber stimulation [47]. At our institution, 44 patients received AAI-R pacemakers during the period January 1986 to May 1990. In only one of these has it been necessary to perform an upgrading to a DDD-R system. After subtraction of the extra hardware costs in this single case, the net savings during this period amount to US$ 72 000 as compared to primary DDD-R implantation in all cases.

Conclusion

AAI pacing is an efficient treatment in selected cases of sinus node disease, producing excellent hemodynamics and a superior clinical course as compared to VVI pacing. With modern atrial leads and multiprogrammable pulse generators, complication rates are low. In a subgroup of patients, the addition of a rate-adaptive function (AAI-R pacing) is of clinical value. In a large number of patients with sinus node disease, treatment with dual-chamber pacing modes (DDD, DDI, DDD-R, DDI-R) is of no benefit over AAI or AAI-R pacing.

References

1. Silverman LF, Mankin HT, McGoon DC (1968) Surgical treatment of an inadequate sinus mechanism by implantation of a right atrial pacemaker electrode. J Thorac Cardiovasc Surg 55:264
2. Amikam S, Riss E (1979) Untoward hemodynamic consequences of permanent ventricular pacing associated with ventriculoatrial conduction. In: Meere C (ed) Proceedings of the VIth world symposium on cardiac pacing. Pacesymp, Montreal, PP 15-6
3. Wirtzfeld A, Himmler FC, Klein G et al. (1982) Atrial pacing in patients with sick sinus syndrome: acute and long-term hemodynamic effects. In: Feruglio GA (ed) Cardiac pacing. Electrophysiology and pacemaker technology. Piccin Medica, Padova, P 651
4. Ausubel K, Furman S (1985) The pacemaker syndrome. Ann Intern Med 103:420
5. Badke FR, Boinay P, Covell JW (1980) Effects of ventricular pacing on regional left ventricular performance in the dog. Am J Physiol 238:H858
6. Askenazi J, Alexander JH, Koenigsberg DI et al. (1984) Alteration of left ventricular performance by left bundle branch block simulated with atrioventricular sequential pacing. Am J Cardiol 53:99
7. Zile MR, Blaustein AS, Shimizu G, Gaasch WH (1987) Right ventricular pacing reduces the rate of left ventricular relaxation and filling. J Am Coll Cardiol 10:720
8. Baller D, Wolpers H-G, Zipfel J et al. (1988) Comparison of the effects of right atrial, right ventricular apex and atrioventricular sequential pacing on myocardial oxygen consumption and cardiac efficiency: a laboratory investigation. PACE 11:394

9. Bedotto JB, Grayburn PA, Black WH et al (1990) Alterations in left ventricular relaxation during atrioventricular pacing in humans. J Am Coll Cardiol 15:658
10. Sutton R, Kenny R-A (1986) The natural history of sick sinus syndrome. PACE 9:1110
11. Rosenqvist M, Brandt J, Schüller H (1988) Long-term pacing in sinus node disease: effects of stimulation mode on cardiovascular morbidity and mortality. Am Heart J 116:16
12. Santini M, Messina G, Porto MP (1985) Sick sinus syndrome: single chamber pacing. In: Comez FP (ed) Cardiac pacing. Electrophysiology and tachyarrhythmias. Grouz, Madrid, P 144
13. Sasaki Y, Shimotori M, Akahane T et al. (1988) Long-term follow-up of patients with sick sinus syndrome: a comparison of clinical aspects among unpaced, ventricular inhibited paced, and physiologically paced groups. PACE 11:1575
14. Alpert MA, Curtis JJ, Sanfelippo JF et al (1987) Comparative survival following permanent ventricular and dual-chamber pacing for patients with chronic symptomatic sinus node dysfunction with and without congestive heart failure. Am Heart J 113:958
15. Greenberg P, Castellanet M, Messenger J, Ellestad MH (1978) Coronary sinus pacing: clinical follow-up. Circulation 57:98
16. Moss AJ, Rivers RJ (1978) Atrial pacing from the coronary vein. Ten-year experience in 50 patients with implanted permanent pacemakers. Circulation 57:103
17. Schüller H, Brandt J (1983) Klinische Erfahrungen mit der Kohlenstoffelektrode SE 412 S in Kammer- und Vorhofposition (465 Patienten). In: Beyer J, Hemmer W (eds) Physiologische Stimulation mit Herzschrittmachern. Thieme, Stuttgart, P 68
18. Bernstein SB, van Natta BE, Ellestad MH (1988) Experiences with atrial pacing. Am J Cardiol 61:113
19. Kleinert MP, Bartsch HR, Mühlenpfordt KG (1983) Comparative studies of ventricular and atrial stimulation thresholds of carbon-tip electrodes. In: Steinbach K et al (eds) Cardiac pacing. Proceedings of the VIIth world symposium on cardiac pacing. Steinkopff, Darmstadt, P 353
20. Brandt J, Attewell R, Fåhraeus T, Schüller H (1990) Atrial and ventricular stimulation threshold development: A comparative study in patients with a DDD pacemaker and two identical carbon-tip leads. PACE 13:859
21. Brandt J, Attewell R, Fåhraeus T, Schüller H (1990) Acute atrial endocardial P wave amplitude and chronic pacemaker sensitivity requirements: relation to patient age and presence of sinus node disease. PACE 13:417
22. Shandling AH, Castellanet MJ, Thomas LA et al. (1990) The influence of endocardial electrode fixation status on acute and chronic atrial stimulation threshold and atrial endocardial electrogram amplitude. PACE 13:1116
23. Brandt J, Fåhraeus T, Schüller H (1988) Far-field QRS complex sensing via the atrial pacemaker lead. I. Mechanism, consequences, differential diagnosis and countermeasures in AAI and VDD/DDD pacing. PACE 11:1432
24. Moss AJ, Rivers AJ Jr, Kramer DH (1974) Permanent pervenous pacing from the coronary vein. Long-term follow up. Circulation 49:222
25. Shandling AH, Castellanet MJ, Thomas L et al. (1989) Impaired activity rate responsiveness of an atrial activity-triggered pacemaker: the role of differential atrial sensing in its prevention. PACE 12:1927
26. Brandt J, Fåhraeus T, Schüller H (1988) Far-field QRS complex sensing via the atrial pacemaker lead. II. Prevalence, clinical significance and possibility of intraoperative prediction in DDD pacing. PACE 11:1540
27. Rosen KM, Loeb HS, Sinno MZ et al. (1971) Cardiac conduction in patients with symptomatic sinus node disease. Circulation 43:836
28. Narula OS (1971) Atrioventricular conduction defects in patients with sinus bradycardia. Analysis by His bundle recordings. Circulation 44:1096
29. Rosenqvist M, Obel IWP (1989) Atrial pacing and the risk for AV block: is there a time for change in attitude? PACE 12:97
30. Sutton R (1989) The natural history of sick sinus syndrome and autonomic disturbances of heart rate control. New Trends Arrhythmias 5:125
31. Abbott JA, Hirschfeld DS, Kunkel FW, Scheinman MM (1977) Graded exercise testing in patients with sinus node dysfunction. Am J Med 62:330

32. Holden W, McAnulty JH, Rahimtoola SH (1978) Characterization of heart rate response to exercise in the sick sinus syndrome. Br Heart J 40:923
33. Vallin H, Edhag O (1980) Heart rate response in patients with sinus node disease compared to controls. Physiological implications and diagnostic possibilities. Clin Cardiol 3:391
34. Simonsen E (1987) Sinus node dysfunction. A prospective clinical study with special reference to true diagnostic value of ambulatory monitoring, exercise testing, and electrophysiologic studies. Thesis, University of Odense, Denmark. CAVI, Odense
35. Johnston FA, Robinson JF, Fyfe T (1987) Exercise testing in the diagnosis of sick sinus syndrome in the elderly: implications for treatment. PACE 10:831
36. Prior M, Masterson M, Blackburn G et al. (1988) Critical identification of patients with sinus node dysfunction for potential sensor-driven pacing. PACE 11:512 (abstr)
37. Kallryd A, Kruse I, Rydén L (1989) Atrial inhibited pacing in the sick sinus syndrome: clinical value and the demand for rate responsiveness. PACE 12:954
38. Rognoni G, Bolognese L, Aina F et al. (1988) Respiratory-dependent atrial pacing, management of sinus node disease. PACE 11:1853
39. Rosenqvist M, Arén C, Kristensson BE et al. (1990) Atrial rate-responsive pacing in sinus node disease. Eur Heart J 11:537
40. Hatano K, Kato R, Hayashi H et al. (1989) Usefulness of rate responsive atrial pacing in patients with sick sinus syndrome. PACE 12:16
41. Brandt J, Fåhraeus T, Schüller H (1990) Rate-adaptive atrial pacing (AAI-R): clinical aspects. In: Barold SS, Mugica J (eds) New perspectives in cardiac pacing, vol 2. Futura, Mount Kisco
42. Winter UJ, Alt E, Zegelman M et al. (1989) Clinical experience with 65 temperature-guided (TP) pacemakers Nova MR in Europe. PACE 12:1567 (abstr)
43. Daubert C, Ritter P, Mabo P et al. (1986) Physiological relationship between AV interval and heart rate in healthy subjects: applications to dual chamber pacing. PACE 9:1032
44. Ruiter J, Burgersdijk C, Zeeders M, Kee D (1987) Atrial Activitrax pacing. The atrioventricular interval during exercise. PACE 10:1226 (abstr)
45. den Dulk K, Lindemans FW, Brugada P et al. (1988) Pacemaker syndrome with AAI rate variable pacing: importance of atrioventricular conduction properties, medication, and pacemaker programmability. PACE 11:1226
46. Pouillot C, Daubert C, Mabo P et al. (1990) The lack of adaptation in PR interval to heart rate: a frequent limitation for AAIR pacing. PACE 13:504 (abstr)
47. Eagle KA, Mulley AG, Singer DE et al. (1986) Single-chamber and dual-chamber cardiac pacemakers. A formal cost comparison. Ann Intern Med 105:264

Follow Up of Patients with Rate-Adaptive Pacemakers

C.P. LAU [1]

Introduction

Rate adaptation to exercise and non-exercise requirements is an important means by which a physiological pacing system can optimise haemodynamics [1, 2], symptomatology [3, 4], quality of life [5], hormonal function [6] and circadian blood pressure variability [7] in patients with bradycardia. However, in order for an implantable sensor to function optimally, judicious programming and follow up of these patients are mandatory. Besides routine assessment of battery and electrode status like the follow up of all conventional pacemaker recipients, special attention to the sensor and algorithms of rate adaptation will be necessary (Table 1).

Clinical Assessment

Symptom assessment is perhaps the most important aspect of follow up of patients with rate-adaptive pacemakers. Adverse symptoms such as palpitations may suggest

Table 1. Follow up of patients with rate-adaptive pacemakers.

Types	Details
Clinical	Symptoms (e.g., palpitations, breathlessness, angina) Well-being Haemodynamics and exercise capacity
Programming	Lower and upper rates Speed of rate adaptation at onset and termination of exercise Matching sensor level to different workloads Choice of AV interval, post-ventricular atrial refractory period and upper tracking rate in DDDR pacemakers.
Special problems	Pacemaker syndrome, myopotential interference, pacemaker- and sensor-mediated tachycardias

[1] Division of Cardiology, Department of Medicine, University of Hong Kong, Queen Mary Hospital, Pokfulam Road, Hong Kong

an inappropriately fast sensor-determined rate and, if this occurs during sleep in a patient with activity-sensing pacemaker, the possibility of sensor activation by the patient lying directly on the activity sensor should be considered [8]. Palpitations can also complicate excessive arm swinging in patients with respiratory-sensing pacemakers [9, 10]. Upgrading a fixed-rate pacemaker to a rate-adaptive pacemaker may result in palpitations, which are likely to improve with time. In patients with ischaemic heart disease, worsening of angina pectoris can occasionally be a problem, but this usually resolves with judicious adjustment of the upper rate [11]. An improvement in exercise tolerance has been documented in rate-adaptive pacemakers because of improved cardiac output at the same rate–pressure product in these patients. Worsening of heart failure [12] and pacemaker syndrome may rarely occur with ventricular rate-adaptive pacemakers in patients in whom atrial transport is particularly important [13] .

Although not an essential part of a clinical follow up, it may also be useful to assess the advantages of rate adaptation over conventional fixed-rate pacing. Symptoms of shortness of breath on exercise and energy during daily activities are likely to improve [5], as well some improvement in the formal quality of life measure [5] . These changes do not necessarily occur immediately on the initiation of rate adaptation, but may take weeks to occur [5]. Haemodynamic and exercise tolerance can be formally tested with either treadmill or cycle ergometry, and a protocol with a gradually increasing workload may be more appropriate for the usual pacemaker recipients [14, 15]. A significant proportion of elderly patients may not be able to perform these exercises [16]. We have found that by measuring the distance covered by these patients during a standard 12-min walking test to be a reproducible and simple means of assessing the benefits of rate-adaptive pacemakers during daily activities. A substantial learning effect occurs between the first and second 12-min walking tests, but thereafter the learning effect is small and the second test can be used as the baseline for future assessment.

Rate-Adaptive Pacemakers Programming

Lower and Upper Rate

The lower rate of a rate-adaptive pacemaker depends on individual fitness, as in general a fitter subject has a lower resting heart rate than those in whom the contractility reserve is reduced. Unlike the case of VVI pacing in which an average rate has to be programmed, the baseline rate becomes less critical in rate-adaptive pacemakers as a higher rate can be achieved by sensor-driven pacing during exercise. A lower pacing rate at sleep is beneficial as tachycardia-mediated symptoms can occur [17]. The ability of some pacemakers to decrease the rate during sleep (determined by the time of the day and absence of sensor activity) allows a closer approximation of the normal variation of the baseline pacing rate to the normal sinus rhythm.

The upper rate is related to the age and activity, and the presence of ischaemic heart disease of the patients. In general, a higher upper rate may be of benefit in the young and in children. Indeed, in a recent review of nine studies on physiological

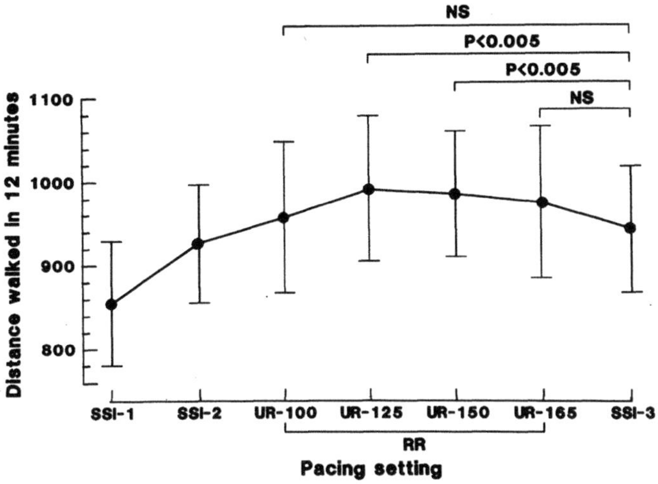

Fig. 1. Distances travelled in 12 min at various programmed upper rates. *SS1-1, 2* and *3* refer to the distances covered during walking at 70 bpm. A substantial learning effect occurs between SS1 and SS2, but not between SS1-2 and SS1-3, so that the latter would be used for comparison. An upper rate (*UR*) of 125 or 150 bpm appeared to be appropriate for maximising exercise capacity. *NS*, not significant. (From [16] with permission)

pacemakers, Nordlander et al. [18] found that the percentage improvement in maximal exercise capacity was linearly related to the maximal rate achieved. However, Holter recordings of patients with complete heart block fitted with VDD pacemakers revealed that the usual pacemaker recipients (mean age 68–70 years) achieved a rate of 150 bpm in less than 0.5% of the time in the day [19]. We have also assessed the effect of upper rate in a group of ten pacemaker recipients of about 70 years old using the 12-min walking tests. We could not find any objective difference between an upper rate of 125 and 150 bpm on the distance covered [16] (Fig. 1). An upper rate of more than 150 bpm was associated with angina and impaired exercise tolerance in this group of patients.

Thus it seems that an upper rate of 125–150 bpm can be chosen for the usual pacemaker recipients. In patients with angina pectoris it is worthwhile performing some form of exercise testing to see if such an upper rate can improve exercise capacity without unduly aggravating angina pectoris. As regards the baseline rate, a recent study [7] using Holter and ambulatory blood pressure recordings has shown that a mean rate of about 60–70 bpm gives the best approximation to the normal variation in rate and blood pressure over the 24-h period. If available in the pacemaker algorithm a further rate drop during sleep should be programmed.

Onset and Termination of Rate Response

At the onset of exercise, the normal heart rate increases almost immediately without significant delay, with over half of the heart rate changes occurring within the first min of exercise [21, 22]. Thus an appropriate speed of rate response is important, especially in patients who exercise only for brief periods of time. Figure 2 shows a

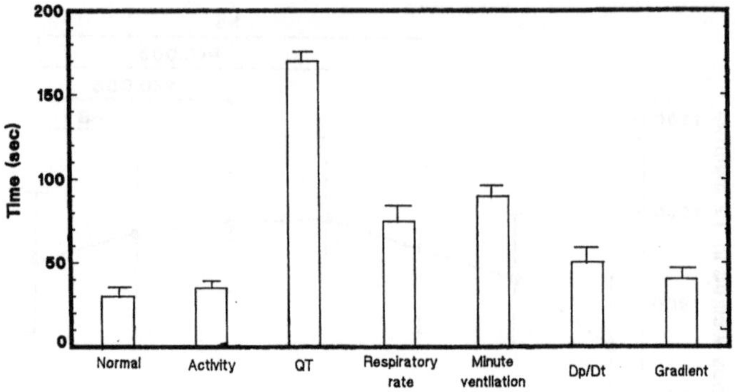

Fig. 2. Delay in the onset of rate response of some currently available rate-adaptive pacemakers. The time delay refers to the time taken for an increase of rate to half of the maximal value during treadmill exercise at 2.5 mph at 0% gradient [26]

comparison of the speed of onset of a number of rate-adaptive pacemakers. Compared with normals, the activity-sensing pacemakers have the best speed of onset of rate response. To some extent, the speed of onset of rate response depends on the algorithm used in relating a change in sensor signal to a corresponding change in rate. In the initial version of the QT sensing pacemaker, a linear relation was assumed between QT shortening and pacing rate change. This was found to be inadequate as the magnitude of QT interval change is small at low heart rate and thus results in a long delay in the onset of rate response. A dynamic slope in which a higher slope is automatically used at the onset of exercise reduces this delay [23]. In activity-sensing pacemakers, the speed of onset is now available as a programmable option. In patients with atrial rate-adaptive pacemakers, sudden rate increase may result in functional AV interval prolongation so that atrial contraction may take place simultaneously with the previous ventricular contraction and may result in pacemaker syndrome [24]. Perhaps a programmable slower speed of rate response may avoid this functional AV conduction problem, especially in patients who are on AV nodal slowing agents [24].

The rate of decay of pacing rate after recovery may also be important. Our recent work [25] suggests that a physiological rate decay may contribute to earlier recovery of haemodynamics and perhaps lower lactate accumulation after exercise (Fig. 3). An appropriate pattern of decrease of pacing rate is necessary, especially in patients who have achieved a high rate at peak exercise. The rate decay pattern is now programmable in a number of rate-adaptive pacemakers. Alternatively, in some sensors such as the sensing of central venous temperature, oxygen saturation and stroke volume, the decay of sensor signal after exercise is related to previous workloads and can be used to modulate the pacing rate recovery after exercise.

Matching Sensor Level to Workload

In an open-loop rate-adaptive system, a certain pacing rate has to be ascribed to a certain sensor level. We [26] and others [27, 28] have used the pacing rate achieved during walking to program the rate adaptive pacemakers. A rate of 90-100 bpm during this exercise was used and this was found to be generally useful. Programming is

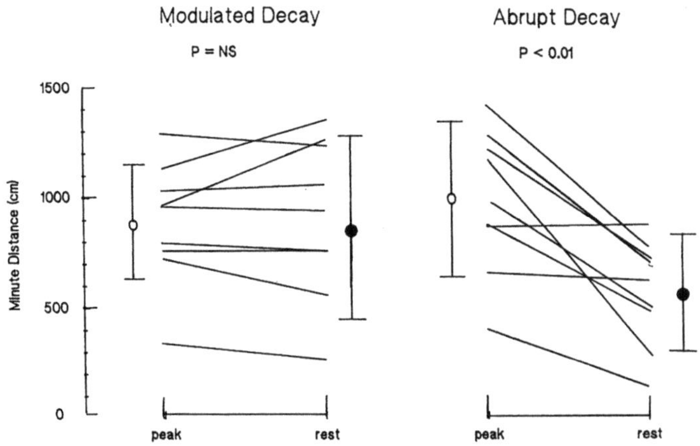

Fig. 3. Changes in cardiac output (represented by Doppler derived minute distance) from peak exercise to the resting state, with the pacing rate falling gradually (*Modulated Decay*) or abruptly (*Abrupt Decay*). An abrupt fall in cardiac output occurred when the pacing rate decreased suddenly on exercise termination [25]. *NS*, not significant

achieved either with the use of ECG telemetry or with built-in rate histograms or Holter in some pacemakers. In the rate histograms, pacing rates are allocated into "bins" of different ranges, and a characteristic "spread" of the percentage of pacing rate in each bin gives an idea of appropriateness of the programming [28, 29]. Built-in "Holters" in some rate-adaptive pacemakers enable the actual rate profile of an exercise to be recorded. In the activity-sensing Relay pacemaker (Intermedics, Inc., Texas, USA), the sensor level after an activity can be remembered and optimised, and the pacing rate at different "slopes" can be redrawn to see if a better rate profile could be achieved with a different slope setting without the need to repeat the exercise ("Activity-Sensing Rate-Adaptive Pacing", this volume, Fig. 7).

It is also important to recognise that although walking is the most common activity, optimisation of the pacing rate for this activity may not necessarily optimise the response during other activities (Fig. 4). This is seen particularly in activity-sensing pacemakers in which the pacing rate achieved is highly dependent on the way in which an activity is carried out [30, 31]. This may be less problematic in sensors which have

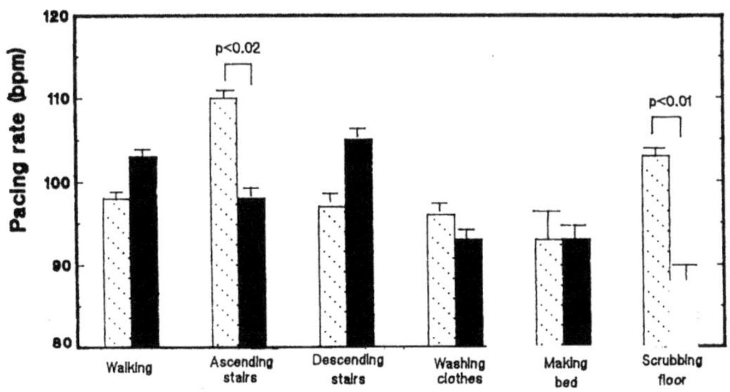

Fig. 4. Comparative evaluation of rate response between an activity-sensing pacemaker (*solid columns*) and the sinus rate (*hatched columns*) during a variety of daily activities. The pacing rates of activity-sensing pacemakers closely mimick the normal rate behavior during lighter activities, but the pacing rate may be insufficient at high work levels especially those involving the upper limbs such as scrubbing floor [31]

a more direct relationship with workloads. Improvement of proportionality of rate response to different types of exercise and non-exercise needs are likely to be realised with sensor combination.

Follow Up of DDDR Pacemakers

Standard DDD pacemakers are programmed in the usual manner. The rate-adaptive function can be programmed in the same way in patients who exhibit chronotropic incompetence during exercise, as sensor-determined AV sequential pacing will occur with moderate levels of activity so that intrinsic rhythm will be suppressed. The main interaction between an implantable sensor and DDD pacemakers is the management of pacemaker mediated tachycardias; for example, in patients with paroxysmal supraventricular arrhythmias in which the upper tracking rate has to be limited. This is circumvened in the Synchrony pacemaker (Siemens, Inc., Sweden) in which a higher sensor rate can be programmed separately. This allows a normal sensor-initiated rate response during exercise but a lower tracking rate during pathological tachycardia [32]. Sensor-initiated DDDR pacing can also result in the smoothing of the upper rate behaviour, so that 2:1 AV tracking with an abrupt rate drop at the upper rate limit can be prevented by the sensor which dictates a more physiological rate [33].

A recently available minute ventilation-sensing DDDR pacemaker (META DDDR Telectronics Pacing Systems, Colorado, USA) also allows for sensor-determined shortening of the AV interval and the post-ventricular atrial refractory period [34]. Because of this automatic shortening of the total atrial refractory period (TARP) as minute ventilation increases during exercise, a relatively long TARP can be used at rest. This has the advantage of avoiding the tracking of retrograde conduction and atrial arrhythmias at rest without compromising a high upper rate to be achieved during exercise (Fig. 5). However, the duration of TARP at baseline has to be tested by a sprint exercise which increases the sinus rate rapidly. The longest TARP at rest corresponds to the longest TARP capable of accommodating the sudden increase in sinus rate and maintaining 1:1 conduction during sprint exercise (Fig. 6).

Another algorithm to avoid rapid ventricular tracking of atrial tachyarrhythmia in DDDR pacemaker is to use an interim rate as the maximum tracking rate in the absence of sensor activation [35]. The sensor is used to diagnose an unphysiological atrial rate, and the pacer can respond only at the so called "conditional ventricular tracking limit". When sensor activation occurs this limit is ignored and normal response to the upper rate can occur. Indications programming of this interior rate B needed to avoid AV dissociation during sinus tachycardia occuring in the absence of sensor activation [36].

Special Problems

Rate-adaptive pacemakers, especially the investigational devices, are sometimes associated with technical problems and new problems of interference such as by

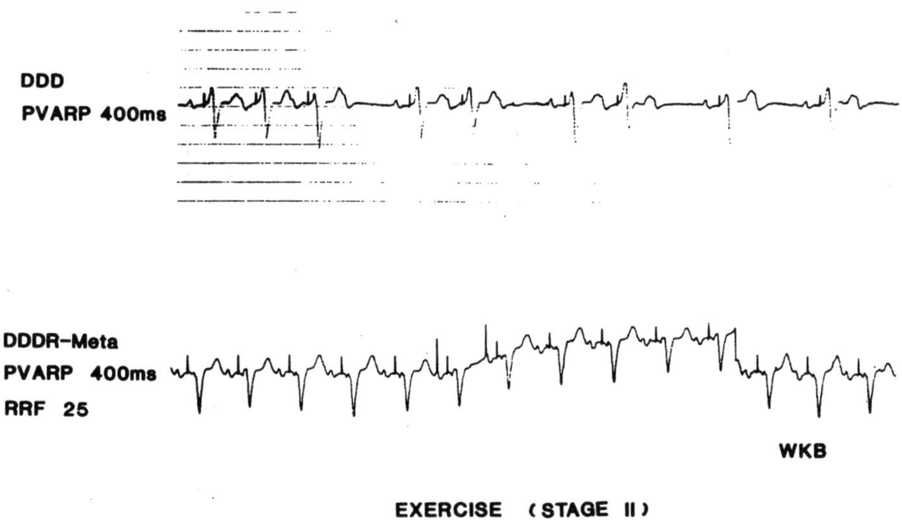

Fig. 5. Adaptation of the total atrial refractory period (TARP) using minute ventilation. *Upper panel*, TARP of 560 ms (AVI = 140 ms, post-ventricular atrial refractory period (*PVARP*) 400 ms) which corresponds only to an upper rate of 107 bpm. Thus, Wenckebach block occurs during exercise in the DDD mode. However, with DDDR pacing, minute ventilation increases during exercise (rate-responsive factor, *RRF*, decreases to 25), the corresponding TARP decreases and a rate of 110 bpm can be reached. Note the intermittent atrial pacing during exercise in the DDDR mode suggesting that the sensor and P wave rates are similar

a

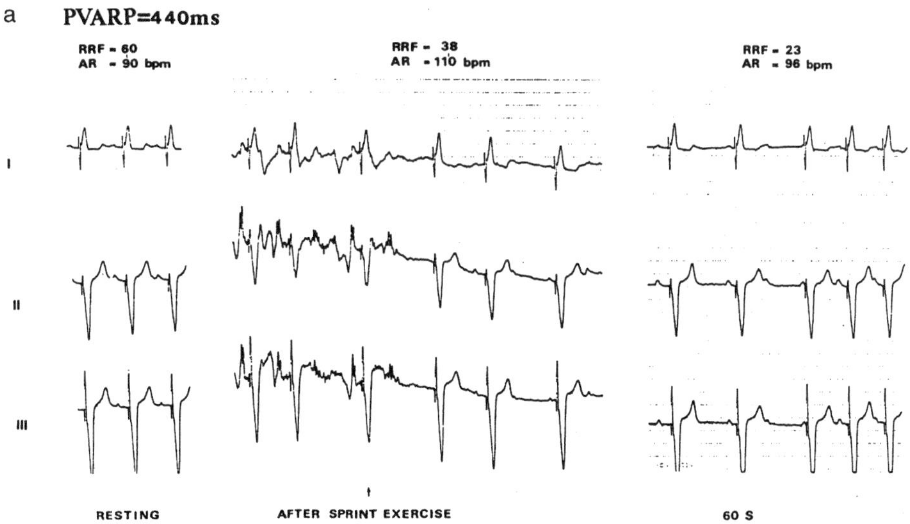

Fig. 6. a Transient AV dissociation associated with a long PVARP (440 ms) in a patients with a DDDR pacemaker. This occurred as the sinus rate increased more rapidly than the increase in minute ventilation during a sudden burst of running.

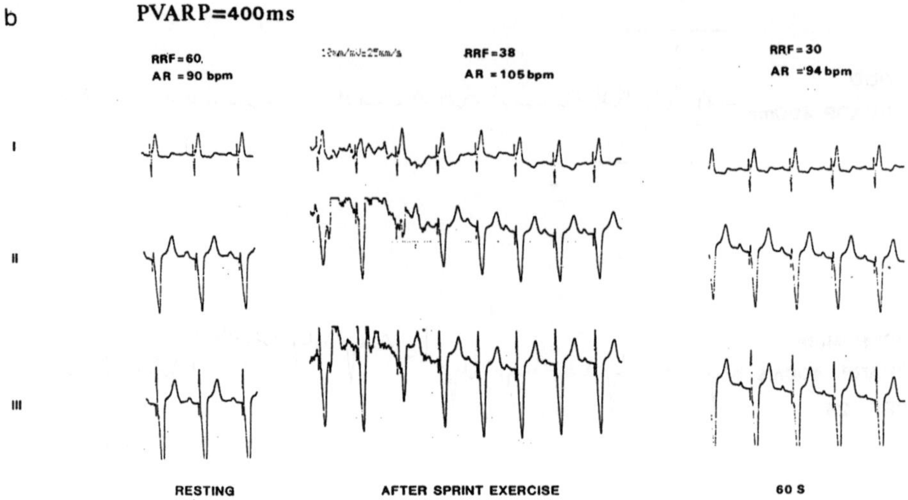

Fig. 6 b This is prevented by using a slightly shorter PVARP (400 ms) at rest. *RRF*, rate-responsive factor; *AR*, atrial rate

Table 2. Reported examples of "sensor-feedback" tachycardias which are self-perpetuating as a positive feedback loop is involved

Sensor	Mechanism	Management
QT interval	QT shortening with exercise increased pacing rate	New software to correct for QT/rate relationship
	Increased pacing rate shortened the QT interval	
Temperature	Diaphragmatic pacing increased temperature	Decrease pacing output
	Increased temperature increased pacing rate	
Activity	Pacemaker "flip" caused pocket pacing	1. Decrease pacing output
	Pocket pacing Increased frequency of vibration increased pacing rate	2. Pacemaker reversal

myopotential and electromagnetic signals (see "New Problems with Rate-Adaptive Pacing: Limitations, Adverse Effects, and Interference." this volume). In addition, pacemaker-mediated tachycardias [37] can occur in single-chamber rate-adaptive pacemakers as a result of inappropriate sensor response or in rare instances can involve a positive feedback loop (Table 2). In the latter, an increase in sensor level triggers off an increase in rate, which in turn results in activation of the sensor and leads to a "sensor feedback tachycardia". DDDR pacemakers are also susceptible to endless-loop tachycardia when functioning in the DDD mode, and occasionally the tachycardia can be terminated by the physician by activating the sensor externally (e.g., by tapping on an activity-sensing DDDR pacemaker) which breaks the endless-loop tachycardia by sensor-mediated AV sequential pacing at a rate higher than the tachycardia [38]. In addition, in patients with rate-adaptive pacemakers undergoing surgery, additional precautions need to taken. It has been shown that general anaesthesia and Caeserean section are safe in activity- [39] and minute ventilation-sensing [40] pacemakers. However, diathermy during cardiac operation close to the pacing electrode in minute ventilation-sensing pacemakers can lead to pacing at maximal rate as the diathermy current can falsely increase the sensed impedance level. In general, programming to the non-rate adaptive mode may be safer during these procedures.

Conclusion

The follow up of rate-adaptive pacemakers involves clinical assessment and an understanding of the sensor involved. The current technological status of rate-adaptive pacing still requires significant time and manpower during the follow up. Follow-up support such as by built-in Holter, rate histograms, and the use of automatic programming may simplify the follow-up procedure substantially in the near future.

References

1. Karlof I (1975) Haemodynamic effect of atrial triggered versus fixed rate pacing at rest and during exercise in complete heart block. Acta Med Scand 10:1215
2. Fananapazir L, Rodemaker M, Bennett DH (1985) Reliability of the evoked response in determining the paced ventricular rate and performance of the QT or rate responsive (TX) pacemaker. PACE 8:701-714
3. Perrins EJ, Morley CA, Chen SL, Gutton R (1983) Randomised controlled trial of physiological and ventricular pacing. Br Heart J 50:112-117
4. Kruse I, Arnman K, Conradson TB, Ryden L (1982) A comparison of the acute and long term hemodynamic effects of ventricular inhibited and atrial synchronous ventricular inhibited pacing. Circulation 65:846-855
5. Lau CP, Rushby J, Leigh-Jones M, Tam CYF, Poloniecki J, Ingram A, Sutton R, Camm AJ (1989) Symptomatology and quality of life in patients with rate responsive pacemakers: a double-blind crossover study. Clin Cardiol 12:505-512
6. Alt E, Zitzmann E, Heinz M, Gastmann U, Matula M, Lehmann M (1990) The effect of rate responsive pacing on exercise capacity, serum catecholamines and other metabolic parameters. PACE 13:531
7. Lau CP, Tai YT, Fong PC, Chung F (1991) The contribution of atrioventricular synchrony and rate responsiveness to the circadian blood pressure. PACE 14:620, A9

8. Wilkoff BL, Shimokochi DD,. Schaal SF (1987) Pacing rate increase due to application of steady external pressure on an activity sensing pacemaker. PACE 10:423 (abstr)
9. Lau CP, Ritchie D, Butrous GS, Ward DE, Camm AJ (1988) Rate modulation by arm movements of the respiratory dependent rate responsive pacemaker. PACE 11:744-752
10. Lau CP, Ward DE, Camm AJ (1989) Single chamber cardiac pacing with two forms of respiration controlled rate responsive pacemakers. Chest 95: 352-359
11. De Cock CC, Paris JHC, Van Eenigl MJ, Roos JP (1989) Efficacy and safety of rate responsive pacing in patients with coronary artery disease and angina pectoris. PACE 12: 1405-1411
12. Moreira LFP, Costa R, Stolf NAG, Jatene AD (1989) Pacing rate increase as cause of syncope in a patient with severe cardiomyopathy. PACE 12:1027-1029
13. den Dulk K, Lindemans FW, Bruguda P, Smiths JLRM, Wellens HJJ (1988) Pacemaker syndrome with AAI rate variable pacing: importance of atrioventricular conduction properties, medication and pacemaker programmability. PACE 11:1226-1233
14. Wilkoff BL, Covey J, Blackburn G (1989) A mathematical model of the cardiac chronotropic response to exercise. J Electrophysiol 3:176-180
15. Alt E (1987) A protocol for treadmill and bicycle stress testing designed for pacemaker patients. Stimucoeur 15:33-35
16. Lau CP, Leung WH, Wong CK, Cheng CH, Tai YT (1989) Adaptive rate pacing at submaximal exercise: the importance of the programmed upper rate. J Electrophysiol 3:283-288
17. Swinehart JM, Recker RR (1973) Tachycardia and nightmares. Nebr Med J 58:314-315
18. Nordlander R, Hedman A, Pehrsson JK (1989) Rate responsive pacing and exercise capacity. PACE 12:749-751
19. Kristensson B, Karlson O, Ryden L (1986) Holter-monitored heart rhythm during atrioventricular synchronous and fixed-rate ventricular pacing. PACE 9:511-518
20. Lee MT, Baker R (1990) Circadian rate variation in rate-adaptive pacing systems. PACE 13: 1797-1801
21. Leoppky JA, Greene ER, Hoekenger DE, Caprihan A, Luft UC (1981) Beat-by-beat stroke volume assessment by pulsed Doppler in upright and supine exercise. J Appl Physiol 50:1173-1182
22. Miyamoto Y (1981) Transient changes in ventilation and cardiac output at the start and end of exercise. Jpn J Physiol 31:149-164
23. Baig MW, Wilson J, Boute W, Begemann MJS, Cobbold JP, Perins EJ (1989) Improved pattern of rate responsiveness with dynamic slope setting for the QT sensing pacemaker. PACE 12:311-320
24. Ruiter J, Burgersdij KC, Zeeder SM, Kee D (1987) Atrial Activitrax pacing: the atrioventricular interval during exercise (abstract). PACE 10:1226
25. Lau CP, Wong CK, Cheng CH, Leung WH (1990) Importance of heart rate modulation on cardiac hemodynamics during post-exercise recovery. PACE 13:1277-1285
26. Lau CP, Butrous GS, Ward DE, Camm AJ (1989) Comparative assessment of exercise performance of six different rate adaptive right ventricular cardiac pacemakers. Am J Cardiol 63:833-839
27. Mahaux V, Waleffe A, Kulbertus HE (1989) Clinical experience with a new activity sensing rate modulated pacemaker using autoprogrammibility. PACE 12:1362-1368
28. Hayes DL, Higano ST (1989) Utility of rate histograms in programming and follow up of a DDDR pacemaker. Mayo Clin Proc 64:495-502
29. Lau CP, Tse WS, Camm AJ (1988) Clinical experience with Sensolog 703: a new activity sensing rate responsive pacemaker. PACE 11:1444-1455
30. Lau CP, Mehta D, Toff W, Stott RJ, Ward DE, Camm AJ (1988) Limitations of rate response of activity sensing rate responsive pacing to different forms of activity. PACE 11:141-150
31. Lau CP, Wong CK, Leung WH, Cheng CH (1989) A comparative evaluation of minute ventilation sensing and activity sensing adaptive-rate pacemakers during daily activities. PACE 12:1514-1521
32. Higano S, Hayes DL, Eisinger G (1989) Advantages of discrepant upper rate limit in a DDDR pacemaker. Mayo Clinic Proc 64:932-939
33. Higano ST, Hayes DL, Eisinger G (1989) Sensor-driven rate smoothing in a DDDR pacemaker. PACE 12:922-929

34. Lau CP, Tai YT, Fong PC, Li JBS, Chung FLW (1990) Clinical experience with a minute ventilation sensing rate adaptive pacemaker: upper rate behavior and the adaptation of PVARP. PACE 13:1201, A50
35. Lau Cp, Tai YT, Forg PC, Li JPS, Levy SK, Chung FLW, Song S (1992) Clinical experience with an accelerometer based activity sensing dual chamber rate adaptive pacemaker. PACE 15:334-343
36. Lau CP, Tai YT, Fong PC, Li JP, Chung FL, Song S (1992) The use of implantable sensors for the control of pacemaker mediated tachycardias: a comparative evaluation between minute ventilation sensing and acceteration sensing dual chamber rate adaptive pacemakers. PACE 15:34-44
37. Lau CP (1991) Sensors and pacemaker mediated tachycardias. PACE
38. Lau CP, Li JPS, Wong CK, Chang CH, Chung FLW (1991) Sensor initated terminating pacemakers mediated tachycardia in a DDDR pacemaker. Am Heart J 121:515-517
39. Anderson C, Oxhoj H, Arnsbo P (1989) Pregnancy and Cesarean section in a patient with a rate-responsive pacemaker. PACE 12:386-391
40. Lau CP, Lee CP, Wong CK, Leung WH, Cheng CH (1990) Rate responsive pacing with a minute ventilation sensing pacemaker during pregnancy and delivery. PACE 13:158-163

New Problems with Rate-Adaptive Pacing: Limitations, Adverse Effects, and Interference

S.S. BAROLD[1]

The widespread use of rate-adaptive pulse generators has created new problems specifically related to the sensor or rate-adaptive function that regulates the pacing rate. Many sensor-driven devices are still investigational and some are not generally available in the United States. This chapter focuses on the limitations, adverse effects, and interference of rate-adaptive pacemakers available in the United States as of the end of 1991. Rate-adaptive pacemakers approved for general use in the United States by the Food and Drug Administration utilize sensor input from activity, minute ventilation volume, and temperature to modulate the pacing rate [1].

Activity

The most commonly used rate-adaptive systems employ a piezoelectric crystal for detecting mechanical forces of vibrations (body movement, but not myopotentials). Deformation or compression of a quartz crystal generates a tiny electrostatic voltage proportional to the applied stress. The frequency (and in some systems also the amplitude) of the vibration signal is eventually translated into an appropriate pacing rate that increases in proportion to the detected vibration. The response depends on the nature of the forces affecting the piezoelectric crystal and the way the pacemaker processes the sensor signal. The piezoelectric crystal is bonded to the inner surface of the pacemaker can and no special lead is required (Fig. 1). There is no metabolic or

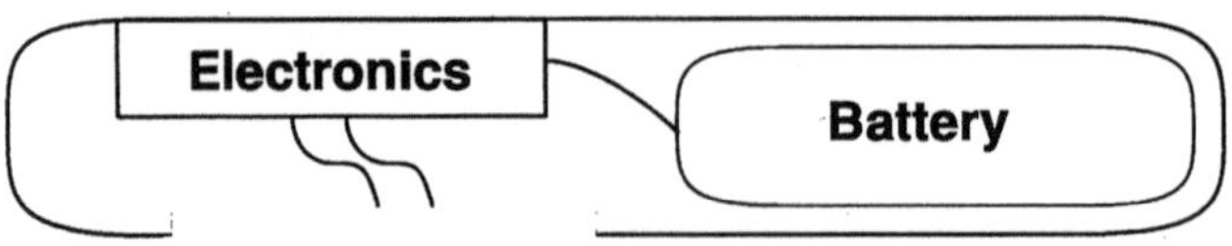

Fig. 1. Pacemaker cross-section showing location of piezoelectric sensor (in *black*) bonded to the inside surface of the pacemaker can. The sensor responds to vibration sensed through tissue contact

[1] Division of Cardiology, Department of Medicine, The Genesee Hospital, University of Rochester School of Medicine and Dentistry, 224 Alexander Street, Rochester, NY 14607, USA

hemodynamic feedback, and the sensor is regarded as nonphysiologic because it does not respond to an increase metabolic demand unrelated to exercise such as emotional stimuli [2]. Indeed, response to emotional stimuli may not be clinically important and may actually be a disadvantage in some patients. Although the "occurrence" of activity is more important than the "strength" of activity [3], this limitation and other idiosyncrasies of piezoelectrically-driven, rate-adaptive systems do not detract substantially from their impressive clinical performance. Activity rate-adaptive single-chamber pacemakers quickly became the largest-selling pacemakers in the world because they are simple and work well in practice in contradistinction to the theoretical advantages of a host of other more sophisticated and specific sensor systems.

The activity system is hermetically sealed, simple, reliable, stable, uses standard lead (any electrode – unipolar or bipolar, atrial and/or ventricular) and exhibits a fast response to brief periods of exercise. Its main advantage is related to the precise detection and rapid response at the onset and end of exercise, important characteristics in older patients who do not perform much exercise and do so primarily in short bursts of physical work such as walking or climbing stairs. The rapid response [4, 5] contrasts sharply with other sensor-driven systems that exhibit a delayed response at the onset of exercise and reach a maximal rate after the end of exercise, making them less desirable for the elderly. However, the plateau response of activity rate-adaptive pacemakers after the initial increase in rate represents a disadvantage. At the end of the exercise, when vibration stops because there is no feedback, an arbitrary setting controls the decay curve and in early models there was an excessively fast rate drop after exercise. Several programmable decay responses are now available but, without feedback, decay times are necessarily either too long or too short. The pacing rate depends on the type of activity and does not correlate well with the level of exertion or the amount of work, i.e., body vibration is not proportional to the level of energy expenditure.

An activity rate-adaptive pulse generator does not respond to isometric exercise such as hand grip or Valsalva maneuver, weightlifting, postural changes (little or not rate change on standing) and to changes in catecholamines [4, 5]. Walking at a faster speed on the treadmill will increase the pacing rate. However, the rate will not increase with a steeper incline, keeping the speed constant, because the steeper incline (at the same speed) requires similar body movements and the number of steps remains the same at each speed, i.e., the input or number of counts generated by the piezoelectric crystal reflects the number of steps [3, 5]. Consequently, jogging in place achieves a high pacing rate. Bicycle riding employs leg motion rather than body vibration. For this reason, bicycle exercise testing is inappropriate to determine optimal settings of the pacemaker and its rate response because it produces inadequate vibration from physical activity [6, 7]. Although the Sensolog (Siemens, Solna, Sweden) pacemaker possesses the same limitations as the Medtronic Activitrax units (Medtronic, In., Minneapolis, Minnesota, USA), it responds better during bicycle because of a different algorithm that integrates vibration waves rather than simply counting peaks of activity [7]. Webb et al. [8] reported an inadequate rate response of the Medtronic Activitrax during swimming (breast stroke, back strokce, and freestyle) when the pulse generator was programmed to produce an increase in rate by approximately 30 beats/minute in response to walking.

An activity-driven pulse generator provides a lesser rate response when walking up stairs compared to going down stairs, the opposite of normal physiology [4, 9–12] and as a rule the rate increase on walking up stairs is inadequate compared to the normal sinus node response. An activity system is more responsive to lower extremity than upper extremity exercise, yet pacemakers implanted in the abdominal wall or subclavian region do not exhibit significant differences in rate response [9]. Simple arm movements such as combing hair or brushing teeth have little effect on the activity pacing rate. Activity pacing produces an appropriate response when making beds or washing dishes and an exaggerated response in rate during tasks involving rapid movement such as scrubbing. Movement of the arm on the side of the implanted activity sensor produces a greater response than movement of the contralateral arm [1]. An excessive rate response occurs in response to lifting a suitcase by the arm on the side of the pacemaker.

An activity system with a piezoelectric crystal is sensitive to pressure on the pulse generator resulting in an increase in the pacing rate, often seen with application of the programmer over the pulse generator [13]. Some patients develop an inappropriate increase in the pacing rate at night when sleeping on the chest or turning in bed, as well as when driving a car with the shoulder seatbelt over the pacemaker site.

Tapping lightly over an activity (piezoelectric) rate-adaptive pacemaker may cause significant increase in the pacing rate that may be useful in certain circumstances: (a) termination of reentrant supraventricular, and ventricular tachycardia – this maneuver is effective only when the tachycardia is relatively slow [14] ; (b) performance of a thallium stress test by increasing the pacing rate not provided by programming the maximal lower rate; (c) termination of endless-loop tachycardia rather than by magnet application [15] ; (d) the rate response can sometimes be used beneficially by patients in anticipation of an increase in cardiac output required with certain activities known to produce an inadequate increase in the pacing rate.

Under general anesthesia, vigorous surgical manipulation may cause a substantial increase in pacing rate, but this is unimportant because of its brief duration [16]. The muscular twitches produced by suxamethonium and the myoclonus resulting from the intravenous administration of anesthetic agents are unlikely to induce an increase in heart rate [16]. Post-operative shivering may cause persistent pacemaker tachycardia [16]. In this respect, Mond and Kertes [17] reported a case of anxiety-provoked shivering that resulted in a pacing rate of 120/min. Epileptic seizures and myotonic jerking with chorea can also increase the pacing rate [18].

Deep implantation, as in the retromammary area in females, may decrease the response to exercise. As a rule, evaluation of an activity rate-adaptive pacemaker to exercise should be performed about 1 month after implantation because fluid in the pacemaker pocket may dampen vibrations and rate response. If programmed too early, there may be an excessive rate response several weeks later, after absorption of fluid in the pacemaker pocket [19]. Occasionally a unipolar pulse generator implanted in the retromammary position or one that flips in the pacemaker pocket may cause local muscle stimulation and create a self-perpetuating mechanism or sensor-mediated pacemaker tachycardia [20–21] (discussed later).

Environmental interference such as riding in a car in rough terrain, in a train, small engine aircraft, helicopter, hovercraft, or on a motorcycle; the use of drills and very loud rock music (large amplifier and ultra-low frequencies near 20 Hz) may cause an increase in the pacing rate that is rarely of clinical significance [22–25]. When bicycling on a paved road, the condition of the road influences the rate response and may provide a better pacing rate compared to the inadequate rate response during stationary bicycle ergometry. Dental drilling represents an important cause of vibrational interference transmitted through a patient with an increase in the rate of activity rate-adaptive pacemakers [6, 26]. In an effort to eliminate false responses due to environmental vibrations and mechanical noise, activity-driven pacemakers are now being designed with an accelerometer (a modified piezoelectric crystal) that reacts primarily to unidirectional forces of acceleration in the anterior-posterior plane (discussed later).

Respiratory-Dependent Systems

Respiratory Rate

This system uses a standard unipolar lead together with an auxiliary lead lying in the subcutaneous tissue across the anterior chest wall and measures electrical impedance between the pacemaker can and the auxiliary lead [27, 28]. The system is unipolar and can therefore be inhibited by myopotentials. The sensor is simple, fairly reliable, but nonspecific so that an increase in pacing rate occurs with swinging arm movements [29–31]. Coughing and hyperventilation can also increase the pacing rate [30]. Dislodgement of the auxiliary lead may occur with loss of function but a new version of the system now incorporates the sensor within the unipolar lead. Pulse generators with a respiratory rate sensor have been used successfully in Europe for several years, but this device is not yet available in the United States.

Minute Ventilation Volume

This system (Meta MV, Telectronics, Englewood, Colorado, USA) determines the minute ventilation volume (total volume multiplied by respiratory rate) by measuring the transthoracic impedance with the injection of a small current (1 mA for 15 ms every 50 ms) between the pacemaker can and the proximal electrode of a standard bipolar lead. This pulse is less than 10% of the threshold required for ventricular capture. Measurement of the transthoracic impedance is performance between the tip electrode and the pulse generator can every 50 ms. The impedance signal consists of two components: respiratory rate and tidal volume, and the pulse generator then derives the minute ventilation volume. The pulse generator ignores impedance changes related to stroke volume by appropriate rate filtering. Signals used for impedance measurement can be seen on an electrocardiogram and can interfere with transtelephonic pacemaker monitoring [18]. The first minute ventilation volume rate-adaptive pulse generator was implanted in 1987 and so far no problems with sensor reliability have been reported [32–34]. The system is highly physiologic. Programming requires a treadmill stress test. Apart from the upper and lower rates, only one other parameter, the rate-responsive factor or slope requires programming and its value is calculated by the pulse generator, producing a suggested optimal slope based on patient response. The system works well and occasionally the reaction to the onset of exercise may be delayed and the rate may be too fast after the end of exercise. The additional current required for sensor function (to measure variation of thoracic impedance) may reduce the life span of the pulse generator. It appears that the tiny pulses required to measure impedance do not interfere with the function of an implanted cardioverter/defibrillator [35].

Hyperventilation, coughing [30] and tachypnea from a chest infection or congestive heart failure can increase the pacing rate [36]. The device is probably contraindicated in patients with chronic obstructive pulmonary disease. Swinging of the arm on the side of the pulse generator and rotating shoulder movements cause displacement of the pacemaker in its pocket and a rate increase secondary to artifactual changes in impedance. The effect of shoulder movement is more marked on the ipsilateral side [37]. The maximal increase in pacing rate occurs with swinging of the arms at 30 cycles per minute even during breath holding [30, 37]. The response of the minute ventilation volume pacemaker is also attenuated by talking continuously during exercise, but this is clinically irrelevant [30, 36]. Electrocautery changes the impedance between the electrode tip and the pulse generator and can cause an increase in the pacing rate to its upper limit [38]. Artificial respiration may also disturb the operation of the pulse generator. The pacemaker can sense its own impedance measurement pulses with reversion to the asynchronous interference mode (loss of rate-adaptive function) but this form of interference can be prevented by improved design, proper programming, and using only recommended leads to match the device [39]. Cheyne-Stokes respiration can also cause an increase in the pacing rate [40]. During general anesthesia, an increase in ventilation can produce a substantial increase in the pacing rate that may cause hypotension [41]. When the respiratory rate exceeds 60 breaths per minute, the rate-adaptive function is deactivated and a paradoxical fall in the pacing rate occurs. The device should be avoided in patients susceptible to hyperventilation, particularly in children with high respiratory rates.

Temperature

An increase in metabolic rate produces heat that is transported in the blood and can be detected in the right ventricle with a small thermistor (capable of detecting temperature change with an accuracy of 1/100° C) totally incorporated into the pacing lead. Clinical experience with such a system has so far been fairly satisfactory [42].

Temperature-sensing rate-adaptive systems have two basic limitations. First, incorporation of a thermistor into the lead itself complicates construction of a reliable system and problems have occured with signal detection. The special lead consumes additional energy, its long-term stability has not yet been established, and acceptability of the system has been disappointing. Such a pacemaker cannot be used for replacement of a non-rate-adaptive unit. The use of temperature sensing at the atrial level is still under investigation. The temperature response at the atrial level may be affected by inadequate venous mixing [43]. Second, the design must deal with the dip in temperature at the onset of exercise. A small decrease in blood temperature occurs at the onset of exercise as the cooler blood returns from the extremities. This temperature dip can delay the rate response of a temperature-based system up to several minutes. However, several designs compensate for this dip by increasing the pacing rate to an interim level when a dip is detected. A paradoxical effect is found in some patients with congestive heart failure due to a temperature profile characterized by a very gradual and prolonged dip that sometimes cannot be detected by the pacemaker, thereby causing a drop in the paced rate during early exercise. Zegelman et al. [44] have demonstrated a dip in only 57% of their patients, while Fearnot et al. [45] found a dip in 91% of their patients ($> 0.1°$ C) at the beginning of exercise. The initiation of exercise in a subject recovering from previous exercise may not produce a dip in temperature [43]. The absence of a dip removes an important early trigger mechanism for accelerating the rate response [44]. In anticipation of exercise, temperature can increase secondary to physiologic influences [44, 45]. Thus, nervousness before exercise can increase the pacing rate and, when exercise is then performed, the faster starting pacing rate prevents a dip response because the algorithm provides no dip response beyond a certain pacing rate [44, 45].

Temperature accurately reflects 0_2 consumption in the middle or late stage of exercise. Central venous temperature is an excellent correlate of metabolic demand at high work loads, but it rises slowly at low work loads. Temperature changes during mild exercise (such as walking) are often very small, usually not exceeding those at rest. Thus, pacemaker rate response may be too slow (latency) and inadequate at low levels of exercise with brief everyday activities [1]. A delayed response causes an increase in rate when activity has already ended [1]. A short exercise time may produce a dip, but no temperature above the baseline to the end of the exercise, especially in patients with congestive heart failure [45]. Increase in heat dissipation during exercise (e.g., swimming) may blunt the rate response [43]. Heat dissipation mechanisms after the end of exercise are often impaired in patients with heart failure. A slow rise in central venous body temperature as a result of fever, emotion, or environmental factors (e.g., high external temperature) generally will not cause a large rate increase because the rate of temperature change is slower than that due to exercise. If they do, the pulse generator will eventually return to the lower rate setting, disregarding the increased temperature. Some algorithms will purposely increase the pacing rate by approximately 12 ppm/° C in an effort to mimic the normal mammalian heart rate response to fever. Likewise, normal hot baths and hot or cold drinks have little effect on temperature-based systems. However, prolonged full-body immersion in a hot tub ($> 38°$ C) coud cause a more rapid increase in body temperature and result in an exercise-type rate increase. Hot tubs $\geq 38°$ C are therefore contraindicated in patients with temperature-responsive pacemakers. Finally, a pulse generator must compensate for circadian temperature fluctuations that may be considerably larger than the changes induced by exercise.

Improvement in Activity Rate-Adaptive Pacing

Numerous studies have demonstrated the significant clinical limitations of can-bonded piezoelectric sensor-based pacemakers: excessively rapid increases in the pacing rate at the onset of exercise, unnecessary rate increase at rest, susceptibility to external sources of vibration and localized pressure on the pacemaker can, and a lack of proportionality to different types and levels of exertion. For this reason, a number of pacemaker manufacturers have incorporated an accelerometer as the activity sensor in rate-responsive pacemakers.

Can-bonded piezoelectric sensors must maintain direct contact with body tissue in order to sense the vibrations or pressure waves produced during physical activity. These pressure waves emanate most frequently from contact of the patient's feet on a hard surface (as in walking or running) and are transmitted throughout the musculoskeletal system. Pressure waves cause microdeflections in the pulse generator can (in a fashion analogous to a stethoscope head), resulting in physical deflection of the can-bonded piezoelectric crystal. Deflections of the crystal, in turn, produce small electrical signals of a frequency, in part influenced by the size of the can (the smaller the can size, the higher the resultant frequency from can deflections) [46], the density of the tissue or fluid surrounding the pacemaker and the intensity of the exercise. Motion in any direction can cause pressure waves that deflect the can so that sensing with can-bonded piezoelectric systems is omnidirectional, i.e., anything that causes deformity or vibration of the can produces an output from the crystal. Various methods in signal processing of the piezoelectric crystal are used to calculate the pacing rate: number of signal crossings above a programmable threshold, area under the output waveform, and combinations of these methods.

To overcome some of the above limitations, some manufacturers have replaced the can-bonded piezoelectric sensor with an accelerometer which itself contains a piezoelectric crystal (Figs. 2, 3). When used as an accelerometer, the piezoelectric crystal may be mounted in a manner that eliminates the effects peculiar to can-mounted sensors, i.e., pressure on the can will not cause a rate response. The accelerometer responds to changes in motion of the pulse generator (not deflections of the can) and is therefore less dependent upon vibration. Acceleration forces due to body motion are strongest in the anterior-posterior and superior-inferior plane and weakest in the lateral plane [47]. Mounting of the accelerometer on the circuit board cannot guarantee that the pacemaker would be oriented in such a way that inferior-superior motion could be detected reliably. Since the pacemaker is, in effect, a flat

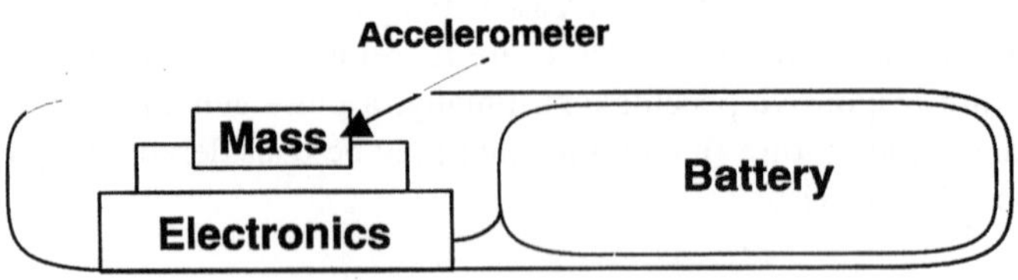

Fig. 2. Accelerometer technology (CPI). Pacemaker cross-section showing location of accelerometer mounted on the electronic circuitry. The accelerometer monitors body motion rather than vibration. (Courtesy of Cardiac Pacemakers, Inc.)

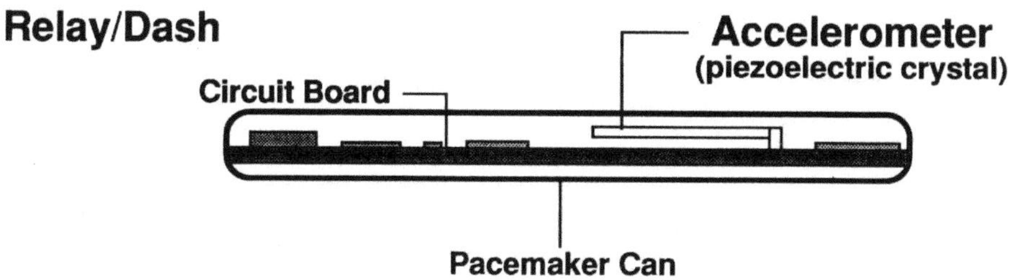

Fig. 3. Accelerometer technology (Intermedics). Pacemaker cross-section showing location of accelerometer mounted on the electronic circuitry. (Courtesy of Intermedics)

object that can be rotated around its radius, the only stable plane of motion is from logo to non-logo side or anterior-posterior because the pacemaker is most commonly implanted parallel to the chest wall (Fig. 4). The sensor mechanism is principally unidirectional because it detects anterior-posterior acceleration forces. As in the can-bonded piezoelectric sensor, signal processing of the accelerometer output can involve frequence and amplitude to determine acceleration and therefore the pacing rate (Fig. 5). Attempts at processing the acceleration signal have produced a better correspondence with normal sinus rhythm [48–50]. Frequencies between 0.5 and 3 Hz are most typical of body motion, and the accelerometer is designed to be most sensitive in this region. In contrast, can-bonded piezoelectric sensors are typically

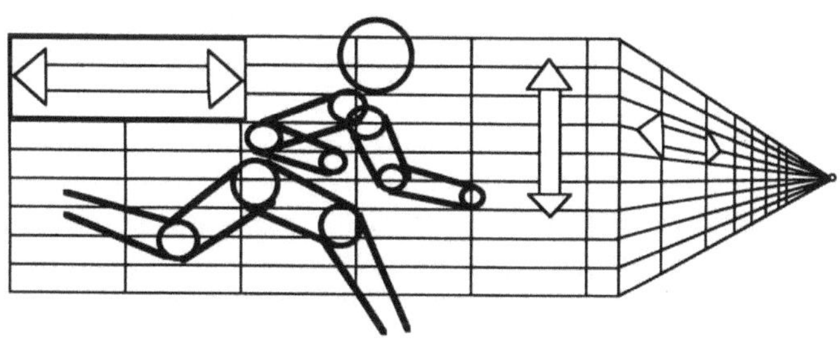

Fig. 4. Direction of acceleration detected by implanted accelerometer-driven devices manufactured by Intermedics. The accelerometer senses acceleration predominantly in the anterior/posterior plane. See text for details. (Courtesy of Intermedics, Inc.)

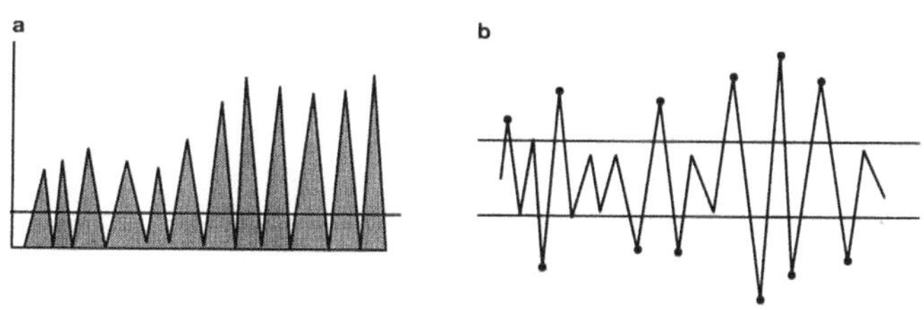

Fig. 5 a, b. Signal processing of accelerometer system **a** and simpler piezoelectric system **b**. Signal processing of the accelerometer signal averages the amplitude of the signal to measure energy content. Signal processing of the piezoelectric crystal counts only the number of times the signal crosses a particular threshold. (Courtesy of Cardiac Pacemakers, Inc.)

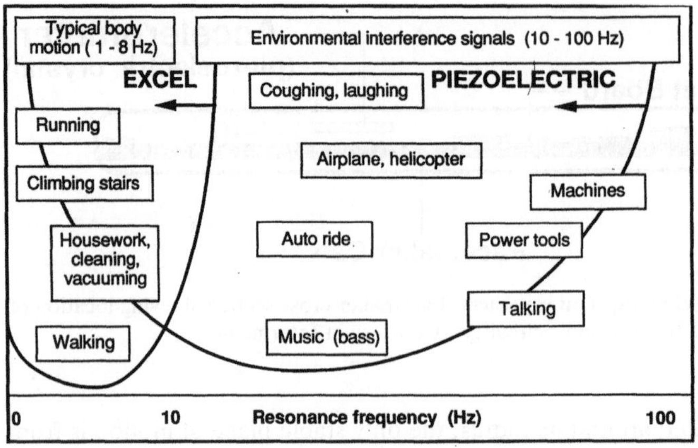

Fig. 6. The band pass filter of the CPI EXCEL Accelerometer rate-adaptive pacemaker on the *left* detects mechanical resonance at frequencies in the 1-8 Hz range associated with typical body motion. While it detects some of the frequencies below 8 Hz, the band pass filter of a typical piezoelectric crystal on the *right* also detects signals in the 10–100-Hz range, not associated with typical body motion. (Courtesy of Cardiac Pacemakers, Inc.)

most sensitive to frequencies in the 5–7 Hz range, beyond the frequencies normally associated with human motion and therefore more likely to mistakenly interpret environmental vibration as body motion (Fig. 6). Patient constitutional factors such as body size, body fat, weight, etc., should have little effect on accelerometer signal so that the sensor settings are less likely to require further adjustment after implantation. In addition, unlike the can-bonded piezoelectric crystals, the nature of the walking surface should have little effect on accelerometer performance since its response does not depend on vibrations created by the impact of the patient's feet on the floor. An accelerometer seems to provide a high discrimination to various work loads, i.e., walking up stairs compared to down stairs, and lower susceptibility to environmental noise [51].

With regard to the Intermedics Dash VVIR and Relay DDDR pulse generators (Intermedics, Freeport, Texas, USA), the accelerometer consists of a piezoelectric crystal in the form of a cantilever (diving board) bonded at one end to its ceramic encasement. The cantilever is free to move at one end (Fig. 2). Thus acceleration forces perpendicular to the lever in the anterior-posterior plane cause displacement of the crystal selectively in response to unidirectional forces. The integrated circuit accelerometer used by CPI (CPI, St. Paul, Minnesota, USA) consists of layers of silicon wafers bonded together to form a sandwich (Fig. 7). The center layer forms the mass suspended by silicon bridges within the cavity in the sandwich. The silicon bridges suspending the mass act as springs. As the mass moves up and down in response to body motions, resistors on each bridge are compressed or expanded producing a sensor signal related to changes in electrical resistance. When there is no acceleration, the mass moves back to its resting position.

Lau et al. [52] compared the sinus rate response on exercise with the response of an activity VVIR pacemaker fitted externally on the chest and with signals measured by an accelerometer in three axes (at 90° to each other, horizontal, vertical, and lateral axes). The correlation between the pacing rate and sinus rate was only fair ($r = 0.51$).

The total root mean square value of acceleration in either the anteroposterior or the vertical axis was found to have a better correlation with sinus rate ($r = 0.8$). Most of the spectral activity during walking or running was found to be between 0.1 and 4 Hz [47, 52] in contrast to the Activitrax that has a broad frequency response with a maximal sensitivity between 10 and 100 Hz [52]. This broad frequency makes the Activitrax unnecessarily susceptible to external vibration. Using a low-pass filter at 4 Hz detracts little from measured acceleration amplitude [52].

Alt et al. [47] also mounted an accelerometer at 90° angles to each other, as did Lau et al. [52]. They documented the frequency of the highest amplitude during walking and found it to be between 1 and 4 Hz. Using a low-pass filter, non-exercise, induced signals can be reduced with enhancement of signal detection of lower amplitude signals such as seen with bicycling [47]. Alt et al. [47] concluded that an accelerometer on the horizontal axis appears to be the best compromise for the various types of exercise.

Matula et al. [51] evaluated nine patients with implanted activity-controlled pacemakers (five Sensolog and four Activitrax) and compared their response with that of the new Intermedics Relay DDDR pacemaker attached to the right upper pectoral region as an external device. The accelerometer-controlled Relay pulse generator showed improved performance with high discrimination to various work loads, walking up and down stairs, and lower susceptibility to environmental noise.

Millerhagen et al. [53] conducted treadmill exercise studies with a CPI Excel VVIR pacemaker (accelerometer based) strapped to the pectoral region of moderately active subjects. The system detects acceleration signals in the anteroposterior axis.

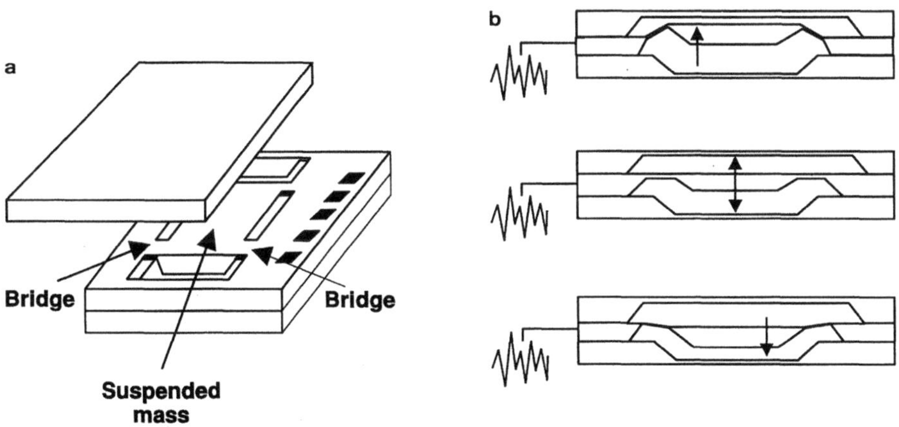

Fig. 7 a, b. Arrangement of silicon accelerometer used in activity rate-adaptive devices manufactured by CPI. **a** Cross-section of the accelerometer. The *arrows* indicate bridges on the silicon structure. **b** As the mass in the center moves upward or downward (*arrows*), the resistivity of the bridges changes. If a constant current is applied to the sensor, the corresponding voltage reflects the change in voltage following acceleration and deceleration of the center mass. (**a** Courtesy of Cardiac Pacemakers, Inc.)

The correlation of accelerometer response to the estimated VO_2 was 0.85, and the correlation between the heart rate provided by the pacemaker and the intrinsic rate was 0.75, far better than what can be expected from can-bonded piezoelectric sensors [54]. Preliminary experience with the implanted CPI Excel pacemaker has demonstrated good discrimination between slow and fast body movements [55].

The performance of motion sensors will continue to improve as signal-processing techniques are modified to eliminate many of the unwanted effects of a nonmetabolic sensor, such as false responses due to environmental vibration and mechanical noise. Preliminary results with accelerometer systems have shown strong correlation between the pacing heart rate and intrinsic heart rate, indicating that an accelerometer-based pacing system will provide adaptive rate response specific to incremental exercise on the treadmill not seen with can-bonded piezoelectric crystals. The target frequency of the motion sensor systems that causes the maximal pacing rate has gradually decreased. While the Medtronic Activitrax had its greatest sensitivity to frequencies around 7 Hz, and the Pacesetter Sensalog system around the 4-5 Hz range, the Intermedics Relay and Dash systems are looking in the 2-3 Hz range. The lower frequency range is more typical of human motion.

Inappropriate Programming and Sensor Idiosyncrasy

Inappropriate programming may cause excessive and rapid increase in the pacing rate with activity leading to unpleasant palpitations and other untoward effects. Overprogramming of rate response is generally not acceptable to patients who often request a change in programming [56] in contrast to underprogramming. As already discussed, rate-adaptive pacemakers are subject to idiosyncrasies related to the type of sensor [18]. For example, in minute ventilation driven pacemakers, hyperventilation with general anesthesia may cause pacemaker tachycardia and hypotension that may be misinterpreted as inadequate anesthesia. Consequently during anesthesia these pulse generators should be programmed to the VVI mode or the magnet applied in the VVIR mode to disarm the sensor and prevent inappropriate increases in the pacing rate.

Sensor Feedback Tachycardia

Occasionally an activity unipolar pacing flips over in the pacemaker pocket and causes local muscle stimulation which in turn increases the pacing rate, thereby creating a self-perpetuating mechanism or sensor-mediated tachycardia (positive feedback loop). Lau [57] has called this phenomenon sensor feedback tachycardia. A rate-adaptive pacemaker implanted in the left retromammary position with possible displacement over the apex of the heart carries the risk of an inappropriate rate response by mechanical stimulation of the heart itself [20]. Similarly, diaphragmatic pacing by a ventricular lead can cause an increase in temperature which in turn increases the heart rate in a self-perpetuating mechanism [58]. With QT rate-adaptive pacemakers, QT shortening with exercise increases the pacing rate and the increase in pacing rate in turn shortens the QT interval [42, 59], but this potential problem has been corrected by appropriate software dealing with the QT/rate relationship.

Problems Related to Underlying Pathology

Inappropriate upper rate programming may precipitate angina in patients with coronary artery disease [18]. Some patients with cardiomyopathie or congestive heart failure may not tolerate high VVIR pacing rates and may develop worsening heart failure, hypotension, and syncope [60]. Excessive adrenergic tone may cause a QT pacemaker to pace at the upper rate limit in the setting of acute myocardial infarction, creating an undesirable response [61, 62].

Induction of Ventricular Tachycardia

The induction of sustained or unsustained ventricular tachycardia by an increase in the ventricular pacing rate is probably an infrequent but important complication of rate-adaptive pacing and should be considered in patients with palpitations or unexplained dizziness, particularly in those with a history of previous ventricular tachycardia [18, 63]. Interestingly, DDDR and DDD pacemakers can actually be used to prevent ventricular tachycardia (possible working best with a relatively short AV interval) with the DDDR mode probably more useful than the DDD mode for exercise-induced ventricular tachycardia [64–67].

Rate-Dependent Overdrive Suppression

Schmidinger et al. [68, 69] emphasized that rate-dependent depression of subsidiary ventricular impulse formation can occur with sudden cessation of ventricular pacing. Thus, sudden inhibition of pulse generator during fast ventricular stimulation may produce a longer period of asystole compared to similar circumstances during relatively slow pacing. The full extent of overdrive suppression and impulse inhibition may not occur if tested after a long duration of pacing at lower rates or after a short period of pacing at faster rates. For this reason, Schmidinger et al. recommended that pacemaker testing should be performed for at least 60 s at each pacing level (followed by abrupt cessation of pacing) to determine the risk of overdrive suppression at a particular level of sensor activity or pacing rate [69].

Response of Rate-Adaptive Pulse Generators to Interference

Endogenous Sources

As a rule, the consequences of myopotential oversensing in unipolar rate-adaptive pacemakers is similar to that seen with non-rate-adaptive devices. Myopotential oversensing may cause inhibition with long pauses and/or reversion to the asynchronous interference mode at a predetermined rate or at the programmed lower rate [34, 70, 71]. The sudden occurrence of myopotential oversensing during exercise can be more dramatic during rapid ventricular pacing in patients with rate-adaptive devices compared to patients with non-rate-adaptive devices. The sudden slowing of the paced rate on exercise in patients with rate-adaptive devices caused by inhibition (with possibly a greater degree of overdrive suppression) or conversion to the slower interference mode can produce serious hemodynamic consequences.

Exogenous Sources

Many sources of interference have been described with standard non-rate-adaptive pulse generators [72]. As yet, relatively little literature exists concerning interference specifically related to sensor function in the rate-adaptive mode.

Lithotripsy rarely affects the sensor function rate-responsive pacemakers. Pulse generators with piezoelectric crystals may be affected if the pulse generator is implanted near the extracorporeal shockwave lithotripsy field (ESWL). Mechanical energy from the lithotripter shock propagates through the tissue, fluid, and bones in the form of pressure waves picked up by the piezoelectric crystal which may increase its rate. The closer the sensor is to the focal point, the more intense the rate response [73, 74]. Therefore, it is recommended that the pacemaker be programmed to the VVI non-activity mode during the procedure and the pacemaker distance from the focal point should be greater than 15 cm. Patients with VVIR pulse generators implanted in the abdomen should probably not undergo ESWL because the procedure may shatter the crystal in the proximity of the focal point [73].

Magnetic resonance imaging (MRI) is contraindicated in patients with implanted pacemakers [72]. However, if MRI is deemed absolutely necessary, the sensor function of the pacemaker should be programmed off before the procedure in the hope of diminishing some of the serious effects of MRI.

Some single- and dual chamber rate-adaptive pulse generators can be reset to a single-chamber non-rate-adaptive mode when exposed to high-level interference such as electrocautery and defibrillation, a response (not malfunction) similiar to the reset behavior of DDD pulse generators to the VVI or VOO mode under the same circumstances [72]. Restoration of the original pacing mode requires reprogramming. Electrocautery can also increase the pacing rate of a minute ventilation sensor-driven pulse generator to its upper rate, presumably by producing spurious signals interpreted by the device as originating from the sensor mechanism [38].

Adverse Hemodynamic Consequences of Rate-Adaptive Pacing

The adverse hemodynamic consequences of single-lead ventricular pacing were first recognized over 20 years ago and called the pacemaker syndrome [75], an entity recently redefined by Schüller and Brandt [76] as follows: "The pacemaker syndrome refers to symptoms an signs present in the pacemaker patient which are caused by inadequate timing of atrial and ventricular contractions." The new definition encompasses the adverse hemodynamic consequences of (a) single-lead ventricular pacing, by far the most common cause of pacemaker syndrome; and (b) other modes of pacing such as single-chamber atrial or dual-chamber modes including sensor-driven (non-P wave) devices because of inappropriate programming or selection of pacing mode.

VVIR-Induced Pacemaker Syndrome

Implantation of a VVIR pacemaker does not protect the patient against the development of the pacemaker syndrome at rest and/or during exercise [77–79]. The behavior of retrograde ventriculoatrial (VA) conduction on exercise has not been studied in detail and it appears that it cannot be predicted individually [80]. Indeed, the pacemaker syndrome may occur on exercise during VVIR pacing in the following circumstances:

1. VA conduction during continuous pacing at rest may persist on exercise [81, 82].
2. Development of atrial chronotropic incompetence after a given level of exercise with the spontaneous sinus rhythm giving way to ventricular pacing and therefore retrograde VA conduction only on exercise and not at rest during normal sinus rhythm.
3. Because VA conduction is dynamic, exercise may occasionally induce retrograde VA conduction when it is absent at rest [80]. Improved and restored VA conduction on exercise under the influence of catecholamines and other factors may cause an exercise-induced VVIR pacemaker syndrome.
4. DDDR pulse generators capable of automatic conversion to the VVIR mode when the atrial rate exceeds the programmed upper rate may precipitate pacemaker syndrome on exercise [83] (Fig. 8). Alternatively, a pacemaker syndrome at rest may actually disappear on exercise if an increase in the ventricular pacing rate blocks VA conduction [84, 85].

Delayed Left Atrial Systole

A DDD pacemaker senses and paces on the right side of the heart. Yet the timing relationships of atrial and ventricular mechanical activity on the left side of the heart determine hemodynamic performance. In the presence of severe atrial disease, increased latency (delay from the onset of pacemaker stimulus to the beginning of an

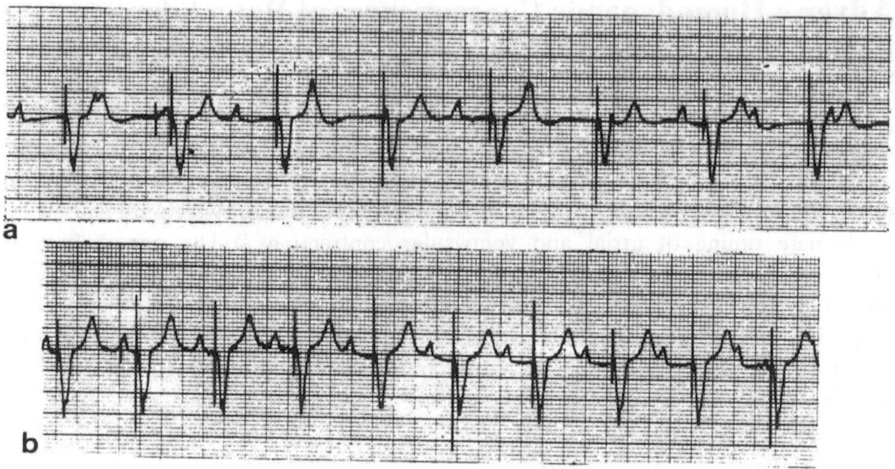

Fig. 8 a, b. Electrocardiogram of a patient who developed the pacemaker syndrome with the DDIR pacing mode. A dual-chamber pulse generator was implanted after His bundle ablation for intractable paroxysmal atrial fibrilation. **a** The DDIR mode at rest functions at the programmed lower rate of 60 bpm, slower than the prevailing sinus rate. Note that sinus P waves march through the cardiac cycle, producing AV dissociation. The P wave following the first ventricular paced beat falls in the 300 ms post-ventricular atrial refractory period and is unsensed, thereby allowing the release of an atrial stimulus at the end of the atrial escape interval initiated by the first ventricular paced complex. **b** On exercise, when the sinus rate is slightly faster than the sensor-driven rate, sinus P waves march through the cardiac cycle, again producing AV dissociation. The pulse generator does not sense the P wave following the first ventricular paced beat because the P wave falls in the post-ventricular atrial refractory period. Therefore the pulse generator release an atrial stimulus at the termination of the sensor-driven atrial escape interval initiated by the first ventricular paced beat

identifiable atrial depolarization) and delayed interatrial conduction can cause delayed left atrial activation following right atrial pacing. In this situation the programmed AV interval may not provide adequate time for effective left atrial systole before left ventricular systole and in extreme cases left atrial systole may actually begin after the onset of left ventricular systole, producing a pacemaker syndrome during apparently normal DDD function [86–88]. A DDDR pacemaker can be programmed to shorten the AV interval (atrial paced-ventricular paced) on exercise automatically according to sensor input. However, when exercise produces little or no associated improvement in latency or interatrial conduction an adequate AV interval (atrial paced– ventricular paced) at rest may paradoxically become inappropriate on exercise and create an exercise-induced pacemaker syndrome if left atrial systole then begins after the onset of left ventricular systole.

DDI and DDIR Modes

The DDI and DDIR modes are useful in some patients with paroxysmal supraventricular tachyarrhythmias, but may cause the pacemaker syndrome if not used or programmed appropriately [89]. The DDI mode provides fixed-frequency ventricular pacing while atrial sensing avoids atrial competition [90, 91]. In the DDI mode a pacemaker cannot follow or track atrial activity faster than the programmed fixed-frequency ventricular pacing rate, i.e., 1:1 AV synchrony at the programmed AV interval cannot occur when the atrial rate is faster than the programmed ventricular pacing rate. In the DDIR mode, the pacemaker increases its rate only in response to sensor input. During episodes of atrial tachyarrhythmias, a DDI (DDIR) system simply paces at the programmed fixed-frequency ventricular rate (or at the sensor-driven rate during DDIR pacing) [92].

In the DDI mode, when the post-ventricular atrial refractory period (PVARP) is relatively short and the spontaneous sinus rate is faster than the programmed lower rate, nonconducted sinus P waves can march through the pacing cycle producing long AV intervals and therefore physiology identical to AV dissociation except when the P wave falls within the PVARP, whereupon the succeeding atrial event will be an atrial paced beat provided the sinus (or atrial) rate is not excessively fast. In the DDI mode, long periods of AV dissociation mimic VVI pacing (release of atrial stimuli are inhibited by the sensed P waves) and may not be tolerated by some patients, i.e., pacemaker syndrome. An identical arrangement may occur in the DDIR mode on exercise when the sinus rate exceeds the sensor-driven ventricular pacing rate, a situation that may precipitate the pacemaker syndrome on exercise (Fig. 8).

Patients with atrioventricular block (either spontaneous or secondary to ablation of AV junction) and intractable paroxysmal supraventricular tachyarrhythmias may receive DDD or DDDR pacemakers programmed to the DDI or DDIR mode to prevent tracking of atrial tachyarrhythmias. Almost continual AV dissociation related to the DDI or DDIR mode with intolerance of pacing can be prevented by implanting a DDD or DDDR pacemaker capable of automatic switching of the pacing mode and/or reduction of the pacing rate upon the detection of a pathologic supraventricular tachycardia. Such a response can be gradual or abrupt with the fallback mechanism to a lower pacing rate with or without a change in the pacing mode [93–95]. In all cases, reversion to the original DDD or DDDR mode of pacing subsequently occurs when the atrial rate drops below the programmed upper rate. In the occasional patient, when a dual-chamber pacemaker (DDD or DDDR) interprets sinus tachycardia on exercise as a pathologic supraventricular tachyarrhythmia, automatic conversion to the VVI or VVIR mode can produce an exercise-induced pacemaker syndrome with severe dyspnea or hypotension, an untoward response often preventable by appropriate programming of the upper rate [93].

Repetitive Non-Reentrant VA Synchrony

In repetitive non-reentrant VA synchrony during DDD pacing, VA synchrony may occur without endless-loop tachycardia (pacemaker-mediated tachycardia) when a

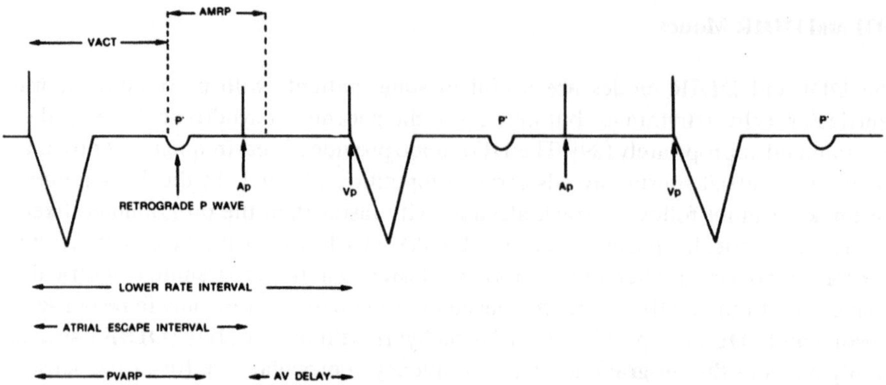

Fig. 9. AV desynchronization arrhythmia (repetitive non-reentrant ventriculoatrial synchrony). There is relatively slow retrograde VA conduction. The retrograde P wave (*P'*) is unsensed because it falls within the post-ventricular atrial refractory period (*PVARP*). At the completion of the atrial escape interval, the pacemaker delivers an atrial stimulus (*Ap*) falling too closely to the preceding retrograde P wave and therefore still within the atrial myocardial refractory period (*AMRP*) engendered by the preceding retrograde atrial depolarization. Ap is therefore ineffectual. Barring any perturbations, this process becomes self-perpetuating, causing repetitive non-reentrant VA synchrony and can lead to the pacemaker syndrome. *VACT*, retrograde VA conduction time; *Vp*, ventricular stimulus. (From [97])

paced ventricular beat engenders an *unsensed* retrograde P wave falling within the PVARP of the pacemaker. Under certain circumstances the process can be self-perpetuating if the pacemaker continually delivers an *ineffectual* atrial stimulus during the atrial *myocardial* refractory period generated by the preceding retrograde atrial depolarization (Fig. 9). This form of VA synchrony has been called "AV desynchronization arrhythmia" (AVDA), repetitive non-reentrant VA synchrony, or non-reentrant VA synchrony arrhythmia [96, 97]. A long AV interval and relatively fast lower rate (or sensor-driven rate with DDDR pacing) favors the development of AVDA. When sustained, AVDA may cause unfavorable hemodynamics similar to the pacemaker syndrome [98]. AVDA should not be an important problem with conventional DDD pacemakers because the duration of the atrial escape and AV interval can be easily controlled. However, DDDR pulse generators may induce AVDA on exercise because the sensor-driven pacing rate increases with resultant abbreviation of the atrial escape interval. Conceivably with DDDR pacing, on exercise a ventricular extrasystole could precipitate AVDA, thereby negating the benefit of AV synchrony and producing a VVIR-like pacemaker syndrome.

Single-Chamber Rate-Adaptive Atrial Pacing

In atrial pacing, a marked delay between the atrial pacemaker stimulus and the onset of ventricular systole may produce atrial systole against closed AV valves and a hemodynamic situation identical to retrograde VA conduction. This form of pacemaker syndrome is unlikely to occur with the pacing rates ordinarily used in the AAI mode. However, VA synchrony may occur in the AAIR mode when the atrial pacing rate is increased. When patients are carefully selected for AAI pacing, the PR interval should shorten (or infrequently remain constant) during exercise [99, 100] as the heart rate increases in contrast to atrial pacing at rest which causes AV conduction delay at faster rates. A fast sensor response in the AAIR mode with an increase in the atrial rate disproportionate to the degree of exercise can lengthen the PR interval before the expected catecholamine surge induces shortening or improvement of AV conduction. The AAIR mode therefore poses the risk of "overstimulation" with rates above exercise requirement that may lead to undesirable paradoxical prolongation of the PR interval. This response usually occurs in patients taking drugs that depress AV conduction [99]. The long PR interval places the atrial paced beat too close to the previous QRS complex, resulting in an exercise-induced pacemaker syndrome with atrial contraction against closed AV valve [101–105].

Consequences of Sensing in the Pacemaker Refractory Period

In the Medtronic Activitrax II [106] and Legend [107] single chamber VVIR (AAIR) pacemakers, the first 125 ms of the ventricular refractory period (or atrial refractory period in the AAIR mode) constitutes the blanking period during which the pulse generator is insensitive to all incoming signals. Sensing may occur during the second part of the refractory period, called the noise sampling period. The consequences of a

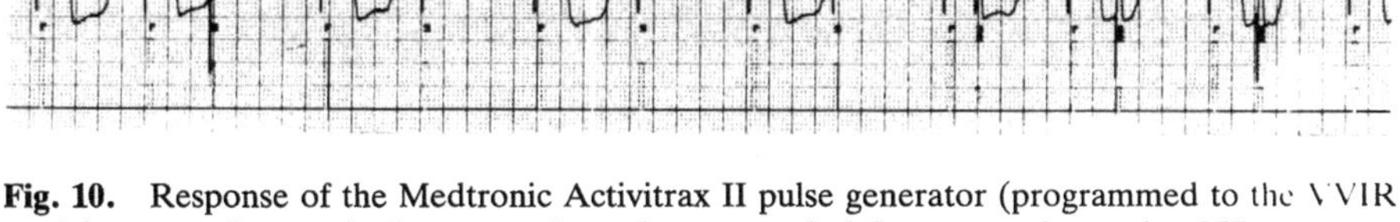

Fig. 10. Response of the Medtronic Activitrax II pulse generator (programmed to the VVIR mode) to sensed events in the pacemaker refractory period. Lower rate interval = 857 ms, upper rate interval = 400 ms, ventricular refractory period = 220 ms. The electrocardiogram was recorded simultaneously with the marker channel at a paper speed of 50 mm/s. The *markers* identify the pacemaker stimulus as *P*, a sensed event as *S*, and a sensed event in the refractory (noise sampling) period as *SR*. Chest wall stimuli (*solid black circles*) were delivered at random at a variable rate. The pacemaker senses chest wall stimuli *1*, *2*, *3*, and *4* well beyond the refractory period and the sensed events initiate a complete sensor-driven escape interval. In contrast, the pacemaker senses chest wall stimuli *5*, *6*, and *7* in the refractory (noise sampling) period, and these refractory sensed events initiate an upper rate interval of 400 ms. The pacemaker then delivers a ventricular stimulus at the completion of the upper rate interval. The interval between the first and second pacemaker stimuli represents the sensor-driven lower rate interval at that particular time

refractory sensed event in the VVIR or AAIR mode (such as ventricular extrasystole, polarization voltage, or farfield R wave) are as follows: (a) no effect on the lower rate timer, i.e., a refractory sensed event does *not* start a new lower rate interval; (b) reinitiation of an entire refractory period (blanking and noise sampling periods); (c) initiation of a new upper rate interval in the activity mode (Fig. 10). The upper rate response was designed to avoid too early a release of a sensor-driven pacing output after a refractory sensed event, a concern during VVIR but not AAIR pacing. In the VVIR mode, a short sensor-driven interval could conceivably allow the release of a ventricular stimulus into the vulnerable period of preceding ventricular extrasystole registered by the pacemaker as a refractory sensed event. Resetting of the upper rate timer by a refractory sensed event guarantees postponement of the subsequent ventricular stimulus beyond the vulnerable period of the refractory sensed beat and avoids the (theoretical) risk of a life-threating repetitive ventricular response. This response is not important in the AAIR mode because delivery of an atrial stimulus into the atrial vulnerable period is unlikely to cause life-threating atrial arrhythmias.

In the Medtronic Activitrax II and Legend pacemakers, when a refractory sensed event (RVs) follows a ventricular stimulus (Vp1), the subsequent ventricular stimulus (Vp2) will occur at the end of one of the following intervals, whichever is shorter: (a) the reinitiated upper rate interval, i.e., (Vp1-Vp2) interval = (Vp1 - RVs) interval + upper rate interval; or (b) the sensor-driven interval initiated by Vp1. In this way the pacemaker never violates its sensor-driven lower rate interval.

In the case of the Medtronic Activitrax II or Legend single-chamber pulse generator programmed with an upper rate to 150 per minute, when sensor activity dictates a pacing rate equal to the upper rate, i.e., sensor-driven interval = upper rate interval (URI) = 400 ms, the repetitive occurrence of a refractory sensed event immediately after the termination of the blanking period (125 ms from the onset of the refractory period) will cause delivery of the stimulus 400 + 125 = 525 ms beyond the preceding stimulus, effectively slowing the maximal rate from 150 to 115 ppm.

The Medtronic Activitrax I rate-adaptive single-chamber pacemaker reacts differently to a refractory sensed event in the VVIR or AAIR mode, with pro-

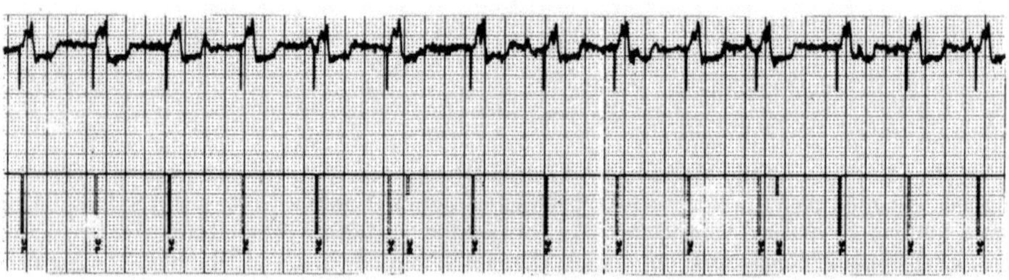

Fig. 11. Afterpotential oversensing by Medtronic Activitrax I pacemaker programmed to the VVIR mode. Lower rate interval = 857 ms, upper rate interval = 480 ms. The sensor-driven interval varies slightly between 720 and 760 ms. The pulse generator was programmed to the maximal output voltage and pulse width, and highest sensitivity. The pacemaker senses the afterpotential in the noise sampling period just beyond the absolute refractory period. The refractory sensed signal (*VR*) prolongs the interval between two consecutive ventricular stimuli (*VP*) by 80 ms, a response characteristic of this particular pulse generator (partial recycling)

longation of the spike-to-spike interval (sensor-driven interval) by 80 ms regardless of the timing of the signal within the noise sampling period (Fig. 11). Thus, repetitive refractory sensed events lengthen the effective URI by 80 ms [108] . A programmed upper rate of 150 ppm yields an effective maximal rate of 125 per minute. As in the Activitrax II and Legend devices, a refractory sensed event by the Activitrax I pulse generator does not initiate a new sensor-driven lower rate interval.

Farfield Atrial Sensing

Farfield sensing of the QRS complex in the atrial electrogram is rare with bipolar systems (unless the lead is in the proximal coronary sinus for atrial pacing), but occurs in about 35% of patients with unipolar atrial leads in conjunction with AAI, AAIR, AAT, and dual-chamber pacemakers programmed to a high atrial sensitivity [109, 110]. In the majority of these cases, farfield sensing can be eliminated by selecting a lower atrial sensitivity that preserves P wave sensing but rejects the farfield QRS complexes. In the remaining cases, prolongation of the absolute atrial refractory period (about 400 ms from an atrial paced event) effectively contains farfield ventricular activity.

The effect of a farfield refractory sensed event on the attainment of the upper rate of Medtronic single-chamber activity-responsive pacemakers is more marked during AAIR than VVIR pacing [108, 111, 112]. Reprogramming atrial sensitivity may allow differential sensing of P and farfield QRS complexes, but when this is not feasible the URI of an AAIR pulse generator decreases by a value equal to the programmed upper rate plus the AV interval (period) from atrial stimulus to the point of farfield sensing). When URI = 400 ms, farfield sensing 250 ms from the atrial stimulus effectively lengthens the URI to 400 + 250 = 650 ms, corresponding to a decrease of the upper rate from 150 to 90 per minute. Therefore, the maximal effective rate varies inversely with the AV delay, i.e., the longer the interval from the atrial stimulus to the conducted QRS complex, the lower the maximal attainable atrial pacing rate.

The Telectronics Meta DDDR pulse generator (Englewood, Colorado, USA) responds in a unique way to farfield atrial sensing during PVARP [113]. The Meta DDDR pulse generator has a common URI (sensor-driven URI = atrial-driven URI). The PVARP shortens with increasing sensor activity on exercise. When a P wave falls in the adapted PVARP, the next atrial stimulus is omitted and any P wave occurring before the next ventricular output will not start an AV delay. The pulse generator is then temporarily operating in the VVIR mode. Thus, in the presence of pathologic atrial tachycardia the pulse generator will continue to function in the VVIR mode as long as the P-P interval is shorter than the adapted total atrial refractory period until slowing of the atrial rate no longer produces P waves within the adapted PVARP, whereupon AV synchrony is restored. Thus, in the unipolar DDDR mode, an atrial refractory sensed event related to the farfield QRS complex will convert the pulse generator to the VVIR mode (Fig. 12).

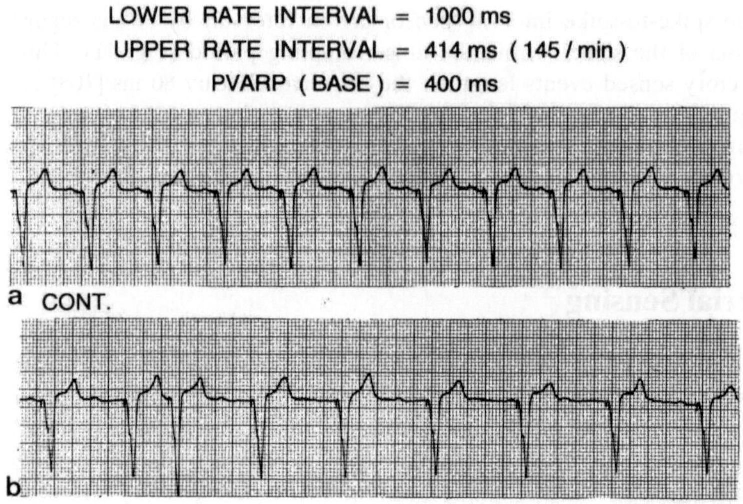

Fig. 12 a, b. Electrocardiogram showing response of Telectronics Meta DDDR pulse generator to farfield sensing. **a** Atrial sensitivity = 1 mV. All the sinus P waves are sensed and followed by a ventricular stimulus. **b** Atrial sensitivity was increased to 0.5 mV, whereupon the atrial channel senses the farfield terminal portion of the QRS complex. The farfield signal occurs in the terminal portion of the post-ventricular atrial refractory period (*PVARP*) and therefore inhibits delivery of the subsequent atrial stimulus, forcing the pulse generator to function in the VVIR mode. In this case there was no sensor activity, and the pulse generator therefore paced at 60 per minute

Oversensing of Polarization Voltage and Crosstalk

During standard VVI pacing, a larger output (voltage and pulse width) and/or high sensitivity increases susceptibility of afterpotential oversensing [114]. When the ventricular pacing rate increases, the polarization voltage at the myocardial–electrode interface (afterpotential) can grow substantially because the shorter pacing cycles provide less time for its dissipation between pacemaker stimuli [115]. Indeed, during VVIR pacing, oversensing of the afterpotential is not uncommon at fast pacing rates with the pulse generator programmed to high output and high sensitivity, particularly in the presence of a short pacemaker absolute refractory period that allows detection of a signal relatively close to the preceding stimulus. Despite the incorporation of a fast recharge pulse after the stimulus to decrease the afterpotential, it should not be surprising that Medtronic single-chamber rate-adaptive pulse generators with a short absolute refractory period (125 ms) can exhibit afterpotential oversensing (in the noise sampling period) during exercise when programmed to respond with a high output and sensitivity [116, 117] (Fig. 11). In this situation, the pulse generator responds in a variety of ways (as already discussed) because it processes the afterpotential signal as a refractory sensed event detected in the noise sampling period (second portion of the pacemaker refractory period). Most cases of afterpotential sensing can be eliminated by appropriate programming.

In a dual-chamber pacemaker (except for VDD and VAT modes), the atrial stimulus generates a small ventricular signal that must be superimposed on any residual afterpotential at the ventricular electrode-myocardial interface. Although a pulse generator may not be able to sense an enhanced afterpotential or the atrial stimulus individually, a relatively large ventricular afterpotential (associated with a fast pacing rate) can set the stage for crosstalk (even in bipolar systems) if the ventricular channel actually sees a large summation signal consisting of the afterpotential and a superimposed, relatively small signal related to the atrial stimulus. Contributions from circuit noise may also play a part in crosstalk and may be design dependent so that data obtained with a particular pulse generator cannot be extrapolated to others [118]. Unipolar DDDR systems are more likely to exhibit crosstalk at faster pacing rates. Byrd et al. [118] studied the incidence of crosstalk in Medtronic 7005 (unipolar) and 7006 (bipolar) DDD pulse generators at rapid paced ventricular rates with the pulse generators programmed to maximal output (volts and pulse width) and high sensitivity of the ventricular channel to mimic DDDR pacing. At 60 ppm, all pacemakers tested negative; 30% of patients with a unipolar pulse generator (54/166) showed crosstalk at pacing rates of 130 per minute, while no crosstalk was seen in 27 bipolar pulse generators under the same circumstances. At 160 ppm, crosstalk was observed in 25% (one of four) and 55% (six of 11) for bipolar and unipolar configurations, respectively. Combs et al. [119] also studied Medtronic 7006 bipolar DDD pulse generators programmed to a maximal output and high ventricular sensitivity and found crosstalk in three of 47 patients at a rate of 130 ppm and none out of 60 patients at rates of 140, 150, and 160 ppm. Crosstalk, when present, was always eliminated when ventricular sensitivity was decreased from 1.25 to 2.5 mV. These observations suggest that testing for crosstalk in unipolar and bipolar DDDR pulse generators for the worst-case situation should be considered in patients with pulse generators programmed to high output, high ventricular sensitivity, and a high upper rate, particularly in unipolar devices.

References

1. Furman S (1990) Rate-modulated pacing. Circulation 82:1081
2. Benditt DG, Milstein S, Buetikofer J, Gornick CC, Mianulli M, Fetter J (1987) Sensor-triggered rate-variable cardiac pacing. Ann Intern Med 107:714
3. Lau CP, Mehta D, Toff WD (1988) Limitations of rate response of an activity-sensing rate-responsive pacemaker to different forms of activity. PACE 11:141
4. Lau CP, Butrous GS, Ward DE, Camm AJ (1989) Comparative assessment of exercise performance of six different rate adaptive right ventricular cardiac pacemakers. Am J Cardiol 63:833
5. McAllister HF, Soberman J, Klementowicz P, Andrews C, Furman S (1989) Treadmill assessment of an activity-modulated pacemaker. The importance of individual programming. PACE 12:486
6. Zegelman M, Kreuzer J, Rahn R, Cieslnski G (1989) Body activity directed pacing Activitrax versus Sensolog. PACE 12:1574
7. Lau CP, Tse WS, Camm AJ (1988) Clinical experience with Sensolog 703. A new activity sensing rate responsive pacemaker. PACE 11:1444
8. Webb SC, Lewis LM, Morris-Thurgood JA, Crick J, Maseri A (1988) Can activity sensing rate responsive pacemakers match the normal heart rate requirements of recreational swimming. PACE 11:514

9. Moura PJ, Gessman LJ, Lai T, Gallagher JD, White M, Morse DP (1987) Chronotropic response of an activity detecting pacemaker compared with the normal sinus node. PACE 10:78
10. Soberman J, McAlister H, Klementowicz P, Andrews C, Furman S (1988) Paradoxical responses in activity-sensing pacemakers. PACE 11:855
11. Sulke AN, Pipilis A, Henderson RA, Bucknall CA, Sowton E (1990) Comparison of the normal sinus node with seven types of rate responsive pacemakers during everyday activity. Br. Heart J. 64:25
12. Lau CP, Wong CK, Leung WH, Cheng CH, Lo CW (1989) A comparative evaluation of a minute ventilation sensing and activity sensing adaptive-rate pacemaker during daily activities. PACE 12:1514
13. Wilkoff BL, Denise D, Shimokochi MS, Schaal SF (1987) Pacing rate increase due to application of steady external pressure on an activity sensing pacemaker. PACE 10:423
14. DenDulk K, Brugada P, Wellens HJJ (1987) Tachycardia termination with a rate responsive pacemaker. Am J Cardiol 59:1424
15. Lau CP, Li JBS, Cheng CH, Wong CK, Chung FLW (1991) Sensor-initiated termination of pacemaker mediated tachycardia in a DDDR pacemaker. Am Heart J 121:595
16. Andersen C, Madsen GM (1990) Rate-responsive pacemaker and anesthesia. A consideration of possible implications. Anesthesia 45:472
17. Mond HG, Kertes PJ (1988) Rate responsive cardiac pacing. Telectronics and Cordis pacing systems, Denver p 23
18. Maloney JD, Vaneiro G, Pashkow FJ (1991) Single chamber rate modulated pacing, AAIR-VVIR. Follow-up and complications. In: Barold SS, Mugica J (eds) New perspectives in cardiac pacing, vol 2. Futura, Mt Kisco, p 429
19. Bana G, Piatti L, Locatelli V (1990) Sensor related PM syndrome in patients with VVIR PM. Rev Eur Technol Biomed 12:23
20. Ahmed R, Gibbs S, Ingram A, Chan SL, Sutton R (1990) Pacemaker mediated tachycardia in the left retromammary implantation of VVIR (activity) pacemakers. PACE 13:1189
21. Lau CP, Tai YT, Fong PC, Cheng CH, Chung FLW (1990) Pacemaker mediated tachycardias in single chamber rate responsive pacing. PACE 13:1573
22. Toff WD, Leeks C, Joy M, Bennett G, Camm AJ (1987) The effect of aircraft vibration on the function of an activity sensing pacemaker. Br Heart J 57:573
23. Toff WD, Leeks C, Bennett JG, Camm AJ (1987) Function of the Activitrax rate-responsive pacemakers during travel by air. PACE 10:753
24. Gordon RS, O'Dell KB, Low RB, Blumen IJ (1990) Activity sensing permanent internal pacemaker dysfunction during helicopter aeromedical transport. Ann Emerg Med 19:1260
25. Stangl K, Wirtzfeld A, Lochschmidt O, Basler B, Mittnacht A (1989) Physical movement sensitive pacing comparison of two activity-triggered pacing systems. PACE 12:102
26. Rahn R, Zegelman M, Kreuzer J (1988) The influence of dental treatment on the Activitrax. PACE 11:499
27. Rossi P (1987) Rate responsive pacing. Biosensor reliability and physiological sensitivity. PACE 10:454
28. Lau CP, Ward DE, Camm A (1988) Rate-responsive pacing with a pacemaker that detects respiratory rate (Biorate). Clinical advantages and complications. Clin. Cardiol. 11:318
29. Lau CP, Ritche D, Butros GS, Ward DE, Camm AJ (1988) Rate modulation by arm movements of the respiratory dependent rate responsive pacemaker. PACE 11:744
30. Lau CP, Ward DE, Camm AJ (1989) Single chamber cardiac pacing with two forms of respiration controlled rate responsive pacemakers. Chest 95:352
31. Webb SC, Lewis LM, Morris-Thurgood JA, Palmer RG, Sanderson JE (1988) Respiratory-dependent pacing: a dual response from a single sensor. PACE 11:730
32. Jordaens L, Berghmans L, VanWassenhove E, Clement DL (1989) Behavior of a respiratory driven pacemaker and direct respiratory measurement. PACE 12:1600
33. Mond H, Strathmore N, Kertes P, Hunt D, Baker G (1988) Rate-responsive pacing using a minute ventilation sensor. PACE 11:1866
34. Lau CP, Antoniou A, Ward DE, Camm AJ (1988) Initial clinical experience with a minute-ventilation sensing rate modulated pacemaker: improvement in exercise capacity and symptomatology. PACE 11:1815

35. Ilvento J, Wilkoff BM, Dorian P, Vidaillet H, Fee J (1991) Favorable interaction between implantable cardioverter defibrillators and impedance based rate responsive pacemakers. PACE 14:629
36. Lau C, Antoniou A, Ward DE, Camm AJ (1989) Reliability of minute ventilation as a parameter for rate responsive pacing. PACE 12:321
37. Seeger W, Kleinert M (1989) An unexpected rate response of a minute ventilation dependent pacemaker. PACE 12:1707
38. VanHamel NM, Hamerlijnek RPHM, Pronk KJ, VanDerVeen EDP (1989) Upper limit ventricular stimulation in respiratory rate responsive pacing due to electrocautery. PACE 12:1720
39. Wilson JH, Lattner S (1988) Apparent undersensing due to oversensing of low amplitude pulses in a thoracic impedance-sensing rate-responsive pacemaker. PACE 11:1479
40. Scanu P, Guilleman D, Groiller G, Potier JC (1989) Inappropriate rate response of the minute ventilation rate responsive pacemakers in a patient with Cheyne-Stokes dyspnea. PACE 12:1963
41. Madsen GM, Andersen C (1989) Pacemaker-induced tachycardia during general anesthesia. Br J Anaesth 63:300
42. Alt E, Heinz M, Theres H, Matula M (1991) Function and selection of sensors for optimum rate-modulated pacing. In: Barold SS, Mugica J (eds) New perspectives in cardiac pacing, vol 2. Futura, Mt Kisco, p 163
43. Lau CP, Camm AJ (1991) Rate-responsive pacing. Technical and clinical aspects. In: El Sherif N, Samet P (eds) Cardiac pacing and electrophysiology, 3rd edn. Saunders, Philadelphia, p 524
44. Zegelman M, Winter VJ, Alt E, Treese N, Kreuzer J, Henry L, Mugica J, Schroeder E, Klein H, Völker R (1990) Effect of different body-exercise modes on the rate response of the temperature-controlled pacemaker, NOVA MR. Thorac Cardiovasc Surg 38:181
45. Fearnot NE, Smith HJ, Sellers D, Boal B (1989) Evaluation of the temperature response to exercise testing in patients with single chamber, rate adaptive pacemakers: a multicenter study. PACE 12:1806
46. Schuchert A, Kuck KH, Bleifeld W (1991) Effects of pacemaker mass on rate response of activity modulated pacemakers. PACE 14:665
47. Alt E. Matula M, Theres H, Heinz M, Baker R (1988) The basis for activity controlled rate variable cardiac pacemakers: an analysis of mechanical forces on the human body induced by exercise and environment. PACE 12:1667
48. Mahaux V, Waleffe A, Mathus F, Kulbertus HK (1990) Preliminary resutls with a new rate modulated pacemaker sensitive to low frequency vibration and acceleration force. PACE 13:1202
49. Silvermint EH, Salo RW, Meyerson SC, Burrell JL, Freudenberg MW, Linder WJ, Maile KR, Nguyen H, Zelkind B (1990) Distinctive characteristics of Excel VR rate-adaptive pacemaker with an innovative activity sensor. PACE 13:1210
50. Hage HJ, Niederlag W (1991) A new concept of data processing for activity controlled rate responsive pacing. PACE 13:1196
51. Matula M, Alt E, Heinz M, Mentrup H, Holzer K (1990) Rate adaptive pacing: comparison between Activitrax, Sensolog, and Relay a new activity based system sensitive to low frequency acceleration. PACE 13:1203
52. Lau CP, Stott JRR, Toff WD, Zetlein MB, Ward DE, Camm AJ (1988) Selective vibration sensing: a new concept for activity-sensing rate-responsive pacing. PACE 11:1299
53. Millerhagen J, Bacharach D, Kelly J, Maile K (1991) An accelerometer based adaptive rate pacemaker. PACE 14:699
54. Millerhagen J, Bacharach D, Street G, Westrum B (1991) A comparison study of two activity pacemakers: an accelerometer versus piezoelectric crystal device. PACE 14:665
55. Erdelitsch-Reiser E, Langenfeld H, Kochsiek K (1991) An acceleration sensor. A new concept in "activity"-controlled pacemaker. Eur Heart J 12:415 (abstr suppl)
56. Sulke N, Dritsas A, Chambers J, Sowton E (1990) Is accurate rate response programming necessary? PACE 13:1031
57. Lau CP (1991) Sensors and pacemaker mediated tachycardias. PACE 14:495
58. Volosin KJ, O'Connor WH, Fabiszewski R, Waxman HL (1989) Pacemaker-mediated tachycardia from a single chamber temperature sensitive pacemaker. PACE 12:311

59. Rickards AF (1985) Rate-responsive pacing. In: Barold SS, (ed) Modern cardiac pacing. Futura, Mt Kisco, p 799
60. Moreira LFP, Costa R, Stolf NAG, Jatene AB (1989) Pacing rate increase as cause of syncope in a patient with a severe cardiomyopathy. PACE 12:1027
61. Edelstam C, Hedman A, Nordlander R, Pehrsson SK (1989) QT sensing rate responsive pacing and myocardial infarction. PACE 12:502
62. Robbens EJ, Clement DL, Jordaens LJ (1988) QT-related rate-responsive pacing during acute myocardial infarction. PACE 11:339
63. Scanu P, Dorey H, Guilleman D, Gofard M, Grollier G, Potier JC (1989) Tachycardies ventriculaires déclencheés par un stimulateur ventriculaire à fréquence asservie. Stimucoeur 17:158
64. Adornato E, Pennisi V, Pangallo A (1990) DDD-R pacemaker in the prevention of ventricular tachycardia. A report on one case. RBM 12:84
65. Adornato E, Pennisi V, Pangallo A (1990) Dual chamber PM in the prevention of ventricular tachycardia – long term follow-up. RBM 12:84
66. Nicolai P, Blache E (1990) Chronic cardiac pacing. A new therapy for severe ventricular arrhythmias? RBM 12:84
67. Sartieaux A, Bohyn P, Deperon R, Bracops CHJ (1990) Dual chamber pacing in the treatment of recurrent ventricular tachycardia. RBM 12:85
68. Schmidinger H, Probst P, Weber H, Kaliman J (1988) Rate dependent depression of subsidiary ventricular impulse formation. Cause of Stokes-Adams attack in a patient with rate modulated pacing. PACE 11:1095
69. Schmidinger H, Probst P, Schneider B, Weber H, Kaliman J (1991) Determinants of subsidiary ventricular pacemaker suppression in man. PACE 14:833
70. Lau CP, Camm AJ, Ward DE (1987) A severe case of myopotential interference in a patient with a respiratory-dependent rate modulated pacemaker. Int J Cardiol 17:98
71. Lau CP, Linker NJ, Butrous GS, Ward DE, Camm AJ (1989) Myopotential interference in unipolar rate responsive pacemakers. PACE 12:1324
72. Barold SS, Falkoff MD, Ong LS, Heinle RA (1991) Interference in cardiac pacemakers. Exogenous sources. In: El-Sherif N, Samet P (eds) Cardiac pacing and electrophysiology, 3rd edn. Saunders, Philadelphia, p 608
73. Cooper D, Wilkoff B, Masterson M, Castle L, Belco K, Simmons T, Morant V, Streem S, Maloney J (1988) Effects of extracorporeal shock wave lithotripsy on cardiac pacemakers and its safety in patients with implanted cardiac pacemakers. PACE 11:1607
74. Fetter J, Patterson D, Aram G, Hayes DL (1989) Effects of extracorporeal shock wave lithotripsy on single chamber rate response and dual chamber pacemakers. PACE 12:1494
75. Ausubel K, Furman S (1985) The pacemaker syndrome. Ann Intern Med 103:420
76. Schüller H, Brandt J (1991) The pacemaker syndrome: old and new causes. Clin Cardiol 14:336
77. Wish M, Cohen A, Swartz J, Fletcher R (1988) Pacemaker syndrome due to a rate responsive ventricular pacemaker. J Electrophysiol 2:504
78. Maloney JD, Vaneiro G, Pashkow FJ (1991) Single chamber rate modulated pacing, AAIR-VVIR. Follow-up and complications. In: Barold SS, Mugica J (eds) New perspectives in cardiac pacing, vol 2. Futura, Mt Kisco, p 429
79. Baig MW, Perrins EJ (1991) The hemodynamics of cardiac pacing. Clinical and physiological aspects. Progr Cardiovasc Dis 33:283
80. Cazeau S, Daubert C, Mabo P, Ritter P, Lelong B, Pouillot C, Paillard F (1990) Dynamic electrophysiology of ventriculoatrial conduction. Implications for DDD and DDDR pacing. PACE 13:1646
81. White M, Gessman L, Morse D, Maranho V, Raman S (1987) Effects of exercise on retrograde conduction during activity sensing rate-adaptive pacing. PACE 10:424
82. Fujiki A, Tani M, Mizumaki K, Asanoi H, Sasayama S (1990) Pacemaker syndrome evaluated by cardiopulmonary exercise testing. PACE 13:1236
83. Vaneiro G, Patel S, Ching E, Simmons T, Trohmam R, Wilkoff B, Castle L, Maloney J (1991) Early clinical experience with a minute ventilation sensor DDDR pacemaker. Pace 14:664
84. Byrd CL, Scala G, Schwartz SJ, Ciraldo RJ, Yahr WZ, Sivina M, Greenberg JJ (1987) Retrograde conduction and rate responsive pacemakers. PACE 10:1208

85. Klementowicz P, Ausubel K, Furman S (1986) The dynamic nature of ventriculoatrial conduction. PACE 9:1050
86. Wish M, Fletcher RD, Gottdiener JS, Cohen AI (1987) Importance of left atrial timing in the programming of dual chamber pacemakers. Am J Cardiol 60:566
87. Wish M, Gottdiener J, Fletcher R, Cohen A (1986) Use of M mode echocardiograms for determination of optimal left atrial timing in patients with dual chamber pacemakers. PACE 9:290
88. Torresani J, Ebagosti A, Allard-Latour G (1984) Pacemaker syndrome with DDD pacing. PACE 7:1148
89. Cunningham TM (1982) Pacemaker syndrome due to retrograde conduction pacemaker. Am Heart J 115:478
90. Floro J, Castellanet M, Florio J, Messenger J (1984) DDI: a new mode for cardiac pacing. Clin Prog Pacing Electrophysiol 2:255
91. Barold SS (1987) The DDI mode of cardiac pacing. PACE 9:480
92. Sutton R, Ingram A, Kenny RA, Vardas P, Travill CM, Bayliss J (1987) Clinical experience of DDI pacing. In: Belhassen B, Feldman S, Copperman Y (eds) Cardiac pacing and electrophysiology. Proceedings of the VIIIth world symposium on cardiac pacing and electrophysiology. Keterpress, Jerusalem p 161
93. VanWyhe G, Sra J, Rovang K, Gilbert C, Akhtar M, Tchou P (1991) Maintenance of atrioventricular sequence after His bundle ablation for paroxysmal supraventricular rhythm disorders: a unique use of the fallback mode in dual chamber pacemakers. PACE 14:410
94. Mugica J, Barold SS, Ripart A (1991) The smart pacemaker. In: New perspectives in cardiac pacing, vol 2. Futura, Mt Kisco, NY, p 545
95. Barold SS, Falkoff MD, Ong LS, Heinle RA (1988) Upper rate response of DDD pacemakers. In: Barold SS, Mugica J (eds) New perspectives in cardiac pacing. Futura, Mt Kisco, p 121
96. Barold SS, Falkoff MD, Ong LS, Heinle RA, Willis JE (1987) AV desynchronization arrhythmia during DDD pacing. In: Belhassen B, Feldman S, Copperman Y (eds) Cardiac pacing and electrophysiology. Proceedings of the VIIIth world symposium on cardiac pacing and electrophysiology. Keterpress, Jerusalem p 117
97. Barold SS, Falkoff MD, Ong LS, Heinle RA (1988) Magnet unresponsive pacemaker endless loop tachycardia. Am Heart J 116:726
98. Chien WW, Foster E, Phillips B, Schiller N, Griffin JC (1991) Pacemaker syndrome in a patient with DDD pacemaker for long QT syndrome. PACE 14:1209
99. Brandt J, Fåhraeus T, Schüller H (1991) Practical aspects of rate-adaptive atrial (AAIR) pacing. Clinical experiences in 44 patients. PACE 14:1258
100. Edelstam C, Nordlander R, Wallgren E, Rosenqvist M (1990) AAIR pacing and exercise. What happens to AV conduction? PACE 13:1193
101. Clarce M, Allen A (1987) Rate responsive atrial pacing resulting in pacemaker syndrome. PACE 10:1209
102. Pouillot C, Mabo C, LeLong B (1990) Bénéfices et limites de la stimulation mono-chambre atriale à fréquence asservie. Arch Mal Coeur 83:1833
103. denDulk K, Lindemans FW, Brugada P, Smeets JLRM, Wellens HJJ (1988) Pacemaker syndrome with AAI rate variable pacing. Importance of atrioventricular conduction properties, medication and pacemaker programmability. PACE 11:1226
104. Daubert C, Mabo P, Pouillot C, LeLong B (1991) Atrial chronotropic incompetence. Implications for DDDR pacing. In: Barold SS, Mugica J (eds) New perspectives in cardiac pacing, vol 2. Futura, Mt Kisco, p 251
105. Ruiter J, Burgersdijk C, Zeeders M, Kee D (1987) Atrial Activitrax pacing. The atrioventricular interval during exercise. PACE 10:1226
106. Medtronic (1989) Technical manual. Activitrax II Models 8412/8413/8413M/8414 multi-programmable rate-responsive (activity) pulse generator. Medtronic, Minneapolis
107. Medtronic (1989) Technical manual. Legend 8416/8417/8418 multiprogrammable rate-responsive (activity) pulse generator. Medtronic, Minneapolis
108. denDulk K, Bouwels L, Lindemans F, Rankin I, Brugada P, Wellens HJJ (1988) The Activitrax rate-responsive pacemaker system. Am J Cardiol 61:107

109. Brandt J, Fåhraeus T, Schüller H (1988) Far-field QRS complex sensing via the atrial pacemaker lead: I. Mechanisms, consequences, differential diagnosis, and countermeasures in AAI and VDD/DDD pacing. PACE 11:1432
110. Brandt J, Fåhraeus T, Schüller H (1988) Far-field QRS complex sensing via the atrial pacemaker lead: II. Prevalence, clinical significance, and possibility of intraoperative prediction in DDD pacing. PACE 11:1540
111. Benditt DG, Dunningan A, Milstein S, Fetter J (1988) Activity-triggered atrial rate-responsive pacing. Importance of polarity and programmable sensivity. PACE 11:802
112. Shandling AH, Castellanet MJ, Thomas L, Rylaarsdam A, Valikai K, Messenger JC, Ellestad MH (1989) Impaired activity rate responsiveness of an atrial activity-triggered pacemaker. The role of differential atrial sensing in its prevention. PACE 12:1927
113. Telectronics (1990) Physician's manual. Meta DDDR Model 1250 multiprogrammable minute volume rate responsive pulse generator with telemetry. Telectronics, Englewood
114. Barold SS, Falkoff MD, Ong LS, Heinle RA (1985) Differential diagnosis of pacemaker pauses. In: Barold SS (Ed) Modern Cardiac Pacing , Futura, Mt Kisco, NY, p 587
115. Barold SS, Roehrich DR, Falkoff MD, Ong LS, Heinle RA (1980) Sources of error in the determination of output voltage of pulse generators by pacemaker system analyzers. PACE 3:585
116. Medtronic (1988) Activitrax II clinical study report. Medtronic, Minneapolis
117. Medtronic (1986) Activitrax clinical study report. Medtronic, Minneapolis
118. Byrd CL, Schwartz SJ, Gonzales M, Ciraldo RJ, Yahr WZ, Sivina M, Greenberg JJ (1988) Rate responsive pacemakers and crosstalk. PACE 11 [June Suppl]:798
119. Combs WJ, Reynolds DW, Sharma AD, Bennett TD (1989) Cross-talk in bipolar pacemakers. PACE 12:1613

Technical Improvements to be Achieved by the Year 2000: Leads and Connector Technology

J. HELLAND[1]

Introduction

During the past 35 years, many technological advantages have been made in cardiac pacemaker leads and in the pulse generator-to-lead connector. Advances have included development of: various coiled wire conductors [1]; new fixation means such as tines, fins, and helix mechanisms [1, 2]; advances in electrodes such as microporous surfaced electrodes, small surface area electrodes, electrodes with special shapes which enhance electrical fields and tissue ingrowth and steroid eluting electrodes [3, 4]; improved insultion such as "high-performance" or "extra tear-resistant" silicone rubbers, and various polyurethanes [5]; and improved, standardized connectors such as the recent "VS-1" and proposed "IS-1" standard connector designs [6]. These advances have improved the performance, reliability, and the ease of implantation of pacemaker leads and pulse generators dramatically. Perhaps however, historically, one of the most significant advances in pacemaking was the development of the transvenous pacemaker lead which made the therapy of cardiac pacing a relatively safe and easy procedure for virtually all patients [7].

There remain, however, numerous areas in leads and connectors, where technological advances continue to occur. Indeed, there are a number of areas where continued clinical needs and problems demand advances in technology. Thus, many of the technical improvements in leads and connectors between now and the year 2000 will be driven by the necessity of solving such problems. Additionally, during the next 10 years, it can also be expected that many technical improvements and advances will by introduced by the pacemaker lead manufacturers as a result of current research and development in an effort to introduce new technical advances to pacemaker therapy.

This report, then, covers some of those areas, where technical advances in bradycardia leads will occur as a result of the need to address these clinical problems and the desire to provide new technologies for various therapies.

[1] Siemens Pacesetter Inc., Sylmar, CA, USA

Pacemaker Lead Technology by the Year 2000

Electrode Technology

Electrode design advances have been dramatic over the past 10 years. During the next 10 years, one can expect continued development. By the year 2000, it is doubtful that any lead's electrode will be simply a polished platinum material. Indeed, it is already common for leads to have electrodes which have a microporous surface. Such a surface increases the real surface area of an electrode by orders of magnitude, resulting in improved electrical efficiency due to reduced electrical polarization [4]. Electrode configuration and macroporosity can also allow for an improved tissue interface where reduced fibrotic tissue response and tissue ingrowth – into the electrode – allow for an improved electrode/tissue interface [1–4], which can enhance both pacing thresholds and sensing.

The microporous surfaced electrodes can be comprised of different materials. Over the next 10 years we can expect to see electrode surfaces with platinized coatings, activated carbon surfaces, titanium nitride coatings, iridium oxide coatings, platinum particles, and other materials or substances, all of which are intended to provide improved electrical efficiency, lower thresholds, and better sensing (Fig. 1). Indeed, because sensing can be enhanced – especially evoked responses – electrodes other than just the tip electrode (cathode) will also become microporous during the next ten years.

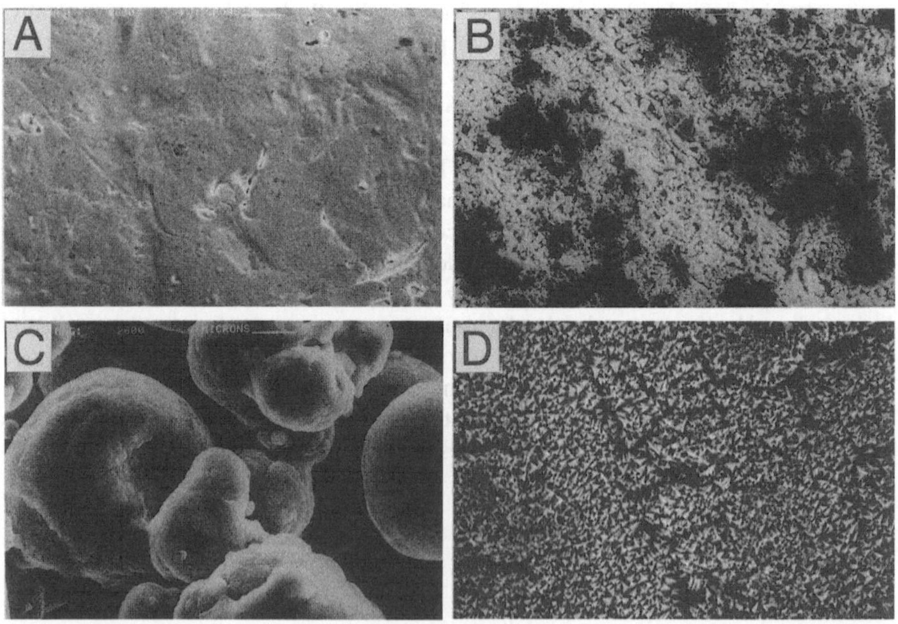

Fig. 1 A-D. SEM examples of microporous electrode surfaces. **A** Activated carbon; **B** platinized platinum; **C** platinum particles; **D** titanium nitride (all at high magnification)

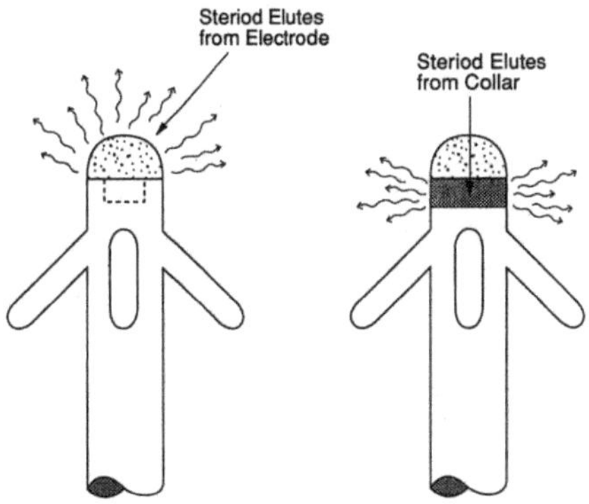

Fig. 2. Two versions of steroid-eluting leads

Another major development in electrodes will be the widespread practice of applying drug-eluting technology at or near the tip of the pacing electrode. Studies have already shown, that the use of glucocorticosteroid elution at or near the pacing electrode can provide lower, more stable pacing thresholds [8] and better, more stable sensing of cardiac signals [9]. Although, up to now, the steroid most commonly used (dexamethasone sodium phosphate) has been located within or adjacent to the cathode electrode (Fig. 2), developments over the next 10 years will likely result in other new methods of delivering steroids or other specialized pharmacological agents to the tissue adjacent to the lead's electrode. Such agents might be used as rate modifiers, antiarrhythmics, or have certain other purposes related to cardiac tissue management.

Lead Fixation Technology

The ability to position the tip electrode of a transvenous lead in an area of the right ventricle or right atrium where low pacing thresholds and good cardiac signal sensing are available is critical to the effectiveness of the pacemaker. Indeed, just as important is the ability to "fix" or keep the tip where it is intended to be, chronically. In the attempt to make fixation of lead tips in proper sites stable, the development of passive fixation means, utilizing tines and fins, for example, occurred. The effectiveness of such fixation means (Fig. 3) has been well established [1, 2].

Both kinds of passive fixation structures appear to work well in the ventrical, though the "fin"-type leads appear to be somewhat easier to maneuver and resposition compared to the tines. The tines tend to "catch" or "snag" more often while being passed through the tricuspid valve. However, in the atrium, many feel the tine may be easier to fix than the fin. Obviously, personal preferences of the implanter will dictate the choice. In either case, these passive fixation designs have been and continue to be very successful. As such, current leads and leads to be developed during the next 10 years will likely continue to incorporate these designs adjacent to the tip for both ventricular leads and atrial leads (which also utilize a distal J-shape portion intended to provide for easier positioning of the tip in the atrial appendage). Passive fixation

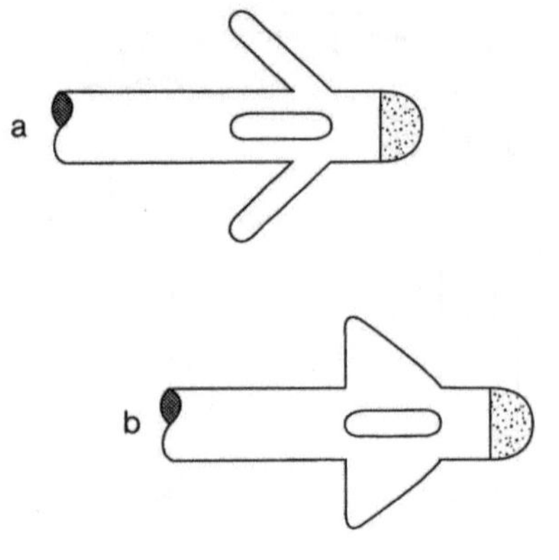

Fig. 3 a, b. Examples of a "tine" (**a**) and "fin" (**b**) fixation means

designs such as the above tines and fins, though being generally effective in preventing lead tip dislodgement, are not always effective. For those patients in whom very little cardiac structure exists to allow the tines or fins to become entrapped, active fixation means have been developed. Active fixation has generally utilized a helical screw which is located at the distal tip of the lead. The helix is either an extendable/ retractable type or it may be a permanently extended type. In either case, it can facilitate the active attachment of the lead tip to the site in the right ventricle or right atrium where it (if it is electrically active) or an adjacent tip electrode shall pace and sense (Fig. 4). This means of fixation is very successful in preventing dislodgements and virtually always assures lead fixation. It will likely continue to be used even more extensively in the next 10 years. Its popularity increase will also be due to the fact that – when used properly – many patients receiving active fixation-type leads can have their pacemakers routinely implanted in outpatient settings – thereby reducing costs and hospital care time [10].

Some key concerns with the active fixation type of leads, however, will need to be addressed over the next 10 years for these leads to make significant gains in usage over passive fixation leads. Some of the current active fixation leads have excellent engineering designs which allow the extension and retraction of the helix. However, the mechanisms necessary to achieve this – especially in bipolar leads – result in relatively larger mass and greater stiffness of the distal portion of the lead than passive fixation leads. The typical clinical implications of these mechanical aspects are higher

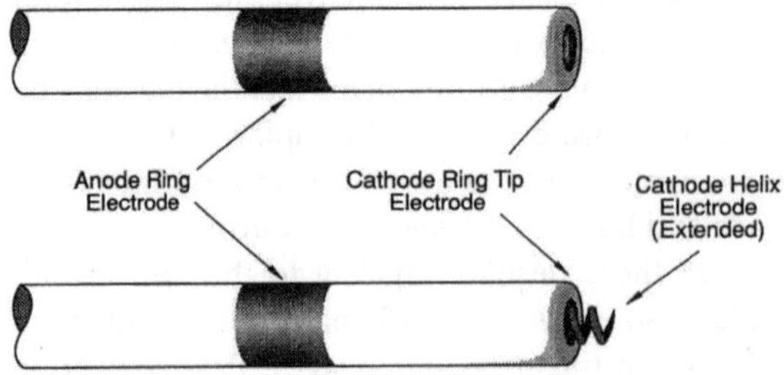

Fig. 4. Example of an active-fixation, bipolar, extendable/ retractable screw-in type lead

thresholds and poorer sensing capability with a higher risk of exit block [11]. As such, new active fixation leads that will be introduced over the next several years will have reduced diameters, smaller distal tip masses, and be much more flexible – all of which will help reduce the greater tissue trauma usually associated with active fixation leads.

In addition, it has not been technically very easy to apply the drug-eluting technologies used so successfully with passive fixation leads to the active fixation leads. As a result, the benefits of the steroid-eluting passive fixation leads during the past several years have not yet been obtainable with active fixation leads. During the next couple of years, however, several manufacturers will be introducing active fixation leads which do incorporate such technology, combined with the more attractive mechanical features noted above. With these advances, the active fixation-type lead will become increasingly popular until, perhaps by the year 2000, active fixation leads will be the predominantly used transvenous leads worldwide.

Improved Durability of Leads

During the first 35 years of pacing, the pacemaker lead has been significantly improved technologically, so that, in general, leads should now be expected to function reliably for the lifetimes of at least two to four pacing implants – perhaps 15-18 years – before the conductor(s) or the insulation could be expected to fail. However, there are leads which have been produced by certain manufacturers which have fallen far short of such standards. The two most well-known problems of the past have been conductor coil fractures due to flex fatigue and failure due to degradation of the insulation in certain leads which have utilized the "80A" version of the Dow Chemical, Inc., Pellathane 2363 polyurethane [12, 13]. As a result of these past problems, most current leads and those which will be developed in the future should benefit from the technical knowledge gained from understanding these shortcomings.

Leads which will be developed during the next decade and, indeed, many current leads are well designed to provide excellent flex fatigue resistance and biostable insulations. However, recent new modes of clinical failure have been reported which will require manufacturers to develop technical solutions. With the widespread use of the percutaneous lead introducer method of lead implantation into the subclavian vein, leads must necessarily pass between the clavicle and the first rib. As a result, certain anatomies and/or patient movements can place excessive crushing stresses on the lead body at the rib – clavicle location. Damage to either the lead's insulation or its conductor coils (or both) can occur [14, 15]. The insulation can be abraded, scuffed, or worn, or it can experience excessive crushing stresses which, in time, can result in stress cracking and eventual failure of the insulation. Additionally, the conductor coils can be severely deformed or crushed, which can ultimately result in a stress fracture of the coil(s). It has been suggested by Byrd [16] and others that a more lateral entry site to the subclavian vein with the introducer may help reduce this problem [16] (Fig. 5). Over the next several years, lead manufacturers will have to develop improved lead bodies – specifically, improved conductor designs and insulations to ensure that not only biostability is assured, but that the mechanical durability of the lead is also assured.

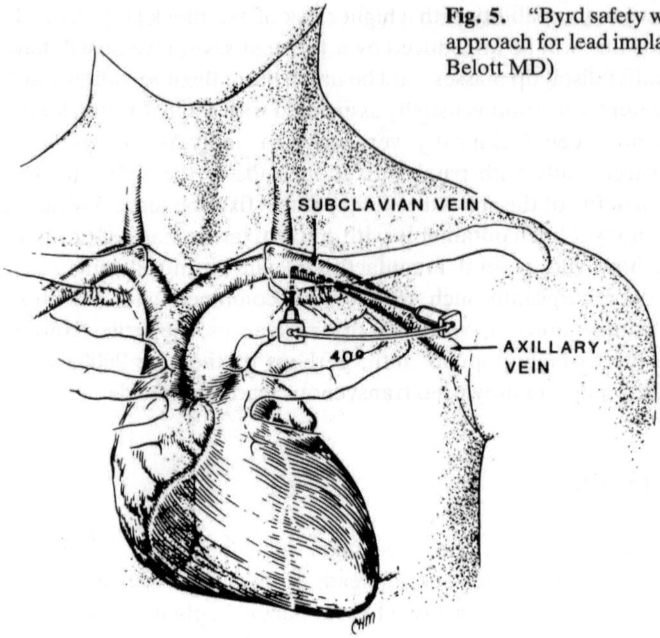

Fig. 5. "Byrd safety window" subclavian approach for lead implantation. (Courtesy of P. Belott MD)

Chronic Removal of Pacemaker Leads

Pacemaker leads must be explanted occasionally, which can be an extremely difficult and potentially risky procedure. Leads are removed typically for only two lead-related reasons: when infection has rendered the implant unmanageable, or when a failure of the implanted lead has occurred, and therefore the need for a new lead requires an explant of the old (i.e., the new lead cannot be effectively implanted due to the presence of the old lead).

A recent development by one manufacturer has been a lead extraction kit, which, when used carefully and properly, can effectively remove chronically implanted leads [17]. The procedure is new and complicated, however, and is currently under clinical usage regulations in the United States. Nevertheless, there is now promise that during the next decade more leads which must be explanted will be able to be removed more effectively and safely than in the past.

As a result of the need for more durable leads and the need to be able to remove leads, manufacturers are developing leads which are stronger and which can withstand greater tensile forces (i.e., stretching and pulling). In addition, there is now and will continue to be a strong emphasis by most manufacturers to develop new leads which are isodiametric – that is, leads which are the same diameter along the entire length of the lead (except for the connector and anchoring sleeve) and which do not have "ridges," "necks," or bulges which can prevent the lead from being more easily and safely retracted, chronically (Fig. 6).

By the year 2000, virtually all transvenous leads should be isodiametric and strongly enough designed to allow safer and easier chronic removal for whatever reason. This one issue alone, with pacemaker leads, is probably one of the most important and in the past has been the cause of some of the greatest patient safety concerns. Thus, new technological development in this area will certainly bring necessary improvements to patient care.

Improved Implantability of Leads

One of the most important aspects of pacemaker leads is the ability of the lead – with respect to its design – to be easily and effectively implanted by clinicians with little implant experience. In addition to the durability of leads being important, transvenous leads must be easily inserted into small veins or small lead introducers, yet be hardy enough not to kink or be damaged by handling and manipulation during the implant.

It can be expected that unipolar, bipolar, and the new multipolar transvenous leads will be developed during the 1990s which will be able to fit in lead introducers of only 4–7 French. As a result, improved lead body designs will be required that achieve the sizes necessary for smaller-size introducers and veins.

One area of critical concern which requires improved technology is the transvenous lead's anchoring sleeve, which is secured to the lead's body with sutures by the implanter. The sleeve is then – in turn – secured to tissue by sutures. The purpose of this anchoring sleeve or "tie-down" sleeve is to secure the lead movement so that the distal tip of the lead does not become dislodged from the atrium or ventricle. Studies show that the forces from an aggressive suture tie on the anchoring sleeve can severely stress and distort the lead's components. This can result in damage to the lead's insulation and/or conductor(s), and result in ultimate failure of the lead (Fig. 7).

Indeed, failure of leads at the anchoring sleeve site is not an uncommon occurrence with leads. In fact, it is likely that some lead failures which are attributed to the rib – clavicle "crushing" are really the result of the severe stresses created by aggressive

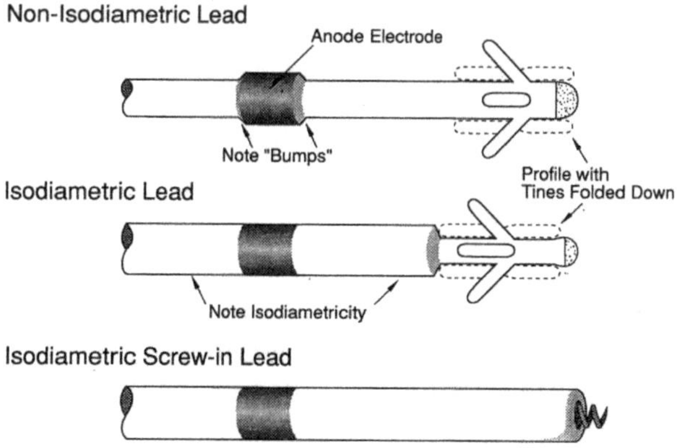

Fig. 6. Examples of nonisodiametric and isodiametric lead design

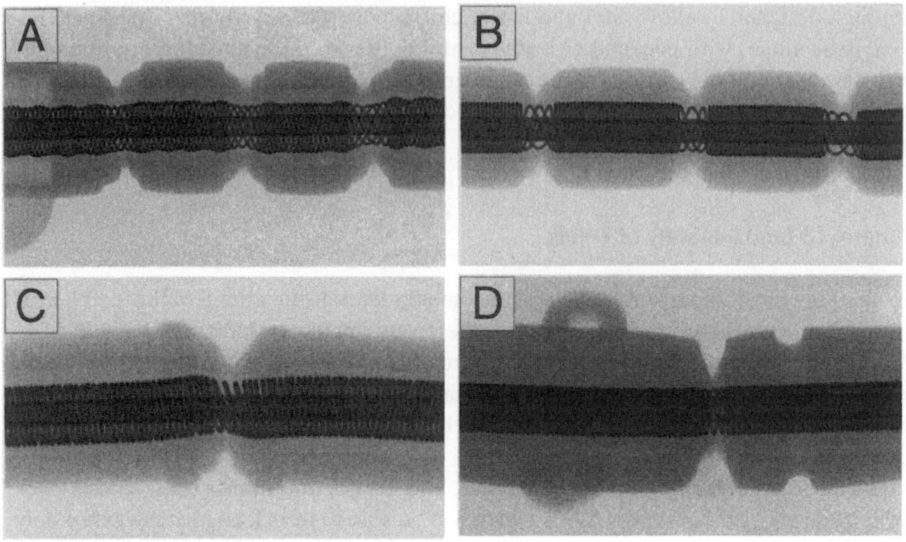

Fig. 7 A-D. X-ray analysis of various leads' anchoring sleeves on bipolar coaxial leads as tested in vitro. **A** Medtronic; **B** Oscor; **C** Intermedics; **D** Siemens-Pacesetter (suture ties made with identical tie forces using 2/0 Prolene suture material)

suture ties which exceed the limits of the protective design of the anchoring sleeve. Whether the ultimate failure is a result of the conductor fracturing, insulation wearing or degrading, or some other problem, the cause is due to the stricture of the anchoring sleeve suture being in excess of what the tie-down sleeve design can safely handle.

As a result, manufacturers must develop new designs of anchoring sleeves which will provide adequate securing of the lead, without the possibility of allowing the sutures to cause damage to the lead body. A number of alternative new designs are in development by various manufacturers at this time.

Improved Myocardial Leads for Pediatric Patients

One of the most neglected segments of lead design over the past couple of decades is the myocardial lead segment – especially for pediatric patients. Although a few advances have been made in this segment, there have been no real breakthroughs. Clearly, the primary reason for this lack of attention is the fact that only a very small fraction of implants are myocardial leads. It is estimated that only 2%–5% of all implants are myocardial leads.

However, those patients who do receive myocardial leads relatively often are patients who are unable to have a transvenous lead implanted. They may have had corrective surgery for congenital defects, valve repair or replacement, or may for some other anatomical reason be poor candidates for a transvenous lead. Many are pediatric patients who require a myocardial lead due to a Fontan or Mustard surgical procedure having eliminated a transvenous lead implant as an option. Additionally, although many centers routinely do transvenous lead implants in even very young and small (< 10 kg) pediatric patients, many implanters still prefer to implant a myocardial lead. This is because the pediatric patient can usually tolerate such a procedure fairly well and a vein – which may be important for use in the future – does not get used up. These young pediatric patients are often problematic and since their possible longevity can be 70+ years, they need special attention from a lead's design perspective. In the past, these young pediatric patients have had to get by with myocardial leads which were designed for adults and therefore have not typically done well with such leads.

During this decade, however, we can expect that with new and recently developed lead technologies several advanced in myocardial lead designs will be developed, especially for the pediatric patient. These designs could be used for adult as well as pediatric hearts and on either the ventricle or atrium. These leads will likely have a very small-sized distal electrode header and have a small, microporous cathode electrode with steroid elution from the electrode or from the material near the electrode. The lead will likely be implanted with use of a simple tool to either "inject" the electrode into the desired location, or to insert the electrode into the myocardium and perhaps staple the lead header in place.

One new design currently being studied clinically by one manufacturer is a suture-on, epicardial steroid-eluting electrode with a 14-mm² porous surface. Another design from a different manufacturer, which is also intended to be studied clinically, is a "suture-in" bipolar myocardial electrode with a 3-mm² microporous cathode electrode, with a steroid-eluting electrode superstructure. In addition, another myocardial lead – also with steroid-elution capability and an advanced electrode design – will be a multipolar lead which can allow sensing of evoked response and other parameters.

Clearly, by the year 2000, the clinical need for effective myocardial leads for the pediatric patient should be met. Indeed, the pediatric patient – probably the most "visible" and concerning pacemaker patient – should finally have viable leads for effective, reliable, state-of-the-art therapy.

Multipolar Lead for Several Functions

Probably the most significant advances in transvenous bradycardia leads during the next 10 years will be the development of multipolar leads. These leads will be able to not only pace or sense in the conventional way (i.e., unipolarly and/or bipolarly), but they will also be able to perform other activities at multiple sites. They will be able to carry sensors such as temperature, pressure, oxygen saturation, and others (Fig. 8). In addition, such leads will be able to have additional electrodes for:

- Sensing atrial electrograms for use in a single-pass lead for VDD pacing
- Sensing evoked responses off passive electrodes for voltage gradient rate adaptation systems or for use in autocapture systems
- Sensing impedance changes off passive electrodes for use in rate-adaptive systems based upon stroke volume, minute respiration, etc.
- Combinations of the above.

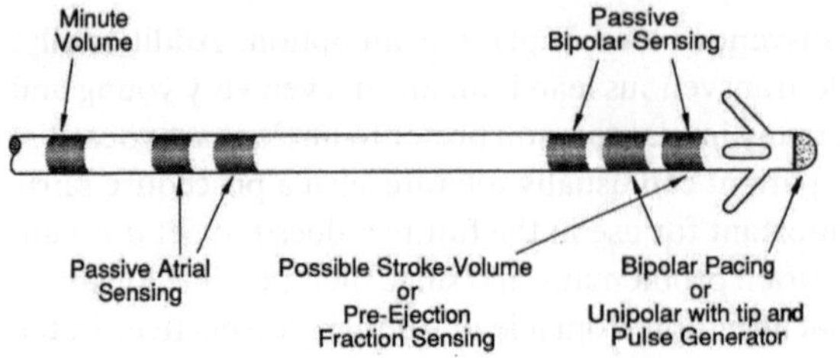

Fig. 8. Example of a multipolar lead with multisensing capability

These multipolar leads will utilize methods of construction which will allow the lead to remain relatively small in diameter, flexible, and be implanted using conventional stylet guidewires for manipulating the leadtip during implant. Such methods include:

- *Multilumen construction:* several different smaller conductors, each having its own lumen situated inside the insulator tube, around or alongside a larger, central lumen which carries the stylet and is continuous to the tip electrode.
- *Coated wire or multiconductor construction:* each individual wire which makes up a conductor coil is individually insulated. As many as four, five, or even six or more wires could be formed into one coil, each of which could service an electrode or sensor (Fig. 9). These multiconductor coils could be used in leads designed for one coil, or coaxial, or triaxial construction, or be combined with other construction variations as well.
- *Multistranded wire construction:* numerous wires are extruded in a spiral fashion within an insulative tubing wall. This tubing can then be used alone or be combined with other types of construction to provide for multipolar capabilities.

The Leads of the Future

As has been discussed previously, the leads of the future will embody numerous advances in technology. Additionally, pulse generators too will experience technological advances which will utilize and take advantage of the new lead technologies. Of course, numerous different types of leads will continue to exist.

What will a typical lead look like by the year 2000? One can only speculate, but it is clear that leads will likely employ the following technologies and features:

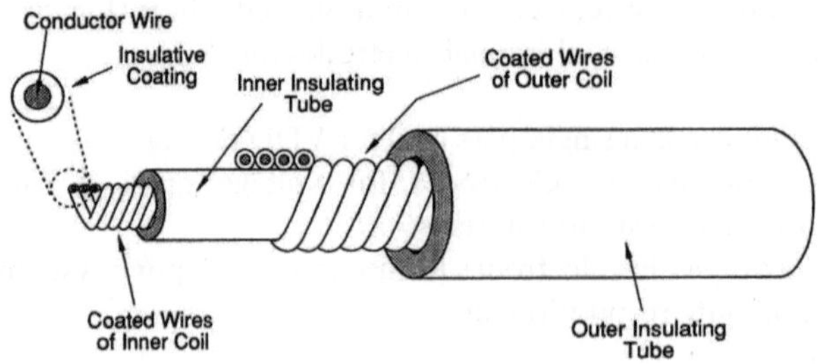

Fig. 9. Example of the construction of a coaxial multipolar lead utilizing coated wire/multi-conductor technology

- Small surface area, microporous, advanced material pacing electrodes (with pacing impedance of 1500–2000 ohms, negligible polarization impedances, and minimized conductor resistances).
- Steroid elution capability to suppress inflammatory responses caused by the electrode.
- Microporous sensing electrode(s).
- Active fixation (nontraumatic implant passage to the heart).
- Multipolar construction with several passive sensing electrodes.
- Sensor(s) utilized for special physiological sensing (i.e., O_2, pressure, etc.).
- Leads will be connected to miniaturized pulse generators by new connector designs.

Perhaps one new type of lead that will be in common use by the year 2000 will be a lead for a VDD pacer with VVIR backup, using a single-pass lead with a snap-on connector (Fig. 10).

Connector Technology by the Year 2000

The connectors utilized for attaching the leads to the pulse generators have not seen a great deal of technical advances over the years. It is likely that by the year 2000 the coming new advances that take place will focus on two key areas: standardized connectors for conventional lead/generator systems, and totally new connectors for the new multipolar lead/generator systems.

The slower rate of advance in connector technology stems, of course, from the need by clinicians and manufacturers to maintain interchangeability and backward compatibility between various leads and generators from any manufacturer. Until recently there has been little attempt to formally standardize between the manufacturers. However, beginning in 1985, and likely concluding in the 1992–1993 timeframe, an attempt to have a standardized connector design will finally become a reality for conventional unipolar/bipolar bradycardia leads.

VS-1/IS-1 Connector Standard Development

In late 1985, a group of manufacturers began to develop a voluntary connector standard that resulted in an agreed-upon set of connector designs providing not only

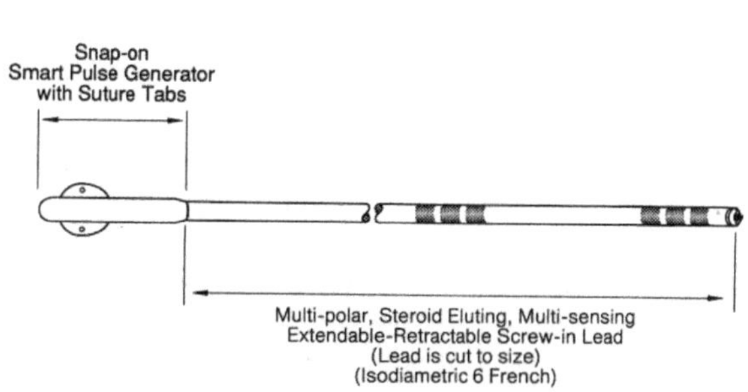

Fig. 10. Future lead for use in a VDD pacer with VVIR backup, using a single-pass lead system

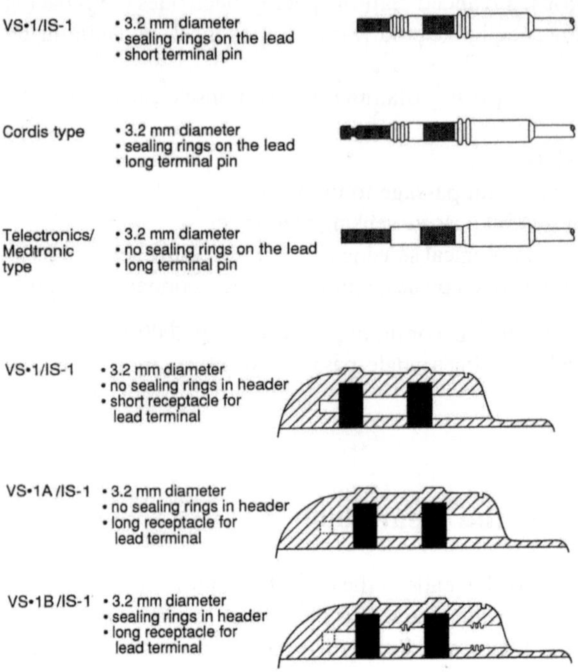

Fig. 11. VS-1/IS-1 lead connector and pacer header combinations. (Courtesy of Telectronics, Ltd.)

for a future or forward looking design, but for backward compatibility as well. This voluntary set of connector designs became known as the VS-1 configuration, which was actually made up of three versions (Fig. 11) [6]. The VS-1, VS-1A, and VS-1B versions of pulse generator connector cavities and their corresponding leads have been utilized since 1986. In 1986, a formal standardization development process was begun through the International Standards Organization (ISO). The results of this effort was the development of the IS-1 proposed connector standard which basically kept the original VS-1 dimensions and added some performance tests. The effect of some manufacturers using VS-1 notation and others prematurely using the IS-1 notations have resulted in a significant amount of confusion for the physician and manufacturers as to what would really (safely) fit what.

One of the key issues related to the proposed IS-1 standard (ISO DIS 5841-2) was whether optional sealing rings should be allowed in the IS-1 pulse generator cavity and, if so, how to specify them and test the design. Disagreement was common among the manufacturers, regulators, and industry experts as to what should be included in the standard.

Recent efforts have resolved the issue as manufacturers and the ISO committee agreed to one standard with one lead connector design (IS-1). The IS-1 compatible pulse generator would be able to accept an IS-1 lead connector (and theoretically a VS-1 lead connector). However, manufacturers will have the option of adding a longer connector pin bore and/or include sealing rings inside the pulse generator's connector cavity. This still allows the connector cavity to be labelled "IS-1" or "IS-1

Compatible" and to be able to connect to some of the pre-IS-1 leads, as shown in Fig. 11.

The standard has now completed its approval cycle, and is currently being utilized by nearly all manufacturers. However, since the standard does not prevent a manufacturer from using the sealing rings inside the pulse generator cavity, it is imperative that implanting physicians check with the IS-1 pulse generators' manufacturer (or their representative) to assure acceptable fit of any lead other than an "IS-1" labelled lead.

In addition, since the unipolar and bipolar IS-1 leads are interchangeable, physicians will have to be careful to not use a unipolar IS-1 lead in a bipolar IS-1 pulse generator (unless the pulse generator can be programmed to unipolar).

Future Connectors

Future connectors will necessarily have to reliably connect multipolar leads to sophisticated pulse generators. Obviously, numerous concepts will be developed and utilized over the next several years. It can be anticipated, however, that the connectors will have to employ new designs compared to those commonly used today. One example of what a future connector may look like is shown in Fig. 12.

Conclusion

Obviously, a great deal of development work and testing is necessary to provide safe, reliable, and effective lead and connector designs for the future. Additionally, it is important to realize that, by the year 2000, pulse generator designs may require other new kinds of technologies which – in turn – may have to be developed for the lead. Whatever the outcome, it is certain that future designs will improve upon the present and offer new options for future pacemaker therapies.

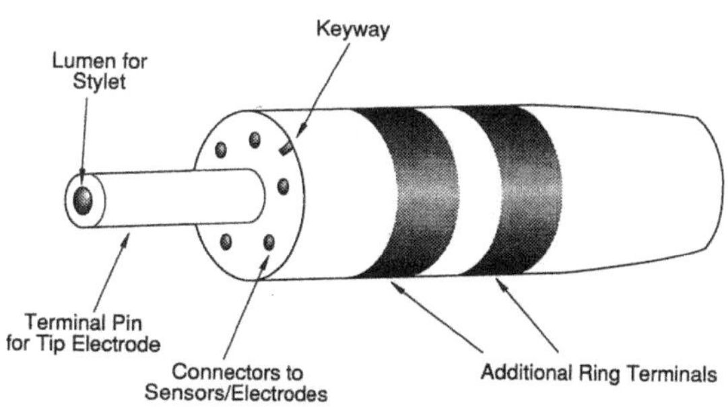

Fig. 12. Future multipolar lead connectors

References

1. Stokes K, Stephenson NL (1982) The implantable cardiac pacing lead – just a simple wire? In: Barold SS, Mugica J (eds) The third decade of cardiac pacing: advances in technology and clinical applications. Futura, Mount Kisco, pp 365-416
2. Timmis GC (1990) The electrobiology and engineering of pacemaker leads. In: Saksena S, Goldschlager N (eds) Electrical therapy for cardiac arrhythmias. Saunders, Philadelphia, pp 35-90
3. Timmis GC, Helland J, Westveer DC et al. (1983) The evolution of low threshold leads. Clin Prog Pacing Electrophysiol 1:313-334
4. Stokes K, Bornzin G (1985) The electrode-biointerface: stimulation. In: Barold SS (ed) Modern cardiac pacing. Futura, Mount Kisco, p 33-77
5. Stokes KB, Church T (1986) Ten-year experience with implanted polyurethane lead insulation. PACE 9:1160-1165
6. Calfee RV, Saulson SH (1986) A voluntary standard for 3.2 mm unipolar and bipolar pacemaker leads and connectors. PACE 9:1181-1185
7. Furman S, Robinson G (1985) The use of an intracardiac pacemaker in the Correction of total heart block. Surg Forum 9:245
8. Mond H, Stokes K, Helland J et al. (1988) The porous titanium steroid eluting electrode: a double blind study assessing the stimulation threshold effects of steroid. PACE 11:214-219
9. Steinhaus DM, Foley LM (1988) Atrial sensing: a continuing problem? PACE 11:A-203 (abstr)
10. Stenzl W, Tscheliessnigg KH, Dacar D et al. (1983) Four years' experience with the bisping transvenous pacemaker electrode. PACE 6:A-58
11. Kleinert MP (1988) Reasons for bipolar electrode lead renaissance. Herzschrittmacher 8:59-66
12. Stokes KB (1988) Polyether polyurethanes: biostable or not? J Biomater Appl 3:228-259
13. Chawla AS, Blais P, Hinberg I et al. (1988) Degradation of implanted polyurethane cardiac pacing leads and of polyurethane. Biomater Artif Cells Artif Organs 16/4:785-800
14. Fyke FE III (1988) Simultaneous insulation deterioration associated with side-by-side subclavian placement of two polyurethane leads. PACE 11:1571-1574
15. Stokes K (1987) A possible new complication of subclavian stick: conductor fracture. PACE 10:A-476, 748 (abstr)
16. Byrd CL (1990) Safe introducer technique. PACE 13:A-26, 501 (abstr)
17. Byrd CL (1990) Use of locking stylets and sheaths as part of an intravascular technique for lead extraction. PACE 13:A-210, 549 (abstr)

V. New Concepts in Rate-Adaptive Pacing

Single-Lead Atrial Synchronous Pacing

S. FURMAN[1]

The restoration of atrial synchrony in the presence of complete heart block has been attempted since the earliest days of cardiac pacing [1]. In the earliest instances the atrial lead was applied by thoracotomy to the surface of the right or left atrium [2]. Later the J-shaped endocardial lead was widely used [3] and presently the passive or active fixation J-shaped lead is usually used either for atrial or dual-chamber pacing [4]. Placement of the atrial lead has been considered as a more difficult effort and one subjected to a higher early and late displacement rate compared to a ventricular lead. Despite the occasional difficulties associated with atrial lead placement, atrial synchrony, with the atrial contribution to cardiac output, avoidance of pacemaker syndrome [5], and the rate modulation which results from sensing the atrial rate has remained an attractive prospect for both single-rate ventricular pacing and rate-modulated ventricular pacing [6]. If the difficulty of placing an independent atrial lead were to be eliminated or reduced, atrial synchrony would likely be a useful and popular pacing mode.

Despite one third of patients having sinus node dysfunction (SND) as an indication for pacing, and about 15% with fixed atrial fibrillation or flutter, many of those with SND and probably a majority of those with AV block have atrial function sufficiently reliable and responsive to provide two requirements, the atrial contribution to cardiac output and rate modulation. Several efforts have been made over the years to develop a lead which would sense atrial activity even if atrial pacing were not possible. Such a lead was the orthogonal lead [7], a special case of a bipolar lead. It may be part of the same lead which stimulates and senses ventricular activity. The orthogonal lead and those which have been subsequently and independently developed, passes through the atrium but does not require contact with the atrial wall to sense the atrial electrogram (EGM) at sufficient amplitude to synchronize ventricular to atrial activity.

An early effort at single-lead atrial synchrony involved the orthogonal lead and the RS4 pulse generator (CPI, Inc., St. Paul, MN, USA). This combination was intended to sense atrial EGM but was designed not to trigger a ventricular response on a basis of one P wave to trigger a ventricular stimulus [8]. The pulse generator was to determine the overall rate of the atrium and gradually bring ventricular stimulation to

[1] Department of Cardiothoracic Surgery, Montefiore Medical Center, Bronx, New York, USA

that rate via the mechanism of a prolonged response time to each P wave. Similarly atrial asystole or one or more unsensed P waves would not return ventricular stimulation to the lower rate limit, but progressive slowing would occur. This design was ultimately unsuccessful, possibly because of inadequate matching of the atrial EGM and pulse generator sensitivity, though the reasons for failure of synchronization have never been fully delineated in the medical literature. Further attempts were to produce 1:1 atrial synchrony in which each P wave produces a ventricular stimulus after a programmed AV delay.

In conventional bipolar leads the ring and tip are circumferential and are separated by length along the lead. In the orthogonal type of lead two or three points or small surface area flat-plate electrodes are spaced around the shaft of the lead, with each electrode separated from the others by space around the lead circumference. One variation places these small electrodes at a single level around the lead, another places several millimeters along the lead between the electrodes. In this later version it is possible to sense two unipolar intrinsic deflection (ID) with the final electrogram as the sum of the two or with both intrinsic deflections entirely independent in the final EGM. In that instance the first of the pair which reaches an amplitude adequate to be sensed triggers the pulse generator. The electrodes are highly directional and, as they are closely spaced bipolar, reject far-field signals very well. Sensing of the atrial EGM is, in general, highly satisfactory. The low level of noise in the EGM allows the setting of a very high level of sensitivity. Movement of the electrode, as the lead moves back and forth within the atrium, causes wide swings of atrial EGM amplitude (Fig. 1).

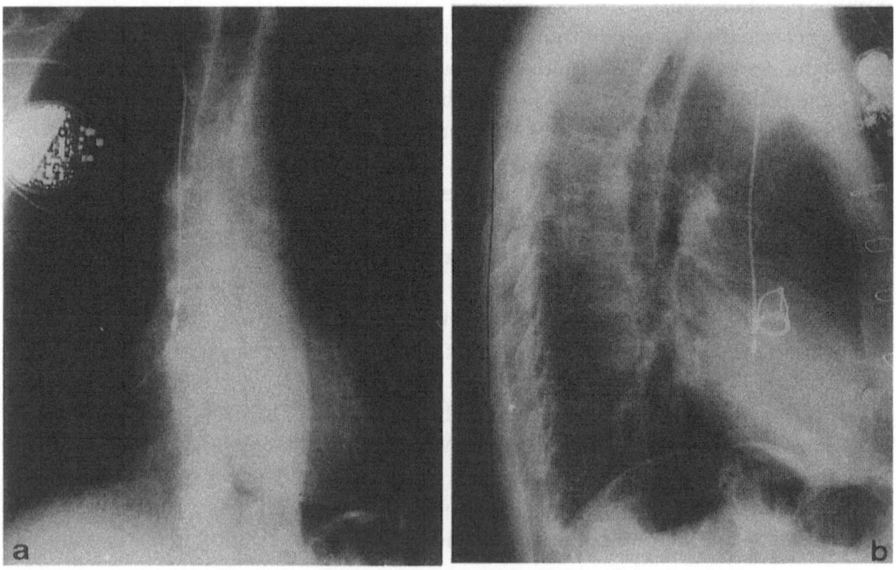

Fig. 1 a, b. PA and lateral of lead "AT" 134 implanted with model 305 via the cephalic vein following open heart surgery for aortic valve replacement

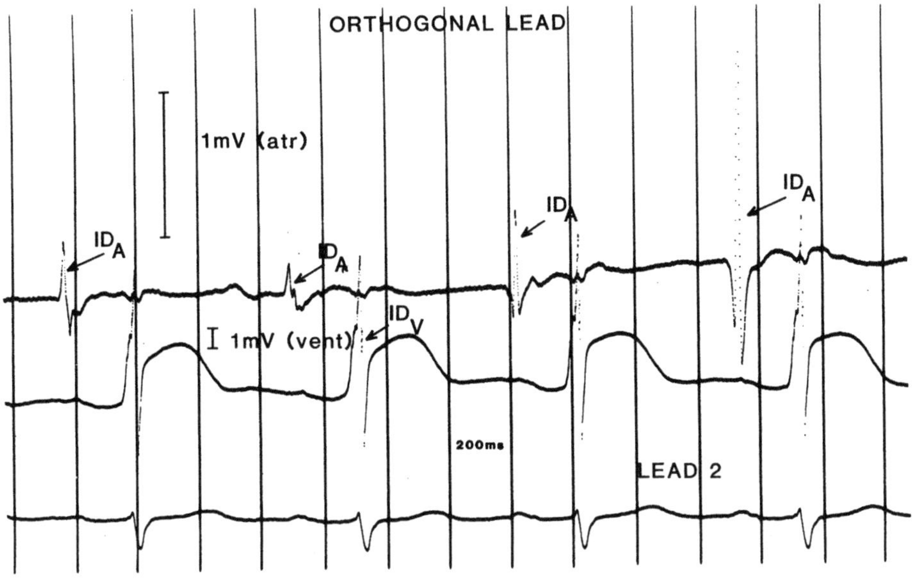

Fig. 2. As the orthogonal lead floats in the right atrium without endocardial contact, the amplitude of the resultant atrial electrogram (EGM) may vary widely with changes in the electrode position within the atrium. The atrial (*atr*) EGM amplitude here varies between 0.3 mV and approximately 3 mV. As the pulse generator sensitivity can be set to 0.3 mV, small EGM amplitudes can be accommodated. *vent*, ventricular; *ID*, intrinsic deflection

Electrogram. Because the electrode is not in contact with the atrial wall and moves within the center of the atrium, its relationship to tissue and orientation continually change. The amplitude of the resulting signal may vary widely. EGM amplitudes of 0.5 mV may alternate with those of 10 mV (Fig. 2). In both instances the slew rate will be greater than that needed to trigger the atrial channel, and triggering will occur if the amplitude is satisfactory. As the electrode is a bipolar variant, sensing is narrow and far-field signals, either the ventricular EGM or noise is not sensed on the atrial channel. This allows a high sensitivity setting without fear of interruption of normal atrial channel function. As two electrodes exist on the lead there are two EGMs derived. Depending on electrode orientation, the two EGMs may interact to produce a single overall resultant ID or two discrete IDs may be detected. Depending on the orientation of the electrode relative to the atrial wall, the resultant EGM may alternate between two IDs and a single ID. Should two IDs exist, the first which reaches an adequate amplitude to be sensed will trigger the atrial channel (Fig. 3).

Pulse Generator. The pulse generator, Model 305 (Cardiac Control Systems, Palm Coast, FL, USA) is lithium iodine powered and hermetically sealed, and has two inputs, one for ventricular sensing and pacing, the second for atrial sensing. Four modes of operation exist, VOO, VVI, VVT, and VDD. In ventricular operation only,

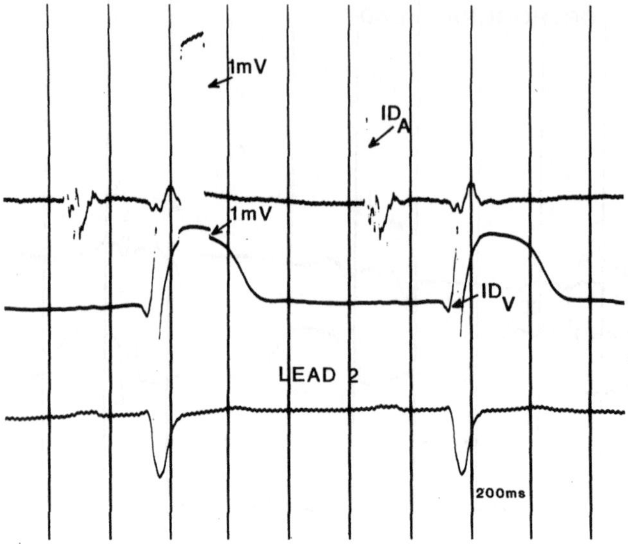

Fig. 3. The orthogonal electrode bears some similarities to bipolarity. Two atrial electrograms (ID_A) are derived and may be additive to produce a single electrogram (EGM) or may be independent, separated by an interval, here about 100 ms. The first ID_A which can be sensed, i.e., sufficient slew rate and amplitude will trigger the pulse generator. *atr*, atrial; *vent*, ventricular

pacing rates of 30–120 bpm can be selected. A pulse duration can be selected between 0.1- and 1.0-ms duration. Output voltage is programmable from 0.4 to 6 V plus 7.5 V. Maximal atrial tracking may be between 65 and 150 bpm, that is atrial refractoriness of 920 – 400 ms, to be set at 20-ms increments. Ventricular sensitivity is 0.5 – 25 mV and atrial sensitivity 0.1 – 5 mV. The AV delay may be set between 60 and 300 ms. Two band passes may be selected for atrial and ventricular sensing: low between 20 and 110 hz and high between 40 and 100 hz.

Lead/Electrode. The ventricular electrode is tined, with passive fixation and otherwise conventional. The atrial electrode is along the shaft of the lead separated either by 13 or 16 cm from the ventricular, allowing preimplant selection of the interatrial position of the atrial electrode. The atrial electrode consists of two semicircular plates facing in opposite directions (i.e., 180° apart) referenced to each other and each 6 mm^2 in surface area.

Implantation Technique. Implantation is conventional with the endocardial lead placed either by cephalic vein cut-down or subclavian puncture. Once the ventricular electrode is in the right ventricular apex, thresholds and EGMs are determined as is usual. The atrial EGM is determined and a further lead is introduced or withdrawn to attempt to have the atrial portion of the lead approach the lateral atrial wall as much as possible. The atrial EGM is then redetermined and the lead is positioned at the site at which the EGM is of greatest amplitude. The lead is secured at the point of entry into the venous system.

Results

Eighteen patients underwent implantation of the single-lead VDD pacemaker at the Montefiore Medical Center. Seventeen were initial implants and one was an upgrade for a patient with renal failure and a ventricular rate-modulated pacemaker but who required atrial synchrony and was hemodynamically substantially improved after VDD upgrade. The minimal atrial EGM amplitude ever recorded was 0.8 mV, the maximum for all patients was 11. mV, mean 3.9 mV. Each had significant variation in EGM amplitude during continuous sensing. The mean level of variation was about 4 mV beat to beat. The mean ventricular threshold was 0.69 mA and 0.47 V at 0.5-ms pulse duration, the mean impedance 461 ohms. The mean ventricular EGM was 12.3 mV and 7.6 mV/ms. The mean fluoroscopy time was 8.8 min, similar to that in our laboratory for dual-chamber placement. The usual atrial sensitivity setting was 0.8 mV. No leads required repositioning or revision. Consistent atrial sensing was present during outpatient follow up and holter monitoring, for all implants, for the duration of follow up (Fig. 4).

Multiple reports [9, 10] of successful atrial sensing and synchronous pacing have appeared over the past several years. Two systems have been successful, one in commercial availability from Medico Italia, Bologna, Italy, with which the author has no experience and the other as above. Thirty-six patients underwent VDD pacemaker implant with universal atrial synchronization and a similar experience [9]. Another 17 patients experienced consistent atrial sensing and ventricular synchronization [10]. The device has just received approval from the Food and Drug Administration for commercial release in the United States (Fig. 5).

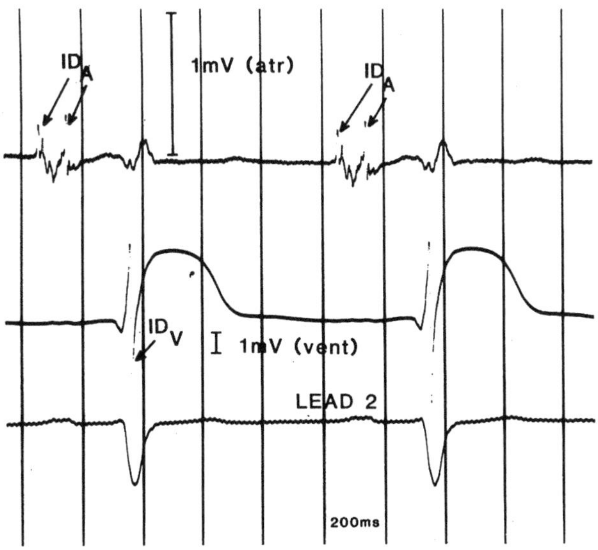

Fig. 4. Despite the possibility of atrial electrogram amplitude variation, the usual circumstance is of amplitude and morphologic stability. *ID*, intrinsic deflection

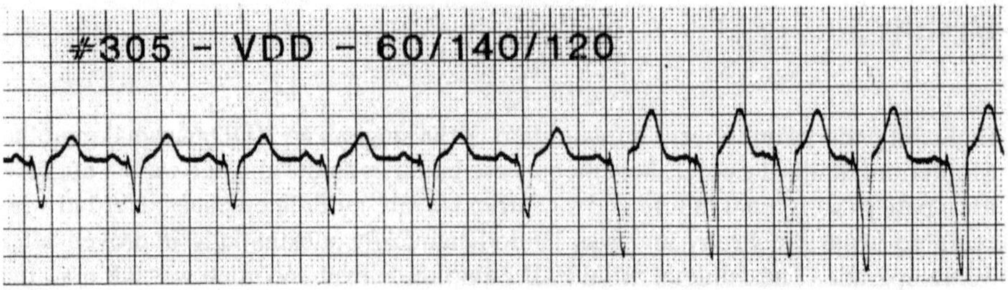

Fig. 5. With change in the amplitude and even the timing of the sensed atrial electrogram, atrial synchronization can, seemingly, change the ventricular complex. In this instance sensing a later portion of the atrial electrogram allows spontaneous conduction and produces ventricular fusion beats (*left*). When an earlier portion of the atrial electrogram was sensed, more conventional stimulation of the ventricle occurred (*right*).

Discussion

The effort at allowing synchronization of ventricular activity with atrial depolarization has occurred over the entire history of cardiac pacing. Initially only one sensing channel was possible, the atrial. With the capability of two sensing channels, atrial and ventricular, atrial sensing and absence of competition with the ventricle was possible. The earliest and even later atrial synchronous pacemakers used a discrete atrial lead through which the atrium could be paced and sensed. Within the past decade evaluation of floating atrial electrodes has been undertaken and systems which provide reliable atrial synchrony have been introduced. The result of this evaluation and others of the same device demonstrate that:

1. Discriminant and reliable atrial sensing with atrial wall contact is possible.
2. Atrial EGM variation occurs and a high sensitivity setting is required.
3. Far-field signals, i.e., the ventricular EGM and muscle noise, are rejected.
4. Long-term atrial synchronous (VDD) ventricular pacing with a single-pass lead is practical.

References

1. Kahn M, Senderoff E, Shapiro J, Bleifer SB, Grishman A (1960) Bridging of interrupted AV conduction in experimental chronic complete heart block by electronic means. Am Heart J 59:548-559
2. Nathan DA, Wu C, Keller W (1963) An implantable synchronous pacemaker for the long term correction of complete heart block. Circulation 27:682
3. Smyth NPD (1985) The J lead. Clin Pacing Electrophysiol 3:435-456
4. Kleinert M (1980) Permanent atrial leads. PACE 3:487-491
5. Ausubel K, Furman S (1985) The pacemaker syndrome. Ann Intern Med 103:420-429
6. Hayes DL, ST Higano, Eisinger G (1989) Utility of rate histograms in programming and follow-up of a DDDR pacemaker. Mayo Clin Proc 64:495-502

7. Goldreyer BN, Aubert AE, Wyman MG, Denys BG, Ector H (1986) Orthogonal atrial appendage sensing. PACE 9:1211-1216
8. Cornacchia D, Fabbri M, Maresta A, Grassi G, Vaiani P (1989) Clinical evaluation of VDD pacing with a unipolar single-pass lead. PACE 12:604-618
9. Longo E, Catrini V (1990) Experience and implantation techniques with a new single-pass lead VDD pacing system. PACE 13:927-936
10. Varriatle P, Pilla AG, Tekriwal M (1990) Single-lead VDD pacing system. PACE 13:757-766

Automatic Pacemakers

T.A. NAPPHOLZ[1]

Introduction

The word automatic is by far one of the most abused terms in all the modern languages. Consequently in the context of this discussion it be used sparingly. Automatic pacemakers are really intelligent pacemakers where the decision-making capability of the device is such as to be able to apply sophisticated "rules" on information it obtains from the biological environment to determine the operation of the device, specific for each individual patient, under all conditions possible throughout the operation of the device.

The most simple example of this concept is the VVI pacemaker. This concept first proposed by Berkovitz [1] ushered in the era of modern cardiac pacemakers. The concept states that the cycle length of the pacemaker is timed either from a pacing pulse or from a natural ventricular depolarization. The "intelligence component," trivial as it may seem, is to use the intrinsic signal from the heart to tell the device how to alter the pacing sequence.

What guides the degree of intelligence in the pacemaker? Is the technology alone or is it our understanding of the biological system? The answer is really "both," and everything inbetween. The availability of the technology spurs on the search for a more thorough understanding of the biological processes, in particular on a long-term basis.

Pillars of the Intelligent Pacemaker

Apart from the simple example given in the introduction, what are the key operations, in a pacemaker, that will benefit from an "injection" of intelligence? They are the following and constitute the topics to be discussed by this treatise:

1. Automatic output regulation (AOR): this is the process of controlling the energy of the pacing stimulus by monitoring the heart's response to this stimulus
2. Automatic sensing threshold: this is the adjustment of the level above which sensing an intrinsic signal is considered valid information

[1] Telectronics Pacing Systems, Research and Development, Denver, USA

3. Automatic setting of refractory time: the setting of the time period, after a depolarization, when sensing is invalid
4. Automatic polarity and chamber determination: this is the process of deciding the configuration and the chamber the electrode is in
5. Automatic rate response factor: this is the process of determining the most suitable relationship between the output of the metabolic indicator and the pacing rate.
6. Automatic sensor selection: this is the process of selecting the correct sensor for a particular activity or life style
7. Automatic AV disassociation (mode switching) in dual-chamber pacing: this is the process of deciding that the atrial function (sinus node) is outside the bounds of physiologically appropriate rates
8. Closed-loop pacing: the process of assuring that the rate at which the heart is paced results in the correct cardiac output for the patient's needs.

Automatic Output Regulation

Automatic output regulation is the most obvious and perhaps the most enigmatic operation to automate. It was discussed extensively nearly 20 years ago [2-17], patented in 1972 by Bowers, tried with a device (Pasys by Medtronic, Minneapolis, USA) in 1982 and by another device (Telectronics/Cordis, Denver, USA) in 1988. The Pasys attempt was aborted as well as the Telectronics/Cordis trials (Prism). In the Prism concept [18, 19] covered by Callaghan [18] the device will only allow AOR with a bipolar electrode in the ventricle. The present Telectronics approach [14] will operate both in the ventricle and atrium with any possible lead. This approach developed independently of Wittkampf [3, 17] but along similar lines is based on a triphasic pulse as shown in Fig. 1 a. The amplitude of the precharge ramp is proportional to the pacing pulse and the post-charge is determined by the remaining charges at the interface. The objective of this modification to the pacing

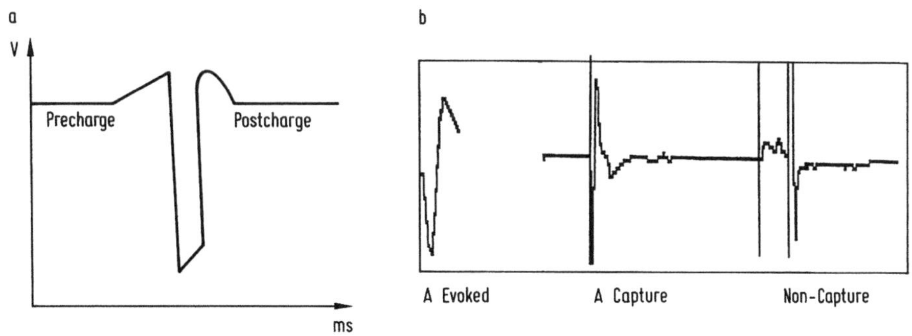

Fig. 1 a, b. Sample of a triphasic pulse morphology (**a**) used for capture detection. This pulse form balances out charges at the metal – electrolyte interface (polarization) and hence enables the detection of the evoked signal from the heart (**b**). The difference in signal shape and configuration between intrinsic (evoked) beats, and captured and noncaptured beats following pacing can be used for automatic output regulation.

pulse is to balance out the charges at the metal – electrolyte interface wihtin 10 ms and hence enable the detection of the evoked signal from the heart. The difference between capture in a patient is shown in Fig. 1. This triphasic pacing pulse is referred to as an active pulse compared to the conventional passive pulse.

The process of balancing a lead is discussed in the following section. The key to this ability is the adjustment of the pre-charge ramp width, which determines the nature of the excess charges at the interface following the pacing pulse. The capability to regulate the pacing output critically depends on the following:

1. Being able to balance out the post-stimulus artifact [10, 15] and being able to verify it, for any electrode, unipolar or bipolar.
2. Knowing the relationship of the residual artifact (deviation from perfect balancing) and the captured signal (the paced depolarization).
3. Being able to operate robustly in the presence of fusion beats.

The Algorithm

To determine capture of the heart, a portion of the evoked electrogram at the pacing site is measured and compared to a threshold value. This portion is called the capture signal. Fig. 2 shows which portion of the electrogram is used to obtain the capture signal.

In order to accurately measure this signal, the charge delivered to the electrode/tissue interface must be balanced. The balancing procedure minimizes the residual artifact so cardiac activity can be monitored. This is achieved, by adjusting the precharge, while an active pulse is delivered, during the refractory period of the heart. The ratio between the capture signal and the residual artifact must exceed a predefined value of eight, for the AOR function to work.

Once the capture threshold (Vthr) has been determined, the pulse generator paces at a voltage level (Vthr + safety margin) so as to assure continued capture of the heart. The objectives of this automatic function are:

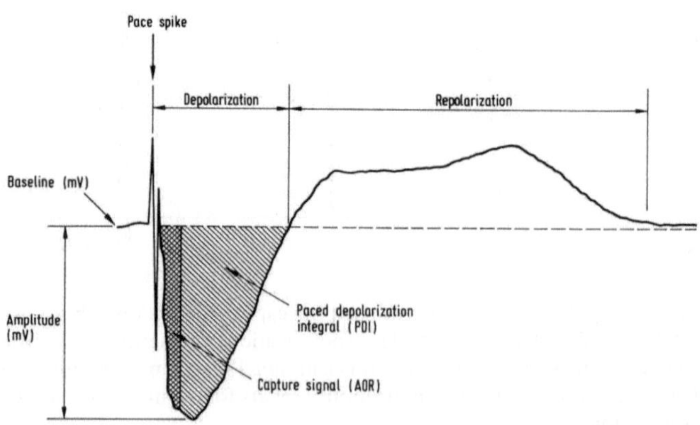

Fig. 2. Morphology of the evoked electrogram is divided into different zones following the pace spike. The correct adjustment of the pre-charge ramp width (Fig. 1a) effects the capture signal detection in the portion of the electrogram immediately following pacing for automatic output regulation

1. To balance the charge at the electrode/tissue interface to ensure that capture of the heart can be effectively discerned.
2. To determine the pacing threshold of the heart.
3. To confirm that capture of the heart is occuring reliably throughout the operation of the product.

These objectives are achieved by running the algorithm in two distinct modes: mode I involves the balancing and threshold determination, and mode II periodically checks that the heart is being captured at the current pacing voltage. Mode I takes place every 36 h or if capture is lost in mode II. Mode I is the standard mode.

Early clinicals, for this function, have highlighted some points of interest;

1. Many high polarization leads make it mandatory to balance at precisely Vthr+margin, to make the artefact acceptable in size.
2. To avoid repeated false negatives for capture, the threshold for capture should be less than 50% of the evoked heart signal.
3. The residual artefact is not modified by the maturation of the lead.

Advantage of AOR

No matter how good an electrode is, in conventional pacing there are always a certain number of exit blocks [20]. This number increases as the demand for smaller pulse generators and hence lower output voltage continues. Hence AOR becomes a safety issue. It is quite obvious that in the large majority of cases the thresholds in the ventricle is < 1 V and in the atrium < 2 V. In the future the energy needed to pace the heart in a dual-chamber pacer will be in the order of 2 μA, total plus about 1 μA for the algorithm. This compares dramatically with 20 μA in the early 1980s (5 V for atrium and ventricle) and the present 12 μA (3.8 V for atrium and ventricle).

Automatic Sensing Threshold

For an implantable pulse generator to be safe it must not only detect intrinsic heart activity but most also be immune to activity, cardiac or otherwise, that is not specifically depolarization of the heart. Consequently the closer the sensing threshold is to the actual depolarization the safer the system.

Even if the sensing threshold is set accurately, the issue of interface modification must be addressed. Myopotentials, although not generally a problem [20], should be considered with a whole slew of electromagnetic interference sources [21]. A number of suggestions in the past [22, 23] were made to combat this problem. The one used in the past [22] is acknowledged to help [21] in repetitive mains (50 or 60 Hz) interference.

Another approach, currently under clinical investigation combines automatic setting of sensing threshold with compensation for background interference. The device measures every intrinsic depolarization and keeps a running average of the last four. The sensing threshold is set to half of this average. If any signals are detected during the refractory period, it uses the amplitude of this signal to increase the

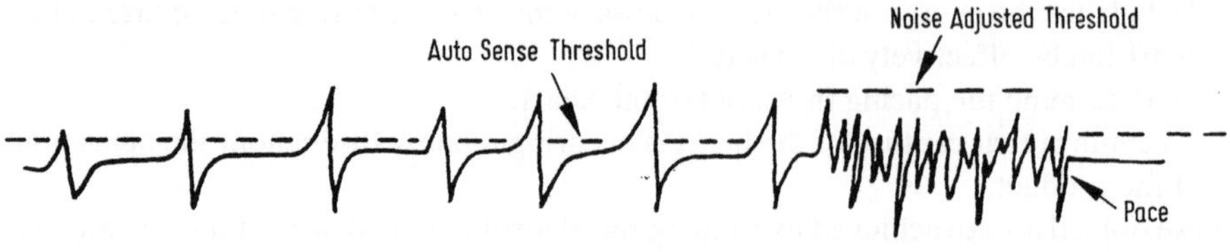

Fig. 3. Every amplitude of intrinsic depolarization is measured and kept as a running average of the last four events. The sensing threshold is set to half of this average. If any signal such as noise is detected within the refractory period, the amplitude of this signal is used to increase the sensing threshold for that single cycle. The increase is noise amplitude + 0.25 of the previous signal, either noise or intrinsic signal, whichever is larger

threshold for that single cycle. The increase is *NOISE AMPL* + 0.25 *PRV*, where *PRV* is either the previous signal or noise, whichever is larger. This concept is shown in Fig. 3.

Automatic Refractory

The concept of automatic refractory has been covered elsewhere [18, 24], and it essentially rests with the determination of the QT interval by sensing the evoked T-wave. In some cases either this value is used with a small positive offset (e.g., 50 ms) or adjustment are made continuously on the basis of rate. From studies done on 17 patients (unpublished data), the coefficient of 1.45 ms/bpm was obtained for this application. Consequently, the measurement of QT at one rate allows reasonable prediction of required refractory period (RP) at all rates. One must, use the more recent modification of Bazetts' relationship [40].

The 1.45 ms/bpm data was obtained by increasing the pacing rate at rest. During exercise, the coefficient is larger: Rickards [25] gives a value of 1.88 ms/bpm. Using the smaller value gives certain safety factors. Another approach is to measure the T wave amplitude and set the sensing threshold above this. Bearing in mind that 'T' wave amplitude is rate dependent. This later approach would oviate the need for an RP and would safeguard against extremely early premature contractions.

Automatic Polarity/Chamber Determination

There are a number of functions in a modern pacemaker that will only operate off a unipolar or bipolar electrode. In many cases a wide range of parameters are only suitable for either atrial or ventricular application. During an implant procedure, it is quite conceivable that errors regarding some of the options are made. To avoid this, and to provide the patient with maximal safety, it is best for the device to make certain decisions continuously during operation.

Lead Polarity Determination

At regular intervals throughout the life of the pulse generator, the microprocessor carries out lead impedance checks. To make this process as short as possible, comprehensive lead testing is done by the processor at implant and the lead type is memorized. For example, if the lead is registered at implant to be unipolar, a bipolar test will be unnecessary. If it is bipolar, the device will do a bipolar impedance test. If the impedance is within the specified bounds, operation will continue as before. If it fails this test, then a breakage is assumed, and the unipolar ring or tip is checked. If the offending pole is isolated, the other one will be paced at emergency energy levels, in life-support mode.

In summary, at "Procedure is Implant" the device determines the electrode configuration. If this is contraindicated at a later stage, during normal operation, emergency action will take place, with priority given to keep the patient supported until subsequent checks have been made from the outside.

At implant, or after disruption by external defibrillator, testing for a bipolar electrode could leave the patient unsupported for one cycle. This can be corrected by either the delivery of a back-up pulse, after the impedance measurement pulse, or by the use of the sense amplifier, to detect an internally generated signal, which remains subthreshold with electrode impedances below 5k (foe example).

Correct Chamber Determination

Correct chamber determination is more difficult as the device must use information from the chamber to decide where it is. The first rule is that, since the device is implanted to prevent bradycardia, decisions must be made from pacing. From all the patient studies to date the atrial evoked signal is about a quarter of that of the ventricle. Hence if the device is only put into a single chamber, it will support the chamber and use the evoked signal as a decision-making parameter. It could confirm this decision by checking in unipolar mode, for the far-field ventricular signal out between 100–250 ms, as part of the automatic refractor determination.

If two leads are placed in the heart, the ventricular lead must confirm the appropriate evoked signal size in comparison with the atrium and the atrium must validate the presence of the far field. In a two-lead system this is easier as the far field should occur immediately following the ventricular pacing pulse. With the above approach sufficiently validated, the dual-chamber pacemaker of the future will not need designated leads for the atrium or the ventricle.

Automatic Rate Response Factor

Most rate-responsive pacemakers operate with the metabolic indicator presenting a signal to be transformed into a corresponding heart rate. This presupposes that a certain signal size for the metabolic indicator always corresponds to a specific heart rate. In a biological environment this assumption is shaky. A better approach is to say that the signal range of the metabolic indicator should map into the desired heart rate range. If, as an example, the physician decides that a patient's heart rate should be between 60 bpm and 140 bpm, then the assumption can be made that over a period of a few months the metabolic indicator will generate the signal range to map into this exact heart rate. This concept has been applied to the minute ventilation pacemaker now undergoing clinical trials.

Previous attempts at automating this relationship [26] always depended on indicating, to the implant, the actual exertion level during exercise. This approach is not warranted in the approach adopted by Callaghan [18] and discussed by Rickards and Boute (this volume). The nature of the paced evoked signal (which is the metabolic sensor) is such that the correct pacing rate is implied in the value of the measurement. That is, when the paced depolarization integral (PDI) is equal to its value at rest, the pacing rate is correct, hence the approach is inherently automatic.

Rate Response Factor

In the minute ventilation system the rate response can be normally adjusted for each patient by means of the rate response factor (RRF). The RRF determines the degree of change in pacing rate that will occur for a given change in minute volume. The larger the RRF, the greater the change in pacing rate for a given change in minute volume.

Fig. 4 shows two typical rate response curves. Two points are emphasized on the X axis: the patient's minimal and maximal minute volume levels. Two points are also emphasized on the X axis: the patients minial and maximal minute levels. Two points are also emphasized on the Y axis: the programmed minimal and maximal pacing rates. One curve shows the response of the pulse generator with an RRF of 20, and the other curve shows the response with an RRF of 27. The RRF of 27 causes minimal rate pacing when minimal minute volume is present and maximal rate pacing when maximal minute volume is present. The RRF of 20, however, does not cause maximal rate pacing when maximal minute volume is present. The RRF of 27 would be recommended because it gives the fullrange of rate response for the full range of minute volume.

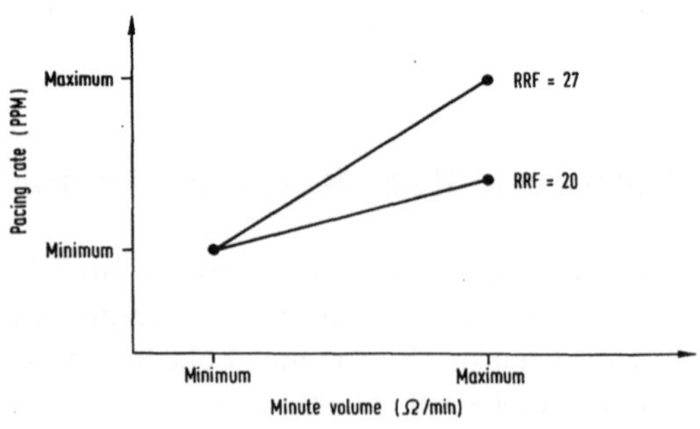

Fig. 4. The patient's maximal minute volume (expressed by changes in ohmic resistance per minute) is shown on the abscissa, the minimal and maximal pacing rate on the ordinate. The rate-responsive factor (*RRF*), also called slope, describe the pacing rate associated with a given ventilation. RRF20 ist too flat to achieve an adequate pacing rate with increased ventilation, RRF27 links maximal ventilation to the maximal achievable pacing rate

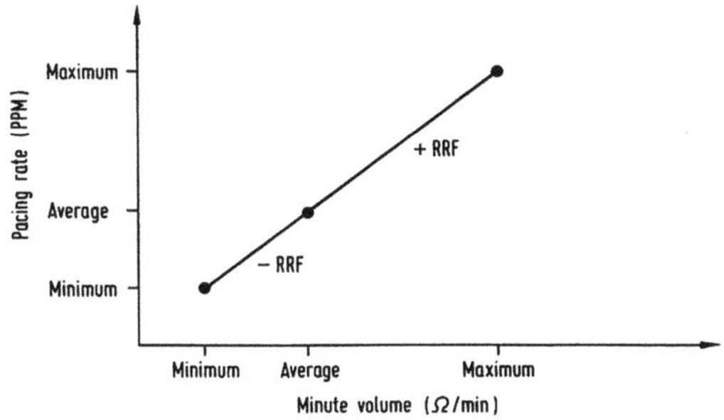

Fig. 5. A typical rate response curve in an automatic RRF mode where the patient's minimal, average, and maximal detected ventilation are taken to determine the two RRF values.

Automatic RRF

Automatic RRF is a mode of operation where the pulse generator continuously monitors the patient's maximal minute volume. On a daily basis, the pulse generator automatically updates the rate response (the RRF) so that the maximal minute volume results in maximal pacing rate. Although the RRF is updated once per day, the pulse generator's estimate of the maximal minute volume only changes gradually, so the RRF changes slowly from day to day.

Following the example in Fig. 4, if automatic RRF was programmed with an initial RRF of 20, but the patient exhibits a maximal minute volume which requires an RRF of 27, the rate-response curve will initially correspond to an RRF of 20. The pulse generator continuously monitors the minute volume and gradually increases the RRF until it is 27. There is simple rule to describe how quickly the RRF increases in automatic RRF mode: to increase the RRF by 7 (e.g., from 20 to 27) requires 36 days.

In automatic RRF mode, the pulse generator is also capable of decreasing the RRF. For example, if the pulse generator is programmed with an initial RRF of 27, but the patient exhibits a maximal minute volume which requires an RRF of 20, over time the pulse generator will reduce the RRF until it is 20. The reduction in the RRF depends on how often the patient exhibits maximal minute volume. The more often the patient exhibits maximal minute volume, the faster the RRF is reduced. The amount of time required to reduce the RRF by 7 (e.g., from 27 to 20) is 6 h given by t (days) = 24/p-1 p is the percentage at maximal rate ($1 < p < 100$).

Pacing Rates in Automatic RRF Mode

The pulse generators will also allow a negative rate response in automatic RRF mode. Negative rate response occurs when the patient exhibits a below-average minute volume. In this case, the pulse generator actually reduces its rate, but not below the programmed minimal rate.

Fig. 5 shows a typical rate response curve in automatic RRF mode. Note that there are three significant points on the X axis: the patient's minimal, average, and maximal minute volumes. These correspond to three points on the Y axis: the programmed minimal, average, and maximal pacing rates.

The pulse generator monitors the patient's average minute volume using a 24-h moving average. Whenever the patient exhibits the average minute volume, pacing occurs at the programmed average rate. If the minute volume is above average, the pacing rate increases above the average rate in accordance with the automatically determined RRF. If the minute volume is below average, the pacing rate decreases below the average rate in accordance with a second automatically determined RRF.

Typical values for the minimal, average, and maximal pacing rates would be 50, 70, and 150 pulses per minute (PPM), respectively. The maximal pacing rate would correspond to peak exercise levels. The physician might elect to set the minimal pacing rate equal to the average pacing rate, in which case the pulse generator would not exhibit negative rate response.

Automatic Sensor Selection

The search for the ideal single metabolic indicator for rate response will culminate with multiple sensors. What criteria can the implantable device use to obtain the correct blend of these sensors? The most obvious approach is to divide exertion into low and high and have sensors appropriate for each segment. At the present time it is recognized that in fact sensors do divide in the same way: fast sensors with higher specificity at low levels of exercise and medium and slow sensors with higher specificity at medium to high levels of exercise. As an example of this concept we can have a cardiac parameter such as PDI=Pacer Depolarization Integral [18, 19] and minute ventilation. The PDI is an indicator of conduction velocity and cardiac volume change, both being very fast indicators of metabolic demand. The PDI is made effective up to only 100 PPM. A compounded response is shown in Fig. 6. Other combinations of sensors being considered are: activity and temperature, activity and QT, and activity and minute ventilation [27–29].

The other approach to sensor selection is to define what the normal rate profile should be for the patient during the day and then select the sensor that comes close to this ideal. A simple example of this would be the criterion that, rates above 100 PPM

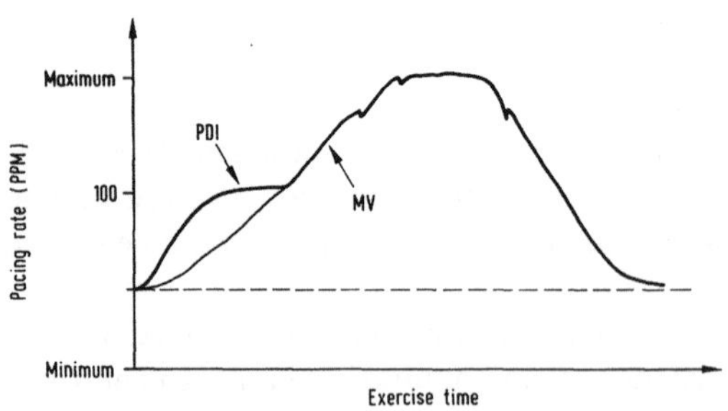

Fig. 6. An additional faster sensor, such as in this example, the pacer depolarization integral (*PDI*) is used as a "quick starter" to increase the pacing rate as soon as possible after commencement of exercise. A more metabolically adequate, but slower parameter, such as in this example ventilation, is used to control the pacing rate with higher and more continuous physical exercise. In other systems of dual-sensor concepts, body activity takes the part of PDI, ventilation can be substituted by, for example QT interval or temperature

should be attained no more than say 5% of the day [31]. If one of the sensors complied it would be selected, with the test applied every few days. The less appropriate sensor would be accumulating data in the background but not controlling the rate until it found acceptance.

Automatic AV Disassociation

Historically the greatest threat to proper atrial synchrony in dual-chamber pacemakers was retrograde conduction which could set up a pacer-mediated tachycardia (PMT) [31–33]. The methods of prevention and termination are also legion [34–36]. With the advent of rate-responsive pacing, it must be obvious that the metabolic sensor can help in the fight against PMT.

The metabolic sensor can serve not only as an indicator of the desired rate, but also as an arbiter for undesirable pathological rates. In the most simple implementation the post-ventricular atrial refractory period (PVARP) is modulated by the metabolic indicator. In this manner it classifies the atrial rate into pathological or physiological. PVARP can start off with a greater value than normally possible and be decreased with metabolic demand, hence giving added protection and avoiding 2:1 block. If a certain number of atrial events occurs during the PVARP, disassociation will occur. Immediately following disassociation, the standby rate is prolonged to allow an atrial pacing pulse to interrupt the PMT. Only after this has been done and pathological rate still persists, disassociation into VVIR will occur. Re-association will take place only after the atrial rate has dropped to a certain value.

Another concept to establish a conditional rate limit for limited tracking of atrial tachyarrhythmias based on the sensor output of an accelerometer has been realized by Intermedic's DDDR Relay pacemaker. If the rate indicated by the sensor is not higher than 20 bpm above the lower rate limit, the atrial tracking rate is limited to 95 bpm. Atrial rates exceeding this limit will result in Wenckebach mode with a maximal achievable ventricular pacing rate of 95 bpm.

Closed-Loop Pacing

The importance of closed-loop pacing lies in the most fundamental nature of cardiac pump mechanics. Cardiac output is not only a function of rate, but also of stroke volume, systemic resistance, and diastolic dimensions. As discussed by Geddes and by Wessale et al. [37], for each level of demand there is an optimal heart rate. Going above or below contradicts the demands of the body or the capabilities of the heart pump. To totally optimize the operation of a pulse generator, knowledge of cardiac output is mandatory

There are certain systems undergoing clinical trials that claim to be closed-loop systems, such as the Prism [19] and the Precept [38]. The Prism is a closed-loop system only to the extent that it has been empirically observed that the PDI is roughly constant in a correctly responding heart. Hence, if PDI is kept constant with the pacing rate, the loop is closed – not quite the same as the hemodynamically defined loop. With the Precept, that ostensibly does measure right ventricular stroke volume (SV), the actual accuracy of this measurement is yet to be proven.

A true closed-loop system must measure cardiac output as true flow in the pulmonary artery or aorta and use this data to continuously meet metabolic demand with a correct balance of SV increase and rate increase. An oxygen saturation-based system [35] is designed to optimize cardiac output at all rates. The problems with this system are the long-term stability and efficacy of the sensor, and the lack of resolution of oxygen saturation at higher levels of exercise.

Conclusion

Intelligent pacemakers are emerging to meet the demands of more comprehensive therapy, continued reliability, and minimal complexity in tailoring to the individual patient's needs. This evolution is vitally important to ensure the preeminence of this therapy in cardiac disease.

References

1. Berkovitz Patent (1964)
2. Mugica J et al. (1973) Pacemaker with automatic adaptation to the pacing threshold. In: Thalen HJT (ed) Cardiac Pacing. Van Gorcum, Amsterdam, p 150
3. Thalen HJT, Rickards AF, Wittkampf FHM et al. (1981) Evoked response sensing (ERS as automatic control of the pacemaker output. Proceedings of the 2nd European symposium on cardiac pacing, Florence, pp 1229-1234
4. Preston TA, Bowers DL (1973) Report of a continuous threshold tracking system. In: Thalen HJT (ed) Cardiac Pacing. Van Gorcum, Amsterdam, p 295
5. Preston TA, Bowers DL (1974) The automatic threshold tracking pacemaker. Med Instrum (Baltimore) 8:322-325
6. Preston TA, Bowers DL (1975) Clinical applications of the threshold tracking pacemaker. Am J Cardiol 36:322-326
7. Boute W et al. (1988) Morphology of endocardial T-waves of fusion beats. PACE 11:1693-1697
8. Auerbach AA, Furman S (1979) The autodiagnostic pacemaker. PACE 2:58-68
9. Donaldson RM, Rickards AF (1983) The ventricular endocardial paced evoked response. PACE 6:253-259
10. Walton C, Gergely S, Economides AP (1987) Platinum pacemaker electrodes: origins and effects of the electrode-tissue interface impedance. PACE 10:87-99
11. Burgess MJ, Steinhaus BM, Spitzer KW, Ershler PR (1988) Nonuniform epicardial activation and repolarization properties of in vivo canine pulmonary conus. Circ Res 62/2:233-246
12. Callaghan F, Vollman W, Livingson A, Birinder B, Abels D (1989) The ventricular depolarization gradient: effects of exercise, pacing rate, epinephrine, and intrinsic heart rate control on the right ventricular evoked response. PACE 12:1115-1130
13. Rickards AF, Donaldson RM, Thalen HJT (1983) The use of the QT interval to determine pacing rate: early clinical experience. PACE 6:346-354

14. Curtis AB et al. (1990) Characteristic variation in evoked potential amplitude with changes in pacing stimulus strength. Am J Cardiol 66:416-422
15. Ripart A, Mugica J (1983) Electrode-heart interface: definition of the ideal electrode. PACE 6:410-420
16. Walton C, Economides AP, Gergely S (1989) Determination of myocardial depolarization and repolarization times using the unipolar ventricular evoked potential: contrasting effects of stimulus interval and isoprenaline in the isolated perfused rabbit heart. PACE 12:784-792
17. Wittkampf FHM et al. (1983) Apparatus for physiological stimulation and detection of evoked response. US Patent 4,3783,531
18. Callaghan FJ (1990) Automatic functions in cardiac pacing. Eng Med Biol 9/2:28-31
19. Paul V et al. (1989) Closed loop control of rate adaptive pacing. PACE 12:1897-1902
20. Watson WS (1985) Myopotential sensing in cardiac pacemakers. In: Barold SS (ed) Modern cardiac pacing. Futura, Mount Kisco, pp 813-857
21. Butrous GS (1983) The effect of power frequency high intensity electric fields on implanted cardiac pacemaking. PACE 6:1282
22. Stein MT (1983) Cardial pacemaker amplifier. US Patent 4,379,459
23. Irnich W (1983) Interference recognition circuit in a heart pacemaker. US Patent 4,516,579
24. Begemann MS (1988) Automatic refractory period. PACE 11:820
25. Rickards AF (1981) Relationship between QT interval and heart rate. Br Heart J 45:56-61
26. Mahaux V et al. (1989) Clinical experience with new activity sensing rate modulated pacemaker using autoprogrammability. PACE 8:1362-1368
27. Alt E, Theres H, Heinz M, Matula M, Thilo R, Blömer H (1988) A new rate-modulated pacemaker system optimized by combination of two sensors. PACE 11:1119-1129
28. Heinz M, Alt E, Theres H, Oelker J, Zimmermann S (1990) Combination of multiple parameters for pacemaker rate control by intracardiac impedance measurement. PACE 13:1197
29. Senden PJ et al. (1989) Clinical study of a dual sensor rate adaptive pacemaker. PACE 12:1574
30. Sulke, N et al (1990) Quantatative analysis of contribution of rate response in three different ventricular rate responsive pacemakers during out of hospital activity. PACE 13:37-44.
31. Den Dulk K, Lindemans FW, Bar FW et al. (1982) Pacemaker related tachycardias. PACE 5:476
32. Furman S, Fisher JD (1982) Endless loop tachycardia in an AV universal (DDD) pacemaker. PACE 5:486
33. Den Dulk K, Lindemans F, Wellens HJJ (1984) Management of pacemaker circus movement tachycardias. PACE 7:346
34. Bertholet M, Materne P, Dubois C et al. (1984) Artificial circus movement tachycardias: incidence, mechanisms, and prevention. PACE 8:415
35. Elmqvist H (1983) Prevention of pacemaker mediated arrhythmias. PACE 6:382
36. Duncan J et al. (1988) Prevention and termination of pacemaker medicated tachycardias. PACE 11:1679
37. Wessale JL et al. (1988) Cardiac output versus pacing rate at rest and with exercise in dogs with AV block. PACE 11:575-582
38. Chirife R et al. (1989) Initial studies on a new rate adaptive pacemaker. PACE 12:1568
39. Stangl K et al. (1988) First clinical experience with an oxygen saturation controlled pacemeter in man. PACE 11/II:1883-1887
40. Lecocq B et al. (1989) Physiologic relationships between cardiac cycle and QT duration in healthy volunteers. Am J Ca, Sept. 1

Combinations of Parameters

K. STANGL and M. LAULE[1]

Introduction

The characterization of the static and dynamic properties of the various parameters makes it clear that no single parameter meets the requirements for an "ideal" command variable. It is therefore useful to combine individual parameters. The particular parameters should supplement one other to provide constant sensitivity throughout the load range and fast dynamic behavior.

Along with these basic physiological conditions, the technical feasibility of useful combinations plays a central part. The various concepts will always be compromises between physiologically optimal solutions and what is technically feasible. Two types of parameter combinations appear fundamentally useful: those with standard leads and those with special sensor leads.

Combinations with Standard Leads

Systems with standard leads (unipolar, bipolar) are the ones that measure parameters (a) electrically via the leads; or (b) via sensors in the pacemaker can.

Figs. 1 and 2 list the parameters that can be detected and combined by systems with standard leads. These systems have some advantages. First, they require no special leads, the systems can be adapted to any implanted standard lead at times the pulse generator is exchange changed. Also, functional disturbances due to sensor failure can be expected less frequently. Finally, the costs for such a total system are definitely lower.

The disadvantages of the majority of these systems are that they don't detect metabolic parameters that reflect hemodynamic effects of the rate variation. These systems therefore only permit control without feedback and hemodynamic optimization. An exception is stroke volume, but it can presumably only be used in combination with other parameters. The diagnostic value of systems with standard catheters must be considered small.

Respiration and Stroke Volume. One possible combination is to use the impedance derived values, respiratory rate/minute ventilation, and stroke volume [4, 5, 6].

[1] First Medical Clinic, Charité, Humboldt University, 1040 Berlin

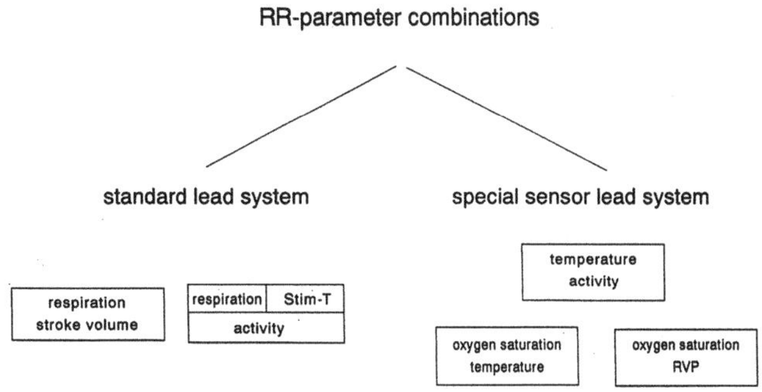

Fig. 1. Measuring methods for rate-responsive (*RR*) parameters. *RVP*, right-ventricular pressure; *RAP*, right-atrial pressure

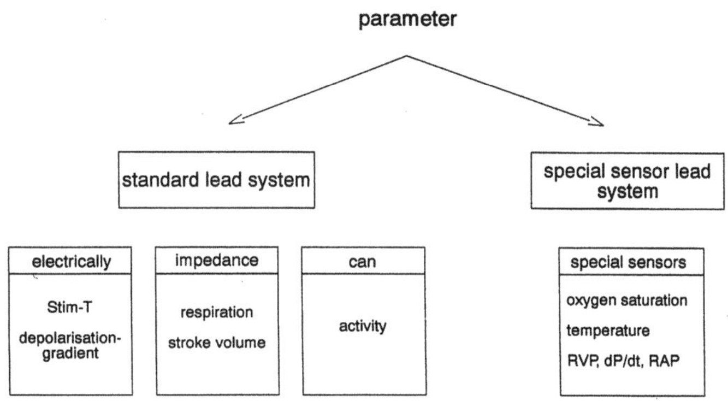

Fig. 2. Parameter combinations. *RVP*, right-ventricular pressure

Respiratory parameters are medium-fast and not very sensitive in the low load range, but show very good correlation to exercise in the higher load range. In combination with stroke volume, respiration is the actual command variable while stroke volume is utilized as a fast-starting trigger signal, in connection with a fixed rate change, and can compensate for the lower sensitivity of the respiratory parameters in the lower load range.

Respiration and Activity. The stroke volume as a trigger signal is replaced here by activity as fast variable that is especially sensitive in the low load range [4, 7]. In this combination, activity commands in the low load range, and respiration in the higher load range. While the mutual balance of the tidal volume and stroke volume components increases the measuring accuracy when impedance signals are used alone, signal processing is more difficult when two different signals such as respiration and activity are used.

Stim-T Interval and Stroke Volume/Activity. The stim-T interval, like respiration, shows sufficient sensitivity only in the higher load range, the dynamic response is slow. As in the combinations described above, the slow dynamics and the lower sensitivity in the low load range can be partly compensated by the additional use of stroke volume or activity [2].

Combinations with Special Sensor Leads

These systems measure parameters by sensors that are additionally integrated in the pacing lead. Figs. 1 and 2 show the measurable variables detected accordingly and possible combinations. Advantages of these systems are the more precise and faster physiological adaptation of the rate. Additionally most parameters have a diagnostic value and can also be used beneficially in antitachycardiac systems. Disadvantages are that a special lead is required and the systems are more susceptible to disturbance, as sensor technology is still under development.

Oxygen Saturation and Temperature. This combination [3] is fast; the decreasing sensitivity of oxygen saturation in the high load range is compensated by the high sensitivity of temperature in this range. Both variables can be detected with an optoelectric sensor since the sensor has an additional temperature response. Oxygen saturation permits hemodynamic self-optimization in a closed circuit. This combination is not only good for pacemaker control but also has possible diagnostic value.

Temperature and Activity. In this combination [1, 4] temperature is the actual command variable. The additional use of activity permits a compensation of the partially low sensitivity of temperature in the lower load range and the slower dynamics. A hemodynamic optimization is more difficult with these variables; the diagnostic value of this combination is low.

Oxygen Saturation, Pressure, Stroke Volume. Aiming at future systems with antibradycardiac, antitachycardiac, and diagnostic properties, one might use combinations of parameters representing the hemodynamics, that thus go far beyond merely antibradycardiac pacing. The combination of pressure, oxygen saturation, and stroke volume can be utilized to detect and discriminate tachyarrhythmias or to control drug therapy, e.g., in future implantable pumps/infusion systems [4]. The problems in terms of the detection and processing of measured values as a result of the use of several sensors are evident.

Conclusion

For selection of the various types of systems, the use of standard systems gives priority to a low-complication detection of measured values at the expense of the need for a more sophisticated algorithm in order to achieve a physiological system response. Systems with special sensor leads approach physiologically optimal solutions while involving a higher technical complication rate for the moment. In accordance with the mentality of the implanting physicians and the patients involved, both types of systems will exist side by side, whereby the choice of system for an individual patient must depend on his or her particular requirements. Cost and size of combination systems will represent an important issue in future pacemakers as well possibly favoring more the combinations with standard lead systems.

References

1. Alt E, Theres H, Heinz M et al. (1988) A new rate-responsive pacemaker system optimized by combination of two sensors. PACE 11:1119
2. Heuer H, Koch T, Isbruch F et al. (1987) Pacemaker stimulation by a two sensor regulation. PACE 10/II:688
3. Stangl K, Wirtzfeld A, Heinze R et al. (1985) Oxygen content and temperature of mixed venous blood as physiological parameters for regulating pacing rate. In: Gomez FP (ed) Cardiac pacing. electrophysiology tachyarrhythmias. Grouz, Madrid, p 810
4. Stangl K, Wirtzfeld A, Heinze R et al. (1988) A new multisensor pacing system using stroke volume, respiratory rate, mixed venous oxygen saturation, and temperature, right atrial pressure, right ventricular pressure and dP/dt. PACE 11:712
5. Alt E (1991) Cardiac and pulmonary physiological analysis via intracardiac measurements with a single sensor. US Patent No 5.003.976 2. April 1991
6. Theres H, Alt E, Zimmermann S, Heinz M, Oelher J,. Huntley S (1991) Intracardiac impedance: an advanced concept for combination of multiple paraneters for pacemaker rate control. PACE 14:692 (abstr.)
7. Heinz M, Alt E, Theres H, Oelher J, Zimmernann S (1990) Combination of multiple parameters for pacemaker rate control by intracardiac impedance measurements. PACE 13:1197

Future Trends

K. STANGL and M. LAULE[1]

Introduction

The continuous detection of biosignals opens up new therapeutic and diagnostic possibilities for both fields of bradyarrhythmias and of tachyarrhythmias. However, the new technologies make high demands on the long-term stability of the sensors, the energy reserve of the system and – in particular – the "intelligence" of the pacemaker.

For the near future one can make out several trends in pacemaker development that can be grouped more or less arbitrarily under the following concepts:

- The smart pacemaker
- Rate-adaptive dual-chamber systems
- Rate-adaptive systems with combinations of parameters
- Hemodynamically self-optimizing systems
- Universal antibradycardiac and antitachycardiac systems

As these developments make immense demands on storage capacity and computing performance, they clearly presuppose the microprocessor-controlled, smart pacemaker. The various development trends shown in Fig. 1 are based on the new computing performance of the intelligent pacemaker alone or on the additional calculation of biological signals.

The Smart Pacemaker

The new developments mentioned above open up new therapeutic and diagnostic possibilities, but they also make exponentially increasing demands on the complete measurement and calculation technology of the pacemaker. The rapid development of chip technology in recent years has permitted complex computation to be performed by microprocessors within tiny spaces, so that these miniaturized functional units with arithmetic and memory functions can be implemented in cardiac pacemakers.

[1] First Medical Clinic, Charité, Humboldt University, 1040 Berlin

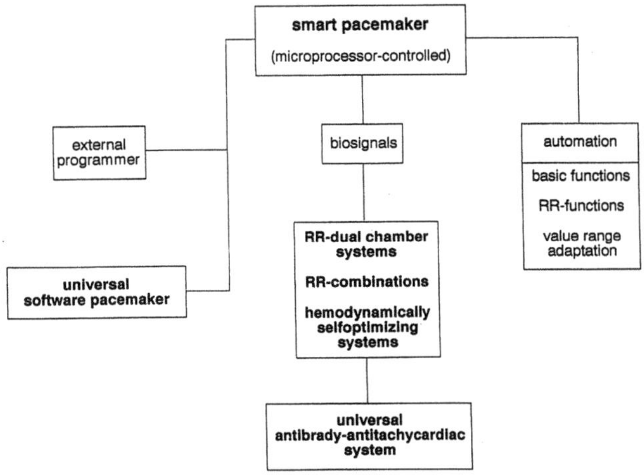

Fig. 1. Future trends in pacemaker therapy. *RR*, rate-responsive

The concept of the smart pacemaker can embrace properties and functions resulting from this new arithmetic and storage capacity. It is useful to distinguish between external and internal intelligence of the system. External intelligence can refer to universal applicability by software control through communication and interaction with the external programmer. Internal intelligence refers to the independent performance of internal functions by the pacemaker. This includes:

- Automation of basic pacemaker functions
- Automation of adaptation of the measuring range
- Storage of diagnostic data
- Hemodynamic self-optimization of rate

External Intelligence: Universal Software Pacemakers

In recent years there has been a trend toward software-controlled pacemakers whose operation can be programmed and modified at will from outside [4, 6, 10]. Software control permits the development of a universal basic model that can be used both as a dual-chamber pacemaker and as a rate-adaptive single-chamber system. The software pacemaker can be adapted with its corresponding special leads to such different trigger signals as the P wave signal, activity, oxygen saturation and pressure, and permits free combination of the detected parameters (e.g., activity with temperature) as command variables.

Software control has the great advantage that any desired programmings and modifications of the mode of operation can be effected for this basic model from outside. A problem of this development trend is that software control is more susceptible to disturbance, so that certain basic functions such as the battery test should still be ensured by hardware for safety reasons.

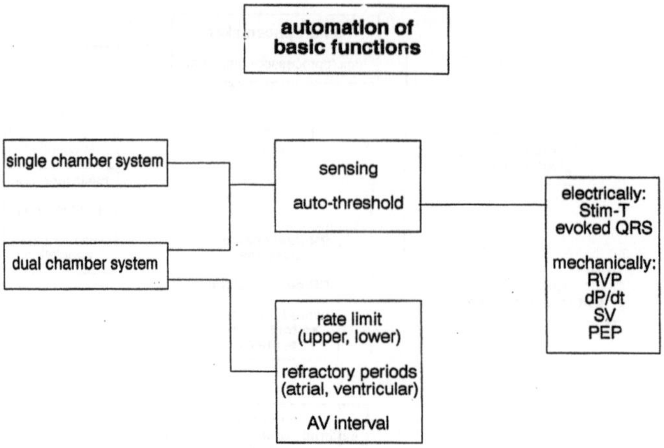

Fig. 2. Automation of basic functions. *RVP*, right-ventricular pressure; *SV*, stroke volume; *PEP*, preejection period

Internal Intelligence: Automation of Internal Functions

The necessity of automating internal functions as far as possible already results from the exponential increase in programming possibilities due to the more widespread use of microelectronics in general and the great number of new rate-responsive functions in particular. The complexity of these systems and the additional time they require from the programming physician have up to now opposed their wider use.

The possibility of automation relates first to basic functions of a system; in rate-adaptive systems and dual-chamber pacemakers further functions can be automated (Fig. 2).

Basic Functions

For the basic functions of a single-chamber system it is possible to automate the sensing function and an independent stimulus threshold determination.

While it appears unproblematic to set the sensing function independently, an automation of stimulus threshold determination (autocapture) is critical. The reliable detection of the stimulus threshold presupposes not only the mere detection of the intracardiac ECG signal but at least one further criterion. This second criterion must report the electric depolarization of the myocardium and/or the hemodynamic effect of a stimulus.

Electric criteria of an effective pacing are the stim-T interval [3] and the ventricular depolarization gradient. Hemodynamic criteria to be used are right ventricular pressure (RVP) dp/dt, and the intraventricular impedance with stroke volume and preejection period [16].

An automation of stimulus threshold determination with a minimization of pacing energy is important in all future developments because the high power consumption in these systems due to sensory analysis, microprocessors, and the higher pacing rates in comparison to fixed-rate systems limits the life of the system. In dual-chamber systems there are additional parameters to the basic functions of the single-chamber system.

It thus appears possible to set the refractory periods of the atrium (and ventricle) [4] automatically in combination with the upper limiting rate and AV interval. The upper limiting rate can likewise be adapted to the individual cardiac situation automatically if one makes use of hemodynamic parameters.

The AV interval itself should be adjusted individually and vary rate dependently in accordance with the physiological conditions. An automatic shortening of the AV interval when the pacing rate increases is already realized technically in some dual-chamber systems [6, 9, 13]. Furthermore, there are already efforts to optimize individually the AV interval, which is important for the hemodynamics, with the aid of hemodynamic parameters (oxygen saturation, stroke volume, RVP).

Rate-Responsive Functions

Along with automation of the basic pacemaker functions, particularly rate-adaptive systems require the rate-responsive (RR) parameters to be set by the system as automatically as possible. This applies to variables valid for all systems, such as the upper and lower limiting rates, and the program points specific to individual command variables (e.g., programmable decay times in activity pacemakers, "dip response" with temperature).

Automatic Adaptation of the Measuring Range

The above possibilities of automation desirably simplify and accelerate the programming process, but they are not obligatory for making rate-adaptive systems operable. By contrast, an automatic adaptation of the measuring range of biosignals appears to be indispensable, particularly in systems with physiological command variables, for several reasons.

Technically speaking, the long-term stability of sensory analysis over year-long periods is the central problem of rate-adaptive systems. Every sensor fundamentally shows a data drift that must be compensated automatically by the system.

Physiologically, most parameters are subject – independently of exercise – to pronounced circadian or other functional fluctuations that can clearly exceed exercise-induced changes in the parameters. Central venous blood temperature and stim-T interval are particularly striking examples of the high exercise-independent range of variation of biosignals.

Data drift and physiological fluctuations mean that the systems only function adequately if the pacemaker is in a position to redefine constantly the measuring range or adapt it to the situation. This means that it is insufficient merely to associate the rate with absolute measured values of the particular parameter. The characteristic of the pacemaker must instead be adapted continuously to the changing range of measured values. A concept for technically realizing automatic rate adaptation that can be transferred in a generalized form to all parameters was recently published by Heinze et al. [11]. The pacemaker continuously stores the maxima and minima of the measured value and reassigns to them in each case the characteristic between the measured value and the pacing rate. If changes in the minima and maxima are registered by the pacemaker, the range is immediately readapted. The system can thus react adequately to slow changes in measured values as in a data drift and to fast, functionally induced changes in the measured value.

Storage of Diagnostic Data

The expansion of computing performance and in particular of storage capacity is the basis for storing and recalling diagnostic data. These data consist, on the one hand, of strictly electric signals that can be grouped under the concept of Holter functions and are already available in some pacemakers in a more or less perfected form. On the other hand, rate-adaptive systems can provide valuable information about the metabolism and/or hemodynamics depending on the diagnostic value of their biosignals.

Holter functions in pacemaker denote memories that continuously record spontaneous and pacemaker rhythm. This is done by measuring each time interval between two events strictly according to time criteria. Owing to the small storage allocation of data acquisition, observation periods of several years are possible. Holter functions fundamentally extend diagnostic and therapeutic possibilities essentially due to the new possibilities they provide for following up a great variety of diseases over long periods and their general screening function for intermittent bradyarrhythmias and tachyarrhythmias and for pacemaker dysfunctions [17].

In the further development of these Holter functions, a crucial advance is to be expected from the integration of a time axis. This will make it possible to produce rate patterns over certain periods. This means a crucial improvement, particularly for rate-adaptive systems, since it will permit the corresponding rate responses to be associated at exactly the right time with certain loads or interference variables [6]. This will make (long-term) ECG controls unnecessary in many cases and substantially simplify the programming and/or correction of the corresponding parameters.

Furthermore, the time axis permits an isolated consideration and analysis of predefined events, such as tachycardias or atrial fibrillation, that were identified beforehand with reference to predefined electric and hemodynamic criteria.

Along with strictly electric events, certain rate-adaptive systems (pressure, oxygen, stroke volume) permit the storage and recallability of hemodynamic data, thereby providing additional useful information. On the one hand, trends and long follow ups of parameters offer diagnostic aid, and, on the other hand, immediate access to current values by means of telemetry may be helpful for differential diagnosis.

Altogether, the evaluation of electric and biological information creates an additional possibility of controlling the pacemaker and of drug and electric therapy [16, 18]. Especially with antitachycardiac pacemakers, the additional utilization of hemodynamic criteria promises to provide a more reliable detection of tachyarrhythmias [5, 7, 8, 14, 16].

Hemodynamically Self-optimizing Systems

It is the basic concern and point of departure for developing rate-adaptive systems to improve the patient's hemodynamics. It cannot suffice to raise or lower the rate within a fixed range without any hemodynamic feedback. The pacemaker's rate response must instead be adapted to the patient's individual cardiac situation that results from the differing contractile myocardial status, the valvular conditions, and the coronary morphology, etc. This means that the rate increase excludes a potential hemodynamic deterioration, e.g., in the case of serious coronary heart disease. The rate variation must therefore take place within limits in which it leads to an increase in cardiac output. A hemodynamic optimization of the pacing rate is therefore only possible with parameters that permit conclusions to be drawn about the effect of the rate change on cardiac output. With most physiological parameters there is a certain hemodynamic feedback, but sufficiently large effects that can be used for pacemaker control are shown only by central venous oxygen saturation [11], RVP, and, with some restrictions, stroke volume.

Rate-Adaptive Dual-Chamber Systems

The extension of atrium-independent rate modulation to dual-chamber systems is a logical development of this therapeutic principle. The development of rate-adaptive dual-chamber systems makes it largely superfluous to discuss the advantages and disadvantages of atrially controlled dual-chamber pacing as compared to rate-adaptive single-chamber pacing (atrial contribution versus rate). The rate-adaptive single-chamber pacing only in the AAIR mode for sick sinus syndrome will reguire intact AV conduction. Rate-adaptive dual-chamber systems extend therapeutic possibilities in the sense that patients with binodal diseases can now also be treated adequately. The extension of the indication for rate-adaptive pacing relates firstly to patients with sick sinus syndrome and accompanying AV conduction defects who cannot be given an AAI system on electrophysiological criteria (e.g., Wenckebach point too low), and, secondly, to patients with higher-grade AV block who additionally show an inadequate sinual rate adaptation [18].

In addition, rate-adaptive dual-chamber systems permit an AV-synchronous pacing with parameters that can only be used in the ventricle as a single-chamber system (stim-T, RVP).

Along with the improvements to be expected from this development trend, rate-adaptive dual-chamber systems are also particularly suitable for accommodating the considerable increase in technical effort, the complexity of future trends, and the necessity of automating as many functions as possible. This is ideally done by systems with hemodynamic self-optimization which are in a position to minimize the programming effort for RR functions to a mere switch-on of the function.

Combinations of Parameters

Numerous studies of the dynamic and static behavior of physiological parameters have shown that no physiological parameter alone meets the conditions of an ideal command variable. It is therefore useful to combine complementary parameters. Two types of combined rate-adaptive systems are emerging: the standard system and the sensor system.

The Standard System

The standard system measures electric signals (intracardiac ECG, impedance) with standard catheters or uses sensors positioned in the pacemaker can. Standard systems can be used to detect the parameters of stroke volume, preejection period, breathing, stim-T interval, evoked QRS, and activity. Useful complementary combinations are:

- Stim-T interval and activity [12]
- Breathing and stroke volume [16]
- Breathing and activity

The Sensor System

This system requires a special sensor catheter. It detects physiological parameters such as the pressure of the right heart, oxygen saturation, and blood temperature. Useful combinations are:

- Oxygen saturation and temperature [15]
- Oxygen saturation and pressure [16]
- Temperature and activity [1, 2]

From a diagnostic point of view, it is useful to combine oxygen saturation, stroke volume, and RVP. This last combination already points toward the presumable end of this line of evolution, namely the development of a universal pacemaker system.

Universal Antibradycardiac and Antitachycardiac Pacemaker

Obviously, the utilization of hemodynamic parameters such as oxygen saturation, RVP parameters, and stroke volume provide possibilities that go far beyond merely antibradycardiac pacing. The pressure parameters are sensitive variables for the preload and the contractility of the right heart.

Furthermore, the very quick change in RVP and stroke volume in the case of tachycardias provides information on the underlying arrhythmia. As an example, Fig. 3 shows the behavior of RVP and right-atrial pressure (RAP) in the case of a

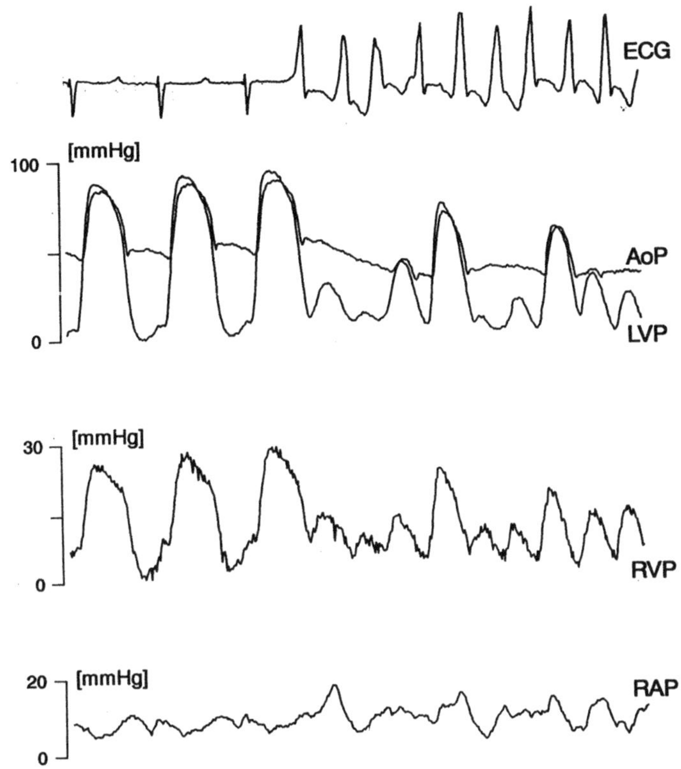

Fig. 3. Behavior of right-ventricular pressure (*RVP*) and right-atrial pressure (*RAP*) at onset of ventricular tachycardia (rates 160/min – 190/min). *LVP*, left-ventricular pressure; *AOP*, aortic pressure

ventricular tachycardia. This of course suggests the use of these hemodynamic parameters in antitachycardiac systems, whose detection and differentiation mechanisms have up to now been based solely on electric criteria.

Since these systems must necessarily have an antibradycardiac "backup" function, the end point of future developments seems to be a universal pacemaker system having antibradycardiac, antitachycardiac, and diagnostic properties. Its complexity and the demands such developments make on technology and the physician are evident.

References

1. Alt E, Theres H, Heinz M et al. (1988) A new rate response pacemaker system optimized by combination of two sensors. PACE 11:1119
2. Alt E (1990) Implantable devices – pending issues and future trends. PACE 13:1079
3. Baig W, Boute W, Wilson J et al. (1988) Use of the paced evoked response in termination of pacing threshold. PACE 11 [Suppl]:822
4. Begeman MJS, Boute W (1988) Automatic refractory period. PACE 11 [Suppl]:820
5. Bennett T, Beck R, Erickson M (1987) Right ventricular dynamic pressure parameters for differentiation of supraventricular and ventricular rhythms. PACE 10:415

6. Boute W, Hamersma M, Vreuls P (1988) AV-delay hysteresis function in dual chamber pacemakers. PACE 11 [Suppl]:815
7. Chirife R (1988) The pre-ejection period: a physiologic signal for rate responsive pacing and tachycardia diagnosis in automatic pacemakers. PACE 11 [Suppl]:821
8. Cohen TJ, Veltri EP, Lattuca J et al. (1988) Hemodynamic responses to rapid pacing: a model for tachycardia differentiation. PACE 11/I:1522
9. Eisinger GE, Winston SA, McGaughey (1988) Rate responsive AV-delay and its effect on upper rate limit performance in DDD pacemakers. PACE 11 [Suppl]:815
10. Garcia JR, Vela JCO (1988) Cardiac pacemakers assisted by computer aids. PACE 11 [Suppl]:793
11. Heinze R, Hoekstein KN, Liess HD et al. (1988) Automatische Anpassung frequenzgeregelter Herschrittmacher an die cardiale Leistungsfähigkeit von Patienten. Biomed Tech (Berlin) 39 [Suppl]:19
12. Heuer H, Koch T, Isbruch F et al. (1987) Pacemaker stimulation by a two sensor regulation. PACE 10/II:688
13. Janosik D, Pearson A, Redd R et al. (1987) The importance of atrioventricular fallback in optimizing cardiac output during physiological pacing. PACE 10:410
14. Shapland JE, Bach S, Baumann L et al. (1988) New approaches for tachycardia discrimination. PACE 11 [Suppl]:821
15. Stangl K, Wirtzfeld A, Heinze R et al. (1985) Oxygen content and temperature of mixed venous blood as physiological parameters for regulating pacing rate. In: Gomez FP (ed) Cardiac pacing. electrophysiology. tachyarrhythmias. Grouz, Madrid, p 810
16. Stangl K, Wirtzfeld A, Heinze R et al. (1988) A new multisensor pacing system using stroke volume, respiratory rate, mixed venous oxygen saturation, and temperature, right atrial pressure, right ventricular pressure, and dP/dt. PACE 11:712
17. Stangl K (1990) Holter-Funktionen. In: Stangl K, Heuer H, Wirtzfeld A (eds) Frequenzadaptive Herzschrittmacher. Physiologie, Technologie, klinische Ergebnisse. Steinkopff, Darmstadt, p 291
18. Wirtzfeld A, Schmidt G, Himmler FC et al. (1987) Physiological pacing: present status and future developments. PACE 10:41

Visionary Concepts on Implantable Devices

P. GORDON[1] and E. ALT[2]

Introduction

Predictions on future implantable devices can be divided into three different areas: (a) the vast majority of all implantable devices will still belong to the group of conventional bradycardia pacing; (b) the group of implantable devices which contain a defibrillator will be of increasing importance, but will not reach the numbers of units of pure pacing devices; (c) a third group of purely diagnostic implantable devices (000) might evolve over the next decade.

Prediction of what is going to go on in the year 2000 can be extrapolated pretty easily, but it is worthwhile to try to extend the vision further into the future, into the twenty-first century, and really look to the day, when not only engineers and technicians but also scientists, and cellular and DNA biologists might discuss the topic of cardiac pacing and of implantable devices. This might remind everybody that the "gestalt" of a pacemaker is inherently an undesirable thing, it is a restorative device, but actually its virtual presence in the body creates a certain morbidity of the cure, so there is a driving force to either eliminate the inorganic pacemaker by replacing it with a true organic pacemaker or to actually cure the disease. So we can look forward maybe into the twenty-first century to going to a museum and seeing in the medical gallery a pacemaker collection right along with the bleeding bowls and iron lungs. That might be the true destiny for the inorganic pacemaker.

Size Hypothesis

Taking that a little further, in the meantime, into the next 2, 3, or 4 decades, what can we do? We are still in the era of the artificial, metallic, silicon-plastic pacemaker. We want to get rid of it as much as we can, so that there is a continued driving force. We put forward the following hypothesis: *given adequate functionality and longevity there is no such thing as an artificial, inorganic pacemaker that is physically too small.*

[1] Medtronic Inc., Minneapolis, MN, USA
[2] First Medical Clinic, Technical University of Munich, 8000 Munich 40, FRG

Even though there has been great progress in reducing the size of the pacemaker, further size reduction will actually map into increased patient quality of life, and we can eliminate morbidity even more.

The conventional bradycardia pacers will only get smaller, and the driving force towards a smaller size will greatly affect what sensors are combined and used in future rate-responsive units and multisensor rate-responsive units.

How can this prediction be made? If we look at modern lead technology we can go through a reasoning process that basically points to a tremendous potential for greater size reduction. There is a whole family of new leads. In the worst case, the peak threshold energy for a modern electrode with for example a porous, platinized steroid-eluting lead is less than half a microjoule for a pacing capture event (Table 1).

If we look at a typical pacemaker today, the nominal pacemaker, we will see that it draws about 18 μA at 70 bpm with one lead at a nominal setting, which is usually 4 – 5 V. This is about 40 μJ per cardiac cycle. So, based on this worst case of peak threshold capture energy, we can conclude that with today's electrode, today's pacemaker is only 1% or 3 % energy efficient. So there is tremendous potential for size reduction by:

1. Coming to terms with safely turning down the amount of energy used for stimulation.
2. Continuing to work on lower current-consuming circuitry.
3. Thus, the "gas tank" of the pacemaker, the battery, which is about the largest thing left inside the pacemaker, becomes quite small.
4. Lastly, new much smaller connectors will evolve.

Pacemaker Lead and Connector

Some succinct predictions about pacemaker leads in the year 2000 can be made (Table 2). Future leads are going to be of a very small diameter, easy to remove, hopefully of variable length – that might simply mean that they will be cuttable, because it is pointless to make a small pacemaker with many turns of wire and a big pocket. IS1 in this context should be history. We need a connector system that is better than IS1, that is more compact. It takes at least one 25 mm dimension to make an IS1 connector. A smaller system with surface contacts needs to be perfected.

This lead will have a worst-case peak threshold of less than 0.7 V, at 0.2 ms. That translates into less than one tenth of a microjoule of capture energy. The

Table 1. Future developments in pacemaker technology

- Modern electrode technology will be the driving force for size reduction
- Worst-case peak threshold energy for a modern electrode (such as the porous, platinized, steroid-eluting type) ≦ 1/2 microjoule
- Typical present pacemaker – total energy consumption per paced cardiac cycle (18 μA, 70 bpm): 40 μJ
- Modern electrodes make today's pacemakers only 1% – 3% efficient!
- Tremendous potential for further size reduction while perfecting rate-responsive pacing

Table 2. Pacemaker leads in the year 2000

- Less than 3 French – easier to remove
- Variable length (cuttable) – no excess loops in pocket
- IS1 will be history
- Worst-case peak threshold < 0.7 V at 0.2 ms (< 1 μJ)
- Pacing impedance 1000 – 2000 ohms – electrode area 2-3 mm^2
- PR-evoked and T wave sensing better than present with source impedance < 5000 ohms
- Nominal pacing pulse – 2.5 V and 0.4 ms into 1000 ohms giving 25-to-1 energy safety margin (1 μA at 60 bpm)
- Anti-inflammatory-eluting electrodes commonly used
- Leads with special sensors rarely used

pacing impedance will be considerably higher than the nominal 500 ohms of todays pacing leads, which helps translate into the lower energy. And yet, there will be at least as good or better PR-evoced and T wave sensing characteristics with reasonably low source impedance.

Batteries

We still believe that we will be using lithium iodine battery technology, because it is really difficult to rationalize a new chemistry. At best, those new chemistries will approach the reliability and track record of lithium iodine, and we really do not need a higher-powered battery for conventional pacing. So a 1/4 A/h (Ah) lithium iodine battery will become the normal "gas tank." That is about half the capacity of the smallest pacemaker that is available today.

Most Common "Special" Pacemaker in the Year 2000

We very much believe that there is a place for a single pass of a VDD unit, particularly one that has rate response, even though the VDDR algorithm can be tricky and in

Table 3. Pacemakers in the year 2000

$SSIR^N$ units	– Under 10 g, < 8 years' longevity
	– 2.5-cm diameter x 4-5 mm thick
	– Total current drain = 3 or 4 μA
	– Circuit current drain < 2 μA
	– 1/4 Ah lithium iodine battery
	– IS1 connector replaced by something better
	– Multisensor rate response, ^{N} typically = 3
	– All sensors work on "normal" leads
$DDDR^N$ units	– Under 13 g, < 8 years' longevity
	– Total current drain = 4 – 6 μA

Table 4. Pacemaker system issues for the year 2000

– Standard connector systems beyond IS1
– Standard sensor leads
– Universal programmer:
Laptop computer and manufacturer supplied wand and software
Laptop – wand interface standard will be needed
– PSA will be history:
"PSA function" at implant will be distributed between programmer and pacemaker
Feedthroughs needed to connect unopened sterile package to lead system
– Special Holter monitor needed:
Direct uplink of pacemaker telemetry, real-time markers, sensor signals, histograms, data dumps, endocardial ECG, etc.
External solid-state unit will always have greater capabilities than pacemaker version

many ways trickier than the DDDR algorithm, since it is not possible to phase-lock the atrium. A multisensor lead should include a sinus sensor, that is floating atrial electrodes, thus making VDDR possible (Table 3).

Fully Implantable "No Lead" Pacer?

Another type of special pacer that is possible is the "button" or "bullet" pacemaker. These are extremely small units that can be directly attached to the mycardium or have a little pigtail lead that connects to the epicardium with some new implant regime. One point is that, as units get small, more implant sites are possible.

Universal Programmer

The universal programmer is an old and mundane subject, but with the price of real estate around the world no hospital can afford a storage room for all the programmers! It seems to us that the laptop computer or the palmtop computer that is evolving with about a half-life of a year or two – mostly in Japan – is basically the universal programmer of the future. We wonder if the universal programmer is nothing more than a laptop with basically a wand and software supplied by each manufacturer. So you simply take out your laptop, load the manufacturer's software and you plug in their wand. Now, that means you have to have a collection of wands. We would like to take this a step further: to see that the wand is not plugged in, to see somehow a wireless link to the laptop, a two-way LED device, or whatever, and the wand would then become what is commonly called in electronics a transponder. Perhaps industry could come up with a two-way communication standard. So then everyone makes their transponder and, of course, it would be desirable to make a nice small one, a little frisbee-type device, that tapes on the patient (Table 4).

Perioperative Stimulation Analyzers

We think the old square box perioperative stimulation analyzers (PSA) will become less and less used and really will not be replaced because there will be so many units with different sensors that somehow at implant the pacemaker and the programmer will work in conjunction with each other to guide the physician through the whole implant process. Perhaps the way to do this would be to package the pacemaker with feed throughs and to have a means to use the packaged generator and programmer as the analyzer for that particular system. Wires could be run over to the candidate lead system. The programmer could have an expert system that really advises the doctor on the status of things. That is not a new idea. It was thought up a long time ago but it makes a lot of sense for the defibrillators of the year 2000 also. Future features of implantable defibrillators in the year 2000 and of the purely diagnostic implantable devices are outlined in Tables 5 and 6.

Conclusion

In no way are small size and advanced rate-responsive pacing two conflicting concepts. We think they can merge completely. There are plenty of sensor systems that can survive size reduction. The implantable devices that include a defibrillator in the future will be the primary vehicle for research to bring physicians and engineers together to solve in collaboration the future challenges of implantable devices: bradycardia pacing, defibrillation, and purely diagnostic implantable devices.

Table 5. Implantable defibrillator in the year 2000

– These devices will become the "Swiss army knife" of implant cardiology
– Even with size reduction, there is still room to add auxilliary functions:
Sensors in unit and on leads
– More robust Holter and data collection than in pacemakers
– On-board expert system
– Likely combination therapies:
PCD + cardiomyoplasty stimulator
PCD + bolus drug pump

Table 6. Diagnostic implantology in the year 2000

– Do pure diagnostic implants make sense medically and economically?
– "000 pacer" for congestive heart failure?
– Monitor transplanted organs?
– Are complex multisensor leads that measure absolute values required?
– Might require external Holter for real-time signal and data processing
– Size might be significantly larger than conventional pacemakers

MIX
Papier aus verantwortungsvollen Quellen
Paper from responsible sources
FSC® C105338

If you have any concerns about our products,
you can contact us on
ProductSafety@springernature.com

In case Publisher is established outside the EU,
the EU authorized representative is:
Springer Nature Customer Service Center GmbH
Europaplatz 3, 69115 Heidelberg, Germany

Printed by Libri Plureos GmbH
in Hamburg, Germany